Beyond Left and Right Handedness

Elke Kraus

Beyond Left and Right Handedness

A Practice-based Approach to Assessing and Analysing Handedness Dimensions and Types

Springer

Elke Kraus
Physiotherapy and Occupational Therapy
Alice Salomon University of Applied Sciences
Berlin, Germany

ISBN 978-3-031-24388-2 ISBN 978-3-031-24389-9 (eBook)
https://doi.org/10.1007/978-3-031-24389-9

Partially based on the German language edition: Zwischen Links- und Rechtshändigkeit: Theorie, Diagnostik und Therapie bei wechselndem Handgebrauch, by Elke Kraus Copyright © 2019 Springer-Verlag GmbH Deutschland, ein Teil von Springer Nature 2021. All Rights Reserved.

This Springer imprint is published by the registered company Springer Nature Switzerland AG
The registered company address is: Gewerbestrasse 11, 6330 Cham, Switzerland

For my beloved Cobus, Kai and Amelie
Thank you!

Manual skill and its complex role differentiation between the hands is an evolutionary phenomenon—one of the wonders of being human. I have been privileged to explore this fascinating issue over the last 30 years. I hope you enjoy the journey with me.

Foreword

A few short years ago, I had the pleasure of writing a Foreword for an important publication on handedness by Dr. E. Kraus titled, *Zwischen Links- und Rechtshändigkeit: Theorie, Diagnostik und Therapie bei wechselndem Handgebrauch* (2019). While I was excited by the book, I was also somewhat disappointed, because, as the title indicates, the book was written in German, and, sadly, only available in German. I had so wanted that the book was also available in English because it offered a wealth of important theory and practice information on a topic that is of great interest to parents and clinicians alike, handedness. I am now extremely pleased to be able to write a Foreword for the English title on the subject of handedness by Dr. Kraus, *Beyond Left and Right Handedness: A practice-based approach to assessing and analysing handedness dimensions and types.*

In preparation for this Foreword, I was privy to the pre-publication manuscript and was delighted to see that this book is not simply an English translation of the German edition, rather, it builds on the content of the German edition and enhances it greatly! This book offers English reading therapists a wealth of information, to inform their work with children who experience issues in the development of functional handedness, considered an important indicator of typical neurodevelopment.

As I noted in the Foreword for the German edition, the literature on handedness is long standing and broad, offering much information, unfortunately, often contradictory in nature, and lacking evidence. In this book, Dr. Kraus provides therapists with a comprehensive and scholarly discussion of the topic, presenting a careful, in-depth description of all aspects of the topic and providing therapists with the necessary, evidence-based tools to address handedness in practice.

In creating *Beyond Left and Right Handedness,* Dr. Kraus has taken into account the differences in practice contexts and has tailored the book to the English-speaking using what she calls a "practice-based" approach to handedness. The result is a three-part book where Parts I and II (Chaps. 1–7) are significantly changed in major aspects while Part III (Chaps. 8–12) are quite similar to the German version. Each part starts with a separate page that has a short introduction on it. In addition, each part ends with a one-page synopsis. The parts are very different, but they are systematically built on each other. The first part, focused on Understanding Handedness, both theory and research, is a critical assessment of the literature on handedness. The second part, focused on the research and practice of the Assessment and Analysis of

Handedness, documents the development of the assessment Dr. Kraus has created and the research around it, as well as a proposed typology of handedness. The third part is focused on Implications for Practice, discussing intervention and presenting case studies that illustrate the implementation of the Handedness Profile that Dr. Kraus has so meticulously constructed.

I congratulate Dr. Kraus on having produced such an excellent English sequel to her German book on handedness. The two editions, together, offer the therapeutic literature an invaluable resource that is well situated in the latest evidence-based understanding of handedness and provides a comprehensive guide to addressing the important development of handedness.

H. J. Polatajko
Department of Occupational Science
and Occupational Therapy
Rehabilitation Sciences Institute,
University of Toronto,
Toronto, ON, Canada

Acknowledgment

There have been many people that have inspired and supported me on my handedness journey, without which this book would not have been possible. Firstly, all the children that were assessed with the Handedness Profile by therapists trained in its use over the last 20 years. They are at the centre of this practice-based approach to handedness. The continuous feedback from these children, their parents and therapists enabled me to remain close to clinical practice, and to develop the Handedness Typology. Also, many mentors and colleagues challenged and supported me, and I have benefitted greatly from their knowledge and experience. In particular, I would like to thank (in alphabetical order): Alexandra Heinzelmann, Barbara Sattler, Bunty McDougall, Carmen Spielbichler, Cornelia Schübl, Erna Schoenthaler, Fritz Buthke, Helen Strebel, Helene Polatajko, Lourdes Bruwers, Heather Mudie, Peter Hufnagl, Susanne Spittel, Theresa Allweiss and Ursula Nagele. Finally, my partner Cobus has been exceptional in his unwavering belief in my abilities, his sharp, critical and analytical mind, and his vision beyond the ordinary. Our children, Kai and Amelie, made valuable inputs and encouraged me over many years. I am immensely thankful to all of you!

Introduction

Why this Book?

Handedness is a fascinating and complex phenomenon. Researchers generally agree that handedness is a multidimensional phenomenon subject to polygenetic and environmental influences. As a result, decades of research have generated an abundance of intriguing but often inconclusive, and even contradictory results.

A major problem is that there is no definition of handedness that is generally agreed upon. The terms handedness, hand preference, hand proficiency and hand performance are often used synonymously. Nor is there a standardised categorisation of handedness groups, making it difficult to compare handedness across different studies. In addition, handedness tests and assessments comprise different items that lead to different results. Furthermore, there is no consensus on which test procedure is the most valid or reliable.

This lack of uniformity complicates *research* and affects clinical *practices* such as occupational therapy, where therapists often work with "mixed-handed"[1] children. When constructs such as handedness lack clear definition, testing and intervention in clinical practice also tend to occur on a rather ad hoc basis. A coherent and systematic basis for assessing, analysing, understanding and treating atypical handedness is required to build evidence-based practice in this area. The absence of a scientific basis prompted me to investigate handedness and develop a differentiated and comprehensive handedness assessment.

As an occupational therapist, I[2] have worked extensively with children with mixed handedness and have researched the topic from a clinical practice perspective since 1995. There seemed to be different reasons why children swap hands during activities. Implementing an appropriate, effective and targeted intervention without understanding these reasons and comprehensively assessing handedness was impossible. In my doctoral research, I developed a

[1]The term "mixed" handedness is used collectively for all handedness types that are not clearly assigned to either *Left* or *Right Handedness*, including unestablished and uncertain handedness. The term will be explored and defined in more detail throughout the book.

[2]For better readability, the book uses the first person (singular) relating to me as the author of the book. The "we-form" refers either to the collective expert experience of myself and other therapists in this field, or to contemplations with the readership.

standardised and normed assessment, the Handedness Profile, that systematically captures various dimensions of handedness, such as preference and proficiency (Kraus 2003). Its development is rooted in the diverse handedness literature and four research studies with 270 typically developed children aged 3–6 years and 67 atypically developed children aged 3–9 years.[3]

The Handedness Profile seeks not only to establish the handedness direction (i.e. left or right) but particularly the handedness degree or extent of handedness. Two defining dimensions of handedness, preference and proficiency, as well as other dimensions, are assessed over seven subtests. In addition, background information on familial handedness and developmental risk factors are documented. Overall, the Handedness Profile enables the categorisation of varying degrees of handedness for left, right and mixed handers, resulting in different profiles corresponding to various handedness types.

Since 2003, I have trained occupational therapists to implement the Handedness Profile in Germany, Austria, Switzerland, Luxembourg and South Africa. Based on their feedback and the data of hundreds of Handedness Profile case studies over the years, I developed additional tools for analysing the results that lead to the proposed *Handedness Typology*. This typology can help to understand likely reasons for variable hand use observed in children and provides direction to subsequent intervention approaches (see also Kraus 2019).

So this book is based on my research and clinical practice on handedness over the last 30 years. Its overall aim is to propose a multidimensional practice-based approach to understanding handedness with implications for research and practice. Whilst my occupational therapy background informs my own approach, I have significantly benefited from research in other disciplines such as neuropsychology, behavioural psychology and neurology. In turn, I hope the book will interest special educators, behavioural psychologists, paediatricians, psychiatrists and researchers dealing with the phenomenon of handedness from various perspectives.

Terminology Used in the Book

Since the handedness literature lacks differentiated and consistent definitions of concepts and processes relating to handedness, the terms used in this book that refer to the Handedness Profile and the Handedness Typology are mainly derived from the literature, explained in the chapters and defined in the Glossary. The latter defines and clarifies essential terms used in the context of the book and the Handedness Profile. All definitions are referenced in the main text at first mention and marked with the symbol ♦. For a better overview, the most important terms are depicted in the Handedness Terminology Map in Fig. 1.

[3]Whilst the Handedness Profile was developed for children and thus particularly deals with the handedness development over the first 6 years of life, it has also been found to be a sensitive assessment for determining degrees of handedness in adults.

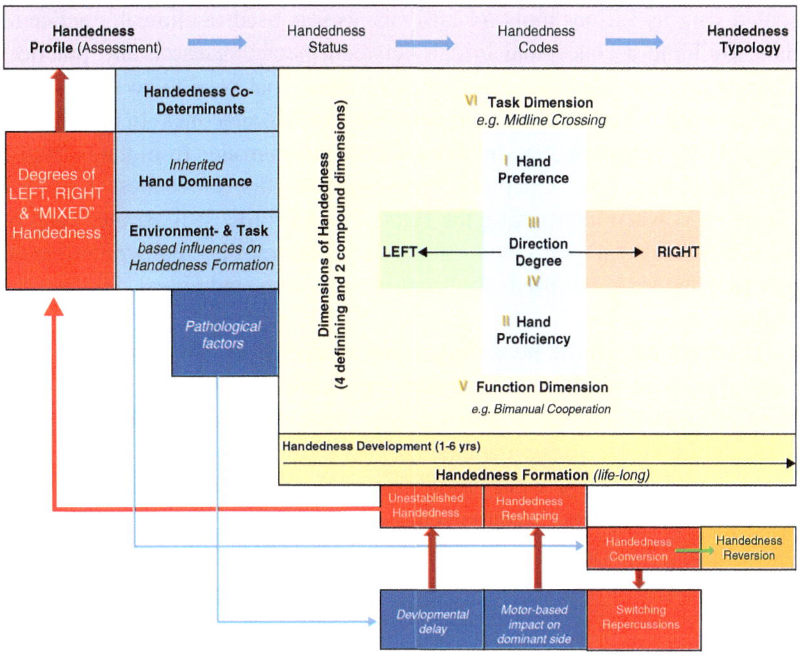

Fig. 1 Map of Handedness Terminology used in this book

Overview of the Book

The book is divided into three parts associated with several aims that are covered in the various chapters.

The first part focuses on **understanding handedness** as a foundation for a practice-based approach. Chapter 1 reviews the emergence of handedness from an evolutionary and developmental research perspective. It also describes handedness in terms of definition, classification and distribution. Chapter 2 looks at neural asymmetries relating to structural, manual and functional asymmetries. Chapter 3 defines reciprocally intertwined co-determinants of handedness: genetic predisposition, motor-sensory impact as a pathological factor and environmental influences. The chapter is critical when capturing background information to a child's handedness. The following two chapters look at research findings on specific handedness groups. Chapter 4 focuses on *Left Handedness* and various groups of left handers. Chapter 5 deals with "mixed" handedness and possible causes for hand use variability. It also explores ambidexterity, converted handedness and pathological handedness, and conditions with reduced lateralisation.

The second part of the book addresses the **assessment and analysis of handedness**. Chapter 6 overviews different methods and measures for assessing handedness, the factors influencing assessment outcomes, and identifying assessment principles. This information is crucial to developing a comprehensive assessment. Chapter 7 demonstrates how the Handedness Profile was developed as a multidimensional assessment and relays the studies supporting its construction. In Chap. 8, the current Handedness Profile 2018 is presented with its various tools for analysis, as it is used in clinical practice to date. Building a conceptual bridge between theory, research and practice, Chap. 9 proposes six dimensions of handedness that need to be assessed by practitioners and correlates the co-determinants of handedness to handedness types. These types are then linked to identified subgroups from the literature and termed Variations. Chapter 10 presents how this Handedness Typology can be used when interpreting the Handedness Profile. It illustrates each of the handedness types with their respective variations, displaying prototypical profiles that can be used for comparison with individual handedness profiles.

The third part of the book, **Intervention and Case Studies**, focuses on clinical practice and looks at relevant implications for assessment and treatment of "mixed" handed children in a practice-based approach to handedness. It draws on the experience of occupational therapists who have implemented the Handedness Profile since 2003. Chapter 11 presents a range of intervention or treatment approaches and principles for addressing handedness cases by relating these to particular handedness variations that typically present in occupational therapy. Chapter 12 then illustrates the application of Handedness Profile and the Handedness Typology by presenting four different handedness cases.

The book closes with reflections on possible implications for practice, theory and research on handedness assessment and intervention.

Further Reading

- Kraus E (2003) The Handedness Profile. The development of a normative profile to determine the extent of handedness in children. Doctoral Thesis. La Trobe University, Melbourne, Australia
- Kraus E (Hg.) (2019) Zwischen Links-und Rechtshändigkeit. Theorie, Diagnostik und Therapie bei Kindern mit wechselndem Handgebrauch. Springer, Berlin

Contents

Part I

Understanding Handedness: Theory and Research

As an occupational therapist, I have worked with children for over 30 years. Occupational therapists enable children to function and participate better in their everyday life, whether at home, school or kindergarten, in sports clubs, playgrounds or wherever they spend their time. So occupational therapists focus on assessing, analysing and optimising children's occupations (e.g. learning to write) together with the children and within their unique environment and context. Many of these occupations require manual skills and practice. When handedness is not established or unclear, children swap hands during activities. Consequently, their manual skills often lack consistent practice and are underdeveloped, impacting their ability to engage in age-appropriate or desired occupations and to participate optimally in their world.

It was against this background back in the 1990s that I started to realise the importance of established handedness and the need for a clear, efficient role division between the hands during manual action. It prompted me to seek to understand handedness better. Fortunately, I was not only a practitioner at the time but also a PhD student and a university lecturer, so my quest to explore handedness was fuelled by clinical practice, research and teaching.

This first part of the book aims to provide theoretical insight on relevant aspects underpinning a practice-based approach to handedness. By looking at various research perspectives and theoretical postulates, we seek to understand handedness as a multidimensional phenomenon.

The Emergence of Handedness

1

Contents

Indeed, one problem with accounting for the evolution of human handedness is the assumption that all aspects of handedness are derived from the same underlying mechanisms and reflect the same phylogenetic history. When explanations for population-level asymmetries of hand-use preference are made, they fail to distinguish between homologous and convergent laterality ... Are traits similar across species or across ontogenetic phases within a species because of homologous (derived from the same ancestral character) or convergent (adapted to similar ecological conditions) evolution? (Michel 2021)

1.1 Introduction

Handedness is more than just an interesting phenomenon: It is a highly complex and intricate construct with various motor, cognitive, psychological and social facets. These affect the functioning of individuals, particularly children who are learning complex manual activities in everyday life and who often present with variable hand use. So it is not surprising that handedness—the most apparent functional asymmetry of the human body—has captivated the attention of many researchers for decades. Why does *Left* and *Right Handedness* exist, and how did it evolve? And how does handedness develop in human beings? These are typical questions confronting those trying to understand handedness.

In this chapter, we briefly look at the evolution of handedness, reviewing some main theories and postulates that propose why handedness exists, i.e. the *ontological emergence of handedness.* I then examine research on the development of individual handedness concerning theoretical postulates, dynamic developmental phases and related processes, i.e. the *individual emergence of handedness.* Knowledge of developmental cascades is important to practitioners working with children of all ages, whose hand preference and hand skills are still developing. Finally, the chapter closes with some formal description of handedness, including its definition, categorisation and distribution, that could be described as the *scientific emergence* of handedness as a construct.

E. Kraus, *Beyond Left and Right Handedness*, https://doi.org/10.1007/978-3-031-24389-9_1

1.2 The Evolution of Handedness

Let us look at the knowledge base around how handedness emerged ontologically. Sidedness, or ♦**laterality**,[1] probably preceded the emergence of handedness. It is not unique to humans and can also be observed in many animal species. In general, the sidedness in animals tends to be fairly equally divided between left and right, and there is not a clear preference for the right side as is the case in humans (Cashmore et al. 2008; McGrew and Marchant 1997). For example, Corballis showed that chimpanzees use their right hand 65% of the time when working with instruments or tools (Corballis 2010).

From an evolutionary perspective, if there is neither a clear left nor a right hand use advantage or disadvantage, a 50–50 distribution would likely have emerged (Christman 2012; Ghirlanda et al. 2009; Prichard et al. 2013). The questions about the origin of human *Left* and *Right Handedness* distribution have been investigated from many different evolutionary and theoretical perspectives. This section will briefly present some of the most common theories on handedness regarding human evolutionary traits: language and gestures, task demands and tool use.

1.2.1 Handedness as an Inherited Evolutionary Trait

The evolutionary perspective on handedness is based on many studies, including those investigating early cave drawings. Several authors have argued that a left-right handed ratio of 10:90 percent may have existed for 10.000 years (Faurie and Raymond 2004; Raymond and Pontier 2004). Forrester and his team studied great apes and suggested that handedness and the underlying hemispheric specialisation may not be an exclusive feature of humans (Forrester et al. 2013). Cashmore and colleagues postulate that Neanderthals had a strong right hand preference (Cashmore et al. 2008). Other researchers describe lateralisation of manual actions as a consequence of the increasing use of tools, which allowed for complex and bimanual movements (e.g. Cochet and Byrne 2013; Uomini 2009). According to Forrester and colleagues, *Right Handedness* has prevailed across time and cultures and is presumed to be an inherited characteristic determined by evolution (Forrester et al. 2013). Overall, evolutionary theories indicate that manual specialisation has been advantageous for human activity and development.

[1]Laterality will be used synonymously with sidedness.

1.2.2 Language and Gestures as Drivers for Hemispheric Lateralisation

Human language is considered a uniquely human trait, probably having evolved from communicative gestures (Corballis 2010). Studies investigating gestures of babies and young children (Cochet and Vauclair 2010) and monkeys (Liebal and Call 2012) showed a strong right-sided asymmetry for non-verbal communication. Corballis argues that the increased use of communicative gestures probably led to brain lateralisation, language development and handedness establishment over time (Corballis 2003, 2010). However, since language developed later than tool use, it has been deemed questionable whether handedness can result from language development alone (Forrester et al. 2013). It also appears unlikely that right-biassed gestural communication is the sole reason for predominantly right-handed humans (Zickert et al. 2021). Since there is scientific evidence for both theories, it is postulated that handedness is an evolutionary trait that developed parallel with communicative and manipulative skills (Cochet and Byrne 2013).

1.2.3 Task Demand, Complexity and Efficiency as Influencing Factors

Some theorists postulate that pre-human upright walking and standing created a “new” precondition that encouraged lateralised hand use (Hopkins et al. 2005; Hopkins and Morris 1993; MacNeilage et al. 1987). This hypothesis was tested by examining hand preference of bonobos (a great ape species) and comparing it to their sitting or standing postures and various task requirements. It was found that body posture did not seem to affect hand preference, but the complexity of the task requirements did: the more difficult the action, the more lateralised the hand use, with a clear tendency to the right (Bardo et al. 2015). The authors argue that more than bipedalism, complex activities contributed to hemispheric lateralisation and *Right Handedness*. Others also found a relationship between the difficulty level of activities and the difference between the hands, such as actions with target accuracy (Bryden and Roy 2005; Bryden et al. 2007).

It is well established that the brain and related movement patterns function the most efficiently, i.e. as fast and accurate as possible, with the least amount of energy expenditure necessary (see (Pool et al. 2014). Michel states that handedness may have developed to meet this need.

> *It is likely that handedness reduces the decision time for the initiation of unimanual tasks (putting food in mouth, throwing or swinging a stick) and for the selection of the different actions in role-differentiated bimanual manipulations (RDBM). During RDBM, the preference efficiently dictates the sequence of the actions of each hand, and the practice of manual actions improves their skill of execution.* (Michel 2021)

1.2.4 The Emergence of Tool Use as a Driver for Handedness Ontogenesis

Several authors focus on tool use and the evolution of manual skills. For example, Legare and Nielsen suggest that these skills were socially transferred from one generation to another (Legare and Nielsen 2015). This may have occurred through imitating and copying behaviour, not only as a product but also as a behavioural process (Schillinger et al. 2015). According to Vaesen, transmitting information via instructions may have been more efficient, thereby contributing to human knowledge and cumulative culture over time (Vaesen 2012).

Zickert and team tested the hypothesis of tool use as a driver for handedness ontogenesis. They examined whether teaching manual skills such as making nautical knots is enhanced when handedness is concordant between teacher and student (Zickert et al. 2021). The team found that learning by imitation is easier when the direction of handedness is matched, whilst the level of activity complexity did not seem to influence the learning process. They conclude that imitation, among other factors, may maintain a right-biassed environment (ibid).

1.3 Development of Individual Handedness

To better understand handedness for a practice-based approach, we now turn to the emergence of handedness across an individual life span, particularly looking at the development of individual handedness. Handedness development is a process that has been typically assigned to the first 6 years of life (Fagard 1987, 1998; Stilwell 1987; Tan 1985) and continues to consolidate up to 12 years (Scharoun and Bryden 2014; Quinn and Geffen 1986). At the same time, there are indications that handedness continues to be formed across the life span (Sivagnanasunderam et al. 2015). In the context of this book, I distinguish between ◆**handedness development** in the first 6 years of life and ◆**handedness formation** across the life span.

Several factors influence the development of handedness, such as the right-handed and right-biassed environment, which are discussed in detail in Chaps. 3 and 4. Historically, research methods of infant handedness have been quite inconsistent. In particular, different types of assessment and criteria were used, compromising the reliability and comparability of the results (Nelson and Gonzalez 2020). Several authors propose that hand preference should be based on longitudinal studies with large samples, where the infants are assessed monthly for 6 months or longer. This enables the trajectories of hand preference development to be characterised, providing a sound basis for rigorous statistical analysis (Campbell et al. 2018; Gonzalez et al. 2020).

In this section, I concentrate on two important approaches to understanding practice-based handedness development, namely the cascading theory and developmental phases and stages.

1.3.1 Cascade Theory on Handedness Development

The *cascade theory* states that the development of handedness resembles a waterfall (cascade), with multiplicative effects due to ongoing interactions between the individual and the environment (Campbell et al. 2015). Preferred hand use evolves over a range of manual actions within the first years of life. These early preferences are linked to preferences in later development, thereby establishing handedness (Harkins and Michel 1988) by linking preferred hand use patterns in early developmental stages with those in later development (Michel 1988). The assumption here is that handedness develops *anew* in each novel task, competency or skill that is being learned rather than being an inherently unchangeable construct of hemispheric specialisation (Babik 2014). Gonzalez describes how increased unimanual reaching results in the repeated use of the same hand during object acquisition. This pattern is later also seen in unimanual and bimanual object manipulation (Gonzalez et al. 2020). The snowball effect of the cascade theory leads to repeated asymmetric motor activities performed with the same hand for a particular task, which in turn affects the hand preference for other tasks and, over time, results in building manual skills.

Moreover, the cascade theory puts forward the hypothesis that the established handedness of a new skill is initially weak, then becomes stronger as the skill is mastered and decreases again when the skill is well established and automated. This pattern emerged from a study with 380 children aged 6- to 14-month-old by Babik and colleagues. They investigated lateralised reaching for age-appropriate objects, such as playing with toys, including unimanual and bimanual manipulations (Babik 2014). Lateralised reaching for toys increased in the period of 6–12 months and after that decreased again. Unimanual as well as role-differentiated bimanual manipulation increased between the 9th and 14th months. In addition, the preferred hand for grasping toys correlated positively with the preferred hand for one-handed manipulation, again indicating a correlation between more complex movements and bimanual role differentiation (Babik 2014). The cascade theory thus challenges the assumption that the observed fluctuation of hand preference in infants and toddlers is a sign of an inherent instability (Corbetta and Thelen 2002; Fagard 1998). Instead, the variability of hand use is attributed to the cascading transformations of handedness across different activities and their demands at various points in time.

Other researchers have focused on identifying trajectories (a chronologically ordered set of dynamical states) to understand early handedness development. Referring to Babik's longitudinal study above, Ferre and colleagues define four latent classes: (1) infants with a very early right-hand preference; (2) infants developing a left preference somewhat later; (3) infants with a late *Right Handedness* and (4) a small group without a preference (Ferre et al. 2020). In another study, three of these trajectories are similarly observed in toddlers aged 18–24 months (Nelson et al. 2017). Ferre and his team conclude that this probably results in different modes of sensorimotor experience, which, in turn, may influence the lateralisation process and interhemispheric communication (Ferre et al. 2020).

Similarly, Michel proposes that a complex cascade of possibilities influences the trajectory of handedness development during infancy. Early prenatal influences such as foetal position and postural asymmetries shape early sensorimotor asymmetries of the upper extremities, which then initiate preferences in reaching and grasping. These early preferences then translate to RDBM around the second year of life, cascading into the general handedness development in the context of the caregiver's handedness and general sociocultural influences (Michel 2021).

1.3.2 Developmental Phases of Handedness

The theories on cascade-like development of handedness encourage us to understand the developmental process as dynamic, highly complex and interrelated with other developmental processes. This theory seems to replace the conventional hierarchical approach to development typically anchored in rather static developmental milestones. However, handedness phases and stages are very useful for practitioners working with children with unclear handedness, when defined broadly and as a dynamic process. Indeed, the cascade theorists also refer to interrelated *phases* and sequences of handedness development. For example, Ferre and colleagues describe the following developmental phases of handedness establishment:

> *Handedness for simple reaching for objects expands into handedness for acquiring objects which, in turn, transfers into hand-use preferences in later-emerging skills such as unimanual manipulation and RDBM… At each phase, self-generated haptic, proprioceptive, kinesthetic, and visual experiences contribute to the transitions in how a hand-use preference is manifested. Moreover, the manifestation of hand-use preferences for a manual skill will vary with the development of each skill; with lateralisation being low at the emergence of the action, increasing as the skill becomes mastered, and then decreasing as the action becomes highly skilled and more automatic*. (Ferre et al. 2020)

These early phases of handedness development described above occur within the first 2–3 years of life. Scharoun and Bryden look at handedness establishment of children between 3 and 12 years, describing three developmental phases:

1. *First phase (3–5 years):* relatively weak and partly inconsistent hand preference (especially in left-handed children)
2. *Second phase (7–10 years):* particularly strong focus on the dominant hand; this hand is used irrespective of the task, object or its positioning in space
3. *Third phase (10–12 years):* development of "adult" handedness: the pronounced use of the dominant hand diminishes somewhat, similar to the differences in performance between the hands (Scharoun and Bryden 2014).

In the context of a practice-based approach to handedness when dealing with children having to decide on a writing hand when starting school, the first 6 years of life is the most crucial developmental phase.[2] In my doctoral thesis, I summarised a range of longitudinal developmental studies on multidimensional handedness guidelines to provide practitioners with guidelines for typical developmental phases. The dimensions include ipsilateral and contralateral reaching as well as unimanual and bimanual actions. I compiled nine dynamic, broadly defined and interrelating stages (rather than static milestones), as shown in Fig. 1.1 (Kraus 2003, 2019; Kraus and Nagele-Hiedl 2019; Allweiss and Kraus 2019). These developmental stages help guide clinical and educational practice with children still establishing handedness, and they are not considered to contradict the cascade theory but rather to provide a complementary developmental perspective for orientation.

As we can see above, the development of crossing the body midline and bimanual coordination not only occur in parallel to handedness development, but they seem intricately and reciprocally linked to one another (Kraus 2003). These relationships are explored in more detail in Sect. 2.4 in the following chapter.

1.3.3 Early Handedness Development and Related Processes

It has been suggested that handedness is helpful as a developmental indicator concerning other

[2]For this reason, I have assigned the term "handedness development" to this phase 0–6 years to differentiate it from "handedness formation", which includes the establishment of handedness across the life span (0–99 years).

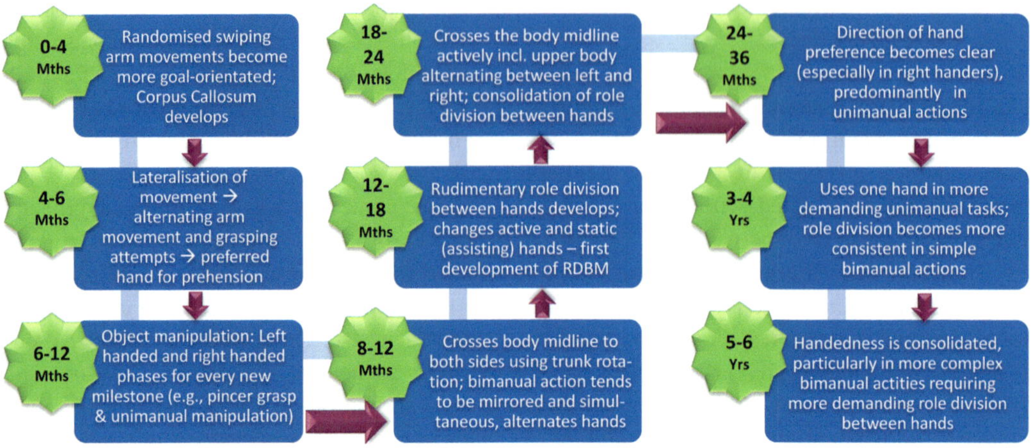

Fig. 1.1 Developmental phases and stages of handedness establishment (Kraus 2003)

developmental processes. They include early development of manual asymmetry and early neuromotor development with particular reference to early bimanual coordination. We will explore these in more detail here.

Early Manual Asymmetry

Hepper and colleagues observed manual asymmetries already during the foetal development stage. Furthermore, they found that this asymmetry tended to be associated with subsequent hand preference during childhood (Hepper et al. 1991, 2005). After birth, infants first exhibit random movements of hand or arm (Fagard 2006). It has been detected that during this early stage of development, the active hand frequently changes, and handedness seems unstable and malleable (Carlson and Harris 1985; Corbetta et al. 2006; Hopkins et al. 2005; Michel et al. 2006). This frequent swapping of hands might partially be due to the newborn's limbs being exposed to gravity in its new environment, making it more difficult to perform movements (Harris 2005). In particular, asymmetrical use of hands has been observed in 6- to 12-month infants in studies investigating unimanual grasping patterns of infants (e.g. grasping for toys or food) and showing a right-sided preference (Michel et al. 2006; Rönnqvist and Domellöf 2006; Sacrey et al. 2013).

During the early development of manual dexterity, children increase their motor control and strength and engage in increasingly demanding and bimanually complex actions such as using a spoon, a hammer or tweezers to manipulate small objects (Harris 2005). Several studies have targeted the development of manual dexterity and its relationship to handedness in infants and toddlers.

On the one hand, some findings indicate more frequent use of the left hand in early years compared to studies with older children. For example, Nelson and colleagues monitored the development of hand dexterity in 23 infants aged 6–24 months. Whilst the sample size is very small, the results indicate that those children without early preferred hand use developed a left- or right-sided preference by 2 years (Nelson et al. 2013). Notably, 65.2% of these children became right handed, 30.5% of the remaining children turned out to be left handed and in 4.4%, hand preference remained unclear (ibid). In their widely cited longitudinal developmental study, Gesell and Ames referred to more frequent left-hand use as "left-handed phases" in the first 2 years (Gesell and Ames 1947).

On the other hand, and similar to Hepper's findings mentioned earlier, there are indications that toddlers' preferred hand use generally coincided with their later handedness (Gonzalez et al. 2015; Isaacs et al. 2006; Nelson et al. 2013). Furthermore, several authors argue that hand preference and the degree of handedness seem to remain the same from childhood to old age (Gonzalez et al. 2015; Gooderham and Bryden 2014).

One explanation for the contradictory results could be that age-related changes in handedness are task-dependent (Sivagnanasunderam et al. 2015), apart from the well-known problem of inconsistent definition, classification and assessment of handedness.

Early Neuromotor Development and Bimanual Coordination

Campbell and colleagues argue that handedness as a developmental trait should not be seen as an isolated phenomenon but as related to neuromotor development processes (Campbell et al. 2018). Based on a number of developmental studies, the authors propose four reasons for examining the relationship between hand preference development and neuromotor development:

1. Hand preference is an aspect of neuromotor development during the rapid neuromotor developmental phase in infancy.
2. Hand preference reflects, and is influenced by, typical developmental locomotor developmental processes.
3. Neuromotor abilities may be a better developmental predictor of hand preference than age during infancy.
4. Early handedness development as an aspect of hemispheric specialisation may be closely related to the development of other neural systems (Campbell et al. 2018).

The early developmental phase of handedness is marked not only by unimanual but also by bimanual hand use. It has been proposed that the acquisition of effective role differentiation between the hands during bimanual action influences handedness development for unimanual actions (Cochet 2016). Cochet argues that this could explain why many children do not display a stable preference for one-handed grasping actions in their first year of life but only when they engage in more bimanual activity as toddlers. However, several authors argue that if a strong hand preference is established very early in the developmental process, this may not be beneficial to the development of bimanual coordination (Babik 2014; Fagard and Corroyer 2003; Goldfield and Michel 1986).

1.3.4 Influencing Factors on Early Handedness Development

Task demands also seem to affect an infant's hand use. For example, hand-to-mouth actions during eating elicit a particularly strong preferential hand use (Gonzalez et al. 2015; Sacrey et al. 2013). Sacrey and colleagues found that children as young as one year showed a clear hand preference in hand-to-mouth actions but not in construction tasks (ibid). Although the task demands of reaching for food and other objects are similar, children appear to perform hand-to-mouth actions with greater precision (Flindall and Gonzalez 2015). The authors explain that there are different end goals for the tasks and that reaching for food is essential since it is necessary for survival (Flindall and Gonzalez 2015; Flindall and Gonzalez 2013). The influence of task demands and the environment appear to be significant even at an early age and are likely to influence the developmental course of handedness establishment. See Chap. 3 for a detailed discussion of these factors.

1.3.5 Handedness Groups in Infants

When examining the neuromotor development of 6- to 14-month-old infants, Campbell and colleagues identified at least four different developmental groups (Campbell et al. 2018):

1. Children with early right-sided preference (32%)
2. Children with early left-sided preference (12%)
3. Children with later right-sided preference (25%)
4. Children with no clear hand preference in this age range (30%)

However, Campbell and colleagues argue that there may be a fifth group of children who later develop a left-sided preference (ibid). The authors postulate that these developmental types may coincide with different degrees of handedness: the lower the degree of handedness, the less likely that a clear preference can be observed within the first 2 years (ibid). Importantly, this categorisation by Campbell indicates that categories based on degrees of handedness can be constructed even in infancy if the assessment of handedness is age-appropriate and comprehensive.

1.4 Describing Handedness

1.4.1 Definition of Handedness

In this section, we look at how definitions and classifications of handedness emerged in the scientific context. There is no consensus in the literature about the exact definition of handedness. It is generally referred to as a functional asymmetry during hand use. In many studies, handedness is "reduced" to the writing hand, but this does not do justice to the phenomenon's complexity and is neither useful in the clinical field nor for researchers trying to get a deeper understanding of handedness.

Researchers generally agree that there are (at least) two aspects or ⧫**dimensions of handedness:** ⧫**hand preference** and ⧫**hand proficiency**. Preference refers to using one hand rather than the other for specific activities—it is about how *frequently* one hand is used compared to the other. Proficiency (or performance) refers to the motor skills and abilities that allow one hand to perform *better* than the other hand in certain activities of the hand for a specific job (see Alphonso et al. 2008). Preference and proficiency are probably both subject to genetic factors (Ocklenburg et al. 2014), as well as being shaped by the environment and the occupations people engage in (e.g. prolonged practice—Peters 1981). In most cases, people perform better with their preferred hand. For example, if a person uses her/his right hand more frequently in everyday tasks (preference), s/he also performs better with that hand (proficiency).

However, the usually assumed correlation between preference and proficiency is not as high as expected (Bryden et al. 1994; Rigal 1992; Tapley and Bryden 1985). This finding has resulted in numerous studies investigating the relationship between preference and proficiency/performance (e.g. (Annett 1970; Brown et al. 2006; Triggs et al. 2000). Some individuals may prefer using one hand for certain tasks but show better performance with the other hand. The relationship between hand preference and proficiency is not yet fully understood. Is there a causal relationship between preference and proficiency? For example, does a superior performance of one hand determine hand preference since the better hand is used more often? Or does preference shape proficiency since the preferred hand is used more and, therefore, becomes more trained?

Researchers have used different approaches to answer these questions and reached different conclusions. Some assume that asymmetries in motor performance influence the development of hand preference (Annett 1985; Triggs et al. 2000). Others argue the opposite: the early preference for hand use influences and shapes motor performance and proficiency (McManus 1991, 1999). Porac and Coren see preference and proficiency as two different phenomena, probably sharing a common origin (Porac and Coren 1981). They base their hypothesis on the different distributions of the two-handedness dimensions in the same population. The distribution of hand preference is usually shaped like a J-shaped curve (see Fig. 1.2a), whilst the distribution of proficiency assumes a bell-shaped curve following a normal distribution (see Fig. 1.2b). These differences also show that preference and proficiency are not the same (Porac and Coren 1981; Corey et al. 2001).

The *level* of proficiency (i.e. how does a particular motor performance compare to the norm) is often neglected in research, as is the *quantified difference* between the hands (i.e. how much better is one hand compared to the other). For example, if both hands show similar performance in a motor test, the inter-hand difference will be slight. However, the inter-hand difference does not convey whether both hands are equally good concerning the norm (i.e. average or above aver-

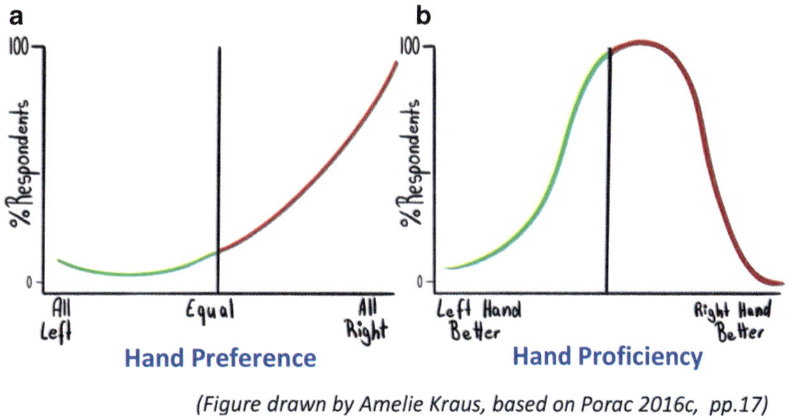

Fig. 1.2 J-shaped distribution of Hand Preference (**a**) and bell-shaped distribution of Hand Proficiency (**b**) (Figure drawn by Amelie Kraus, based on Porac 2016b, pp 12)

age performance) or similarly poor (i.e. sub-average performance)

In the end, preference and proficiency are often considered different dimensions of handedness, even though the debate as to which of the two-handedness dimensions is pivotal or decisive remains inconclusive. In this book, hand preference and hand proficiency will be considered as equally important dimensions of handedness. In addition, a further distinction is frequently made between the direction and the degree of handedness. The ♦**direction** of handedness makes a binary distinction whether a person is left or right handed. The ♦**degree** (or extent) of handedness indicates the extent of handedness, or how strongly established a person's handedness is (Biddle and Eales 1996; Bryden et al. 2000; Dassonville et al. 1997; McManus 1999).

For example, a person with a high degree of *Right Handedness* will display a strongly established and consistent performance pattern with the right hand. Conversely, a person with a mild degree of *Right Handedness* will be more inconsistent, use the left hand more frequently in preference tasks and perform better with the left hand than a strongly established right-handed person. In the context of this book and the Handedness Profile, degrees of handedness are measured as inter-hand differences using the ♦**laterality quotient**. Some authors critically reflect that research studies tend to neglect degrees of handedness, which may have contributed to research results being often contradictory and diverse (Prichard et al. 2013).

Papadatou-Pastou suggests in her article that the primary focus on hand preference in the handedness research may result in inconclusive results, also because differentiating according to degrees of handedness is neglected. She proposes that in addition to hand preference, hand proficiency and the degree of handedness need to be incorporated when relationships between handedness and cognitive abilities are investigated (Papadatou-Pastou 2018).

In the context of this book, I define handedness direction and degree as two further dimensions of handedness. So how can we conceptually combine these four defining dimensions: preference, proficiency, direction and degree? First, let us assume that a person's degree of *Left* or *Right Handedness* will be apparent in both preference and proficiency. This can result in several possible combinations, even if one assigns only two categories to the degree (strongly and mildly established) of either *Left* or *Right Handedness* (see Fig. 1.3).

However, handedness is rarely defined to incorporate all these aspects. Usually, preference and performance are both mentioned in definitions but referred to as either-or, as seen in the following definition:

> *A preference for using one hand rather than the other, or a tendency to use one hand more skillfully or comfortably than the other, depending on which cerebral hemisphere is dominant for motor control, approximately 90 percent of people showing right handedness or left hemisphere dominance for motor control* (Colman 2015)

A more comprehensive definition will be attempted in Chap. 7, regarding the four defining dimensions, task and environmental demands.

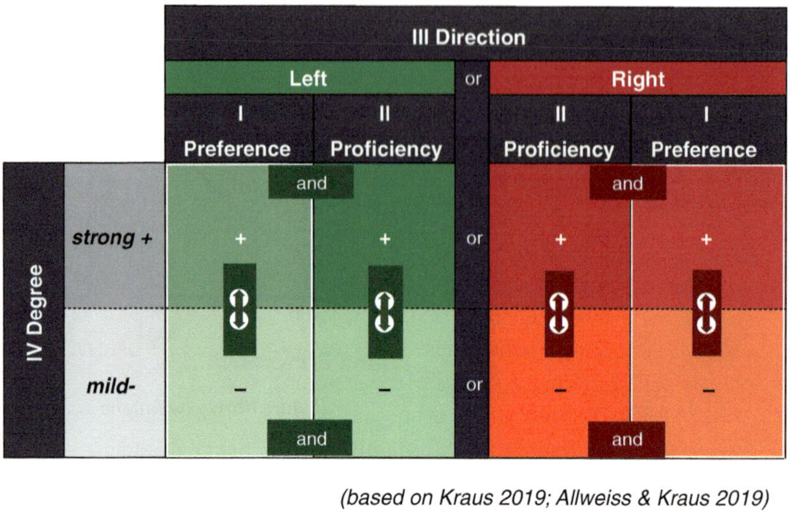

Fig. 1.3 Four defining dimensions of handedness (indicated with Roman numbers) (based on (Kraus 2019; Allweiss and Kraus 2019)). The arrows between the strong+ and mild− degrees of handedness indicate continuums. Note also that there could be differences in degree between preference and proficiency in the same person (e.g. strong proficiency and mild preference)

1.4.2 Classification of Handedness

Handedness can be classified differently, depending on whether we want to assess only the direction or the degree of handedness. Classifications range from a binary distinction between *Left* and *Right Handedness*, measuring only the direction, to classifications ranging between 3 and 8 subgroups, measuring the degree, usually in combination with the direction. An alternative (or addition) to categorising handedness is mapping it as a continuum (Denny and Zhang 2017; Hardyck and Petrinovich 1977) as shown in Fig. 1.4. Different terms are used to describe the degree of handedness, such as "strongly/weakly established", "variable", "mixed", "inconsistent", "unestablished", "unclear", "uncertain" handedness, or "to a lesser extent", "to a low degree" *Left* or *Right Handedness* (see also Christman 2012; Prichard et al. 2013). In the context of this book, I will consistently use the term ⧫**degree of handedness** together with "explicit", "moderately" and "mildly established" handers. The term ⧫**mixed handedness** is used collectively when the direction is not clear or no further differentiation is made. However, mixed handedness is a place-holder category, with the assumption that it is not a true category but mildly established left or right handers that have not been clearly identified (see also McManus 2002).

This diversity in possible handedness classifications with different cut-off points makes studies extremely difficult to compare. It is compounded by the diverse definitions of handedness whereby "handedness" may only consist of hand preference *or* hand proficiency, and seldom both, and numerous disparate test procedures. In fact, some authors have observed that different classification instruments produce different results, whereby the introduction of "consistent" and "inconsistent" handedness categories resulted in more differentiation (Budisavljevic et al. 2021). In addition, the category of mixed handedness is particularly diffuse and even less clearly defined than *Left* and *Right Handedness*. For example, McManus argues that mixed handedness is not a natural category but instead constitutes "weak" *Left* and *Right Handedness* together (McManus 2002). McManus proposes to use four groups of handedness to represent the degree of handedness more clearly. However, this does not solve the problem of the highly inconsistent cut-off point between the categories. "Strongly established" (or "consistent") handedness in some studies refers to hand use, in which all tasks are performed with the dominant hand. "Mildly established" (or "inconsistent") handedness might refer to performing at least one task up to just over half of the tasks with the non-dominant hand (Prichard et al. 2013). In Chap. 6, we look at classifying handedness in more detail.

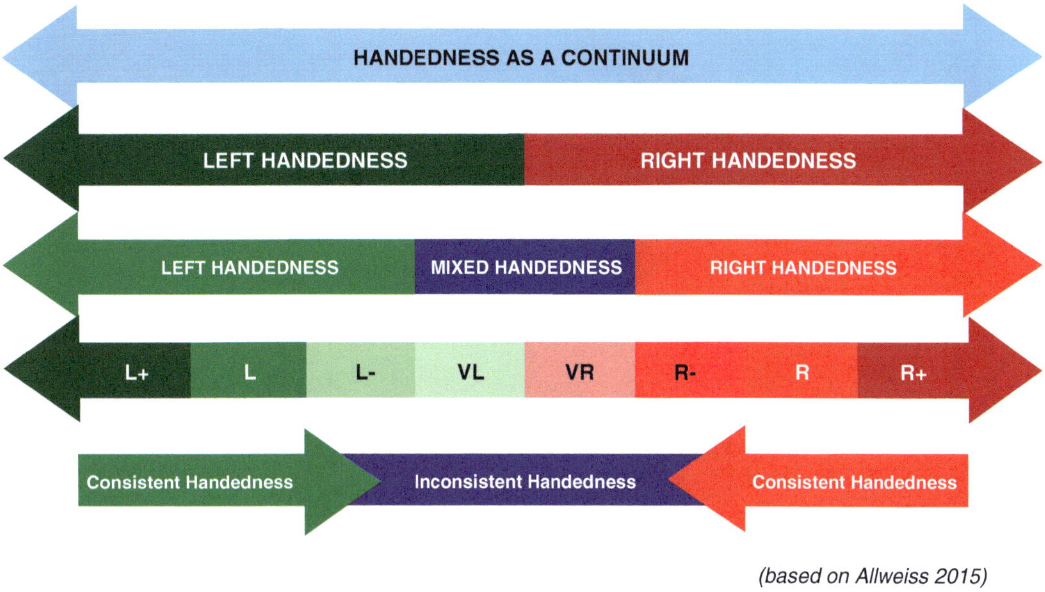

Fig. 1.4 Handedness classifications (based on (Allweiss 2015). This figure does not display the distribution of handedness in the population. *L+* explicit *Left Handedness*, *L* moderate *Left Handedness*, *L−* mild *Left Handedness*, *VL Variable Left Handedness*, *R+* explicit *Right Handedness*, *R* moderate *Right Handedness*, *R−* mild *Right Handedness*, *VR Variable Right Handedness*

1.4.3 Distribution of Handedness

In the literature, it is typically assumed that a ratio of 10:90 percent reflects the average proportion of *Left* and *Right Handedness* in normal populations (Christman 2012; Corballis 2003, 2010; Willems et al. 2014). For example, Papadatou-Pastou and colleagues looked at five meta-analyses on hand preference where the prevalence of *Left Handedness* was found to be between 9.3 and 18.1%, depending on the criteria of *Left Handedness*, with an overall average of 10.4% (Papadatou-Pastou et al. 2020).

When considering the degree in addition to the direction of handedness, the distribution patterns seem to change. For example, Annett argues that the degree of handedness is generally much lower in left-handed than in right-handed persons and that 60% of right handers were consistent, compared to only 4% of left handers and 36% less pronounced "handers" as depicted in Fig. 1.5 (Annett 2004).

In developmental research, some studies find that the incidence of left handers far exceeds the presumed 10% in children in their first 2 years of life (Babik 2014; Marschik et al. 2008; Prichard et al. 2013). Similarly, some studies found a significantly higher number of left handers. For example, Sovák hypothesised in the 1960s that "latent" (or weakly) established left handers, together with strongly established left handers, account for about 50% of the population based on measures such as folding arms and hands (Sovák 1962; Sovak 1974). However, Porac argues that such measurements do not differentiate between laterality/sidedness and handedness. This is problematic since they appear to be two separate two phenomena that do not correlate highly and should thus not be used synonymously (Porac 2016a, 2016b).

One could conclude that the typically cited 10:90 ratio of *Left-to-Right Handedness* is questionable - the incidence of *Left Handedness* may considerably exceed the proposed 10%. Not only are the findings determined by the definition and the methods of assessing handedness, but they are also influenced and skewed by the right-biassed physical and socio-cultural environments. For a practice-based approach,

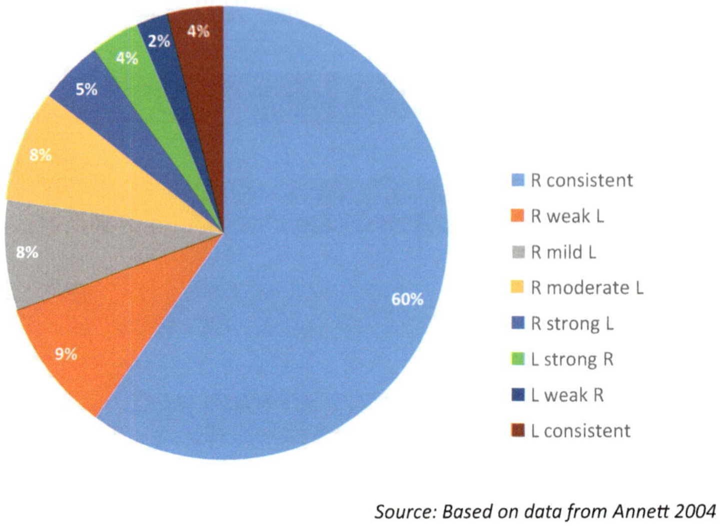

Fig. 1.5 Eight Handedness Categories based on hand preference (Source: Based on data from Annett 2004). A total of 2388 subjects (5–63 years old; 949 males, 1439 females) were examined for their handedness and divided into 8 categories based on their results. Hand preference was assessed by observing the 12 activities of the "Annett Hand Preference Questionnaire" (Annett 1970). The terms weak, mild, moderate and strong refer to the use of the other hand. The higher proportion of females in the study may have resulted in a slight overrepresentation of *Right Handedness*. *L* left, *R* right

practitioners need to be informed about the possibility of a higher *Left Handedness* incidence and understand the importance of implementing both an evidence-based and non-biassed approach when assessing and treating handedness.

1.5 Concluding Remarks

In this chapter, we looked at three perspectives on the emergence of handedness. **Evolutionary theories** increase our understanding of how handedness came to exist in the first place. However, they do not provide compelling or coherent arguments for the typically cited higher prevalence of *Right Handedness* in contemporary society. **Individual handedness development** is characterised by general principles of dynamic cascade-like development, which are highly individual, multidimensional and lifelong. Moreover, it provides valuable insights into the complexity of the diverse environment and task demands in which handedness develops. In addition, some developmental phases can be roughly identified, which are useful for practitioners working with children with unestablished or unclear handedness. The **description and definition** of handedness in the scientific context are indeed complex and without consensus in the research community. Broadly speaking, handedness is best described as a *multidimensional* and *polygenetic* phenomenon consisting of hand preference and proficiency and it can be measured in terms of direction and degree.

In addition to the evolutionary and developmental handedness research perspectives presented in this chapter, the next chapter explores handedness from an anatomical and physiological angle to expand our understanding of this complex phenomenon. It deals with a neural perspective on handedness, revealing some central underlying mechanisms in terms of neuro-anatomical, neuro-behavioural and neuro-functional asymmetries.

References

Allweiss TC (2015) The digitalised handedness profile: reliability and measurement error of the digital and the conventional methods of analysis. Masterthesis. Hochschule für Angewandte Wissenschaften Hamburg, Hamg

Allweiss T, Kraus E (2019) Grundlagen der Händigkeit. In: Zwischen Links-& Rechtshändigkeit. Springer, 9–46

Alphonso K, Roy EA, Bryden PJ, Balkowski B, Mayer M, Kuehner Z (2008) Preference and performance measures of handedness: the effect of task complexity. Brain Cogn 67:11. https://doi.org/10.1016/j.bandc.2008.02.014

Annett M (1970) A classification of hand preference by association analysis. Br J Psychol 61(3):303–321. https://doi.org/10.1111/j.2044-8295.1970.tb01248.x

Annett M (1985) Left, right, hand, and brain. The right shift theory. L. Erlbaum Associates, London

Annett M (2004) Hand preference observed in large healthy samples: classification, norms and interpretations of increased non-right-handedness by the right shift theory. Br J Psychol 95(3):339–353. https://doi.org/10.1348/0007126041528130

Babik I (2014) Development of handedness for role-differentiated bimanual manipulation of objects in relation to the development of hand-use preferences for acquisition. Dissertation. The University of North Carolina at Greensboro, Greensboro

Bardo A, Pouydebat E, Meunier H (2015) Do bimanual coordination, tool use, and body posture contribute equally to hand preferences in bonobos? J Hum Evol 82(11):159–169. https://doi.org/10.1016/j.jhevol.2015.02.015

Biddle FG, Eales BA (1996) The degree of lateralization of paw usage (handedness) in the mouse is defined by three major phenotypes. Behav Genet 26(4):391–406. https://doi.org/10.1007/BF02359483

Brown S, Roy E, Rohr L, Bryden P (2006) Using hand performance measures to predict handedness. Laterality 11(1):1–14. https://doi.org/10.1080/13576500542000000440

Bryden PJ, Roy EA (2005) Unimanual performance across the age span. Brain Cogn 57(1):26–29. https://doi.org/10.1016/j.bandc.2004.08.016

Bryden MP, Singh M, Steenhuis RE, Clarkson KL (1994) A behavioral measure of hand preference as opposed to hand skill. Neuropsychologia 32(8):991–999. https://doi.org/10.1016/0028-3932(94)90048-5

Bryden PJ, Pryde KM, Roy EA (2000) A performance measure of the degree of hand preference. Brain Cogn 44(3):402–414. https://doi.org/10.1006/brcg.1999.1201

Bryden PJ, Roy EA, Rohr LE, Egilo S (2007) Task demands affect manual asymmetries in pegboard performance. Laterality 12(4):364–377. https://doi.org/10.1080/13576500701356244

Budisavljevic S, Castiello U, Begliomini C (2021) Handedness and White matter networks. Neuroscientist 27(1):88–103. https://doi.org/10.1177/1073858420937657

Campbell JM, Marcinowski EC, Babik I, Michel GF (2015) The influence of a hand preference for acquiring objects on the development of a hand preference for unimanual manipulation from 6 to 14 months. Infant Behav Dev 39:107–117

Campbell JM, Marcinowski EC, Michel GF (2018) The development of neuromotor skills and hand preference during infancy. Dev Psychobiol 60(2):165–175. https://doi.org/10.1002/dev.21591

Carlson DF, Harris LJ (1985) Development of the infant's hand preference for visually directed reaching: preliminary report of a longitudinal study. Infant Ment Health J 6(3):158–174. https://doi.org/10.1002/1097-0355(198523)6:3<158::AID-IMHJ2280060307>3.0.CO;2-X

Cashmore L, Uomini N, Chapelain A (2008) The evolution of handedness in humans and great apes: a review and current issues. J Anthropol Sci 86:7–35

Christman SD (2012) Handedness. In: Ramachandran VS (Hg.) Encyclopedia of human behavior. Elsevier Academic Press, Amsterdam, pp 290–296

Cochet H (2016) Manual asymmetries and hemispheric specialization: insight from developmental studies. Neuropsychologia 93(2):335–341. https://doi.org/10.1016/j.neuropsychologia.2015.12.019

Cochet H, Byrne RW (2013) Evolutionary origins of human handedness: evaluating contrasting hypotheses. Anim Cogn 16(4):531–542. https://doi.org/10.1007/s10071-013-0626-y

Cochet H, Vauclair J (2010). Pointing gesture in young children: Hand preference and language development. Gesture 10(2–3);129–149

Colman AM (2015) A dictionary of psychology: Oxford quick reference

Corballis MC (2003) From mouth to hand: gesture, speech, and the evolution of right-handedness. Behav Brain Sci 26(2):199–208; discussion 208–60. https://doi.org/10.1017/s0140525x03000062

Corballis MC (Hg.) (2010) Handedness and cerebral asymmetry. An evolutionary perspective. MIT Press, Cambridge

Corbetta D, Thelen E (2002) Behavioral fluctuations and the development of manual asymmetries in infancy: contributions of the dynamic systems approach. Handbook of Neuropsychology 8(1), 311–330

Corbetta D, Williams J, Snapp-Childs W (2006) Plasticity in the development of handedness: evidence from normal development and early asymmetric brain injury. Dev Psychobiol 48(6):460–471. https://doi.org/10.1002/dev.20164

Corey DM, Hurley MM, Foundas AL (2001) Right and left handedness defined: a multivariate approach using hand preference and hand performance measures. Neuropsychiatry Neuropsychol Behav Neurol 14(3):144–152

Dassonville P, Zhu XH, Uurbil K, Kim SG, Ashe J (1997) Functional activation in motor cortex reflects the direction and the degree of handedness. Proc Natl Acad Sci U S A 94(25):14015–14018. https://doi.org/10.1073/pnas.94.25.14015
Denny K, Zhang W (2017) In praise of ambidexterity: how a continuum of handedness predicts social adjustment. Laterality 22(2):181–194. https://doi.org/10.1080/1357650X.2016.1153107
Fagard J (1987) Bimanual stereotypes: bimanual coordination in children as a function of movements and relative velocity. J Motor Behav 19(3):355–366. https://doi.org/10.1080/00222895.1987.10735417
Fagard J (1998) Changes in grasping skills and the emergence of bimanual coordination during the first year of life. In: Conolly KJ (ed) 18986831
Fagard J (2006) Normal and abnormal early development of handedness: introduction. Dev Psychobiol 48(6):413–417. https://doi.org/10.1002/dev.20159
Fagard J, Corroyer D (2003) Using a continuous index of laterality to determine how laterality is related to interhemispheric transfer and bimanual coordination in children. Dev Psychobiol 43(1):44–56. https://doi.org/10.1002/dev.10117
Faurie C, Raymond M (2004) Handedness frequency over more than ten thousand years. Proc R Soc Lond B 271(suppl_3):S43–S45. https://doi.org/10.1098/rsbl.2003.0092
Ferre CL, Babik I, Michel GF (2020) A perspective on the development of hemispheric specialization, infant handedness, and cerebral palsy. Cortex 127:208–220. https://doi.org/10.1016/j.cortex.2020.02.017
Flindall JW, Gonzalez CLR (2013) On the evolution of handedness: evidence for feeding biases. PLoS One 8(11):e78967. https://doi.org/10.1371/journal.pone.0078967
Flindall JW, Gonzalez CLR (2015) Children's bilateral advantage for grasp-to-eat actions becomes unimanual by age 10 years. J Exp Child Psychol 133(1):57–71. https://doi.org/10.1016/j.jecp.2015.01.011
Forrester GS, Quaresmini C, Leavens DA, Mareschal D, Thomas MSC (2013) Human handedness: an inherited evolutionary trait. Behav Brain Res 237(6):200–206. https://doi.org/10.1016/j.bbr.2012.09.037
Gesell A, Ames LB (1947) The development of handedness. Pedagogical Semin J Genet Psychol 70(2):155–175
Ghirlanda S, Frasnelli E, Vallortigara G (2009) Intraspecific competition and coordination in the evolution of lateralization. Phil Trans R Soc B 364(1519):861–866. https://doi.org/10.1098/rstb.2008.0227
Goldfield EG, Michel GF (1986) The ontology of infant bimanual reaching during the first year. Infant Behav Dev 9:81–89
Gonzalez CLR, Flindall JW, Stone KD (2015) Hand preference across the lifespan: effects of end-goal, task nature, and object location. Front Psychol 5(82):641. https://doi.org/10.3389/fpsyg.2014.01579
Gonzalez SL, Campbell JM, Marcinowski EC, Michel GF, Coxe S, Nelson EL (2020) Preschool language ability is predicted by toddler hand preference trajectories. Dev Psychol 56(4):699
Gooderham SE, Bryden PJ (2014) Does your dominant hand become less dominant with time? The effects of aging and task complexity on hand selection. Dev Psychobiol 56(3):537–546. https://doi.org/10.1002/dev.21123
Hardyck C, Petrinovich LF (1977) Left-handedness. Psychol Bull 84(3):385–404. https://doi.org/10.1037/0033-2909.84.3.385
Harkins DA, Michel GF (1988) Evidence for a maternal effect on infant hand-use preferences. Dev Psychobiol 21(6):535–541
Harris LJ (2005) Handedness. In: Hopkins B, Barr RG, Michel GF, Rochat P (Hg.) The Cambridge encyclopedia of child development. Cambridge University Press, Cambridge, pp 321–326
Hepper PG, Shahidullah S, White R (1991) Handedness in the human fetus. Neuropsychologia 29(11):1107–1111. https://doi.org/10.1016/0028-3932(91)90080-r
Hepper PG, Wells DL, Lynch C (2005) Prenatal thumb sucking is related to postnatal handedness. Neuropsychologia 43(3):313–315. https://doi.org/10.1016/j.neuropsychologia.2004.08.009
Hopkins WD, Morris RD (1993) Handedness in great apes: a review of findings. Int J Primatol 14(1):1–25. https://doi.org/10.1007/BF02196500
Hopkins B, Barr RG, Michel GF, Rochat P (Hg.) (2005) The Cambridge encyclopedia of child development. Cambridge University Press, Cambridge
Isaacs KL, Barr WB, Nelson PK, Devinsky O (2006) Degree of handedness and cerebral dominance. Neurology 66(12):1855–1858. https://doi.org/10.1212/01.wnl.0000219623.28769.74
Kraus E (2003) The handedness profile. The development of a normative profile to determine the extent of handedness in children. Doctoral thesis. La Trobe University, Melbourne
Kraus E (Hg.) (2019) Zwischen Links-& Rechtshändigkeit. Theorie, Diagnostik & Therapie bei Kindern mit wechselndem Handgebrauch. Springer, Berlin
Kraus E, Nagele-Hiedl U (2019) Fallbeispiele aus der Praxis. In: Kraus E (Hg) Zwischen Links-& Rechtshändigkeit. Springer
Legare CH, Nielsen M (2015) Imitation and innovation: the dual engines of cultural learning. Trends Cogn Sci 19(11):688–699
Liebal K, Call J (2012) The origins of non-human primates' manual gestures. Phil Trans R Soc B 367(1585):118–128. https://doi.org/10.1098/rstb.2011.0044
MacNeilage PF, Studdert-Kennedy MG, Lindblom B (1987) Primate handedness reconsidered. Behav Brain Sci 10(2):247–263. https://doi.org/10.1017/S0140525X00047695
Marschik PB, Einspieler C, Strohmeier A, Plienegger J, Garzarolli B, Prechtl HFR (2008) From the reaching behavior at 5 months of age to hand preference at preschool age. Dev Psychobiol 50(5):511–518. https://doi.org/10.1002/dev.20307

McGrew WC, Marchant LF (1997) On the other hand: current issues in and meta-analysis of the behavioral laterality of hand function in nonhuman primates. Am J Phys Anthropol 104(S25):201–232
McManus IC (1991) The inheritance of left-handedness. In: Ciba Found Symp 162, 251–67; discussion 267–81. https://doi.org/10.1002/9780470514160.ch15
McManus IC (1999) Handedness, cerebral lateralization and the evolution of language, p 194–217
McManus C (2002) Right hand, left hand. The origins of asymmetry in brains, bodies, atoms, and cultures. Harvard University Press
Michel GF (1988) A neuropsychological perspective on infant sensorimotor development, p 1–38
Michel GF (2021) Handedness development: a model for investigating the development of hemispheric specialization and interhemispheric coordination. Symmetry 13(6):992
Michel GF, Tyler AN, Ferre C, Sheu C-F (2006) The manifestation of infant hand-use preferences when reaching for objects during the seven- to thirteen-month age period. Dev Psychobiol 48(6):436–443. https://doi.org/10.1002/dev.20161
Nelson EL, Gonzalez SL (2020) Measuring infant handedness reliably from reaching: a systematic review. Laterality 25(4):430–454. https://doi.org/10.1080/1357650X.2020.1726367
Nelson EL, Campbell JM, Michel GF (2013) Unimanual to bimanual: tracking the development of handedness from 6 to 24 months. Infant Behav Dev 36(2):181–188. https://doi.org/10.1016/j.infbeh.2013.01.009
Nelson EL, Gonzalez SL, Coxe S, Campbell JM, Marcinowski EC, Michel GF (2017) Toddler hand preference trajectories predict 3-year language outcome. Dev Psychobiol 59(7):876–887. https://doi.org/10.1002/dev.21560
Ocklenburg S, Beste C, Arning L (2014) Handedness genetics: considering the phenotype. Front Psychol 5(9):221. https://doi.org/10.3389/fpsyg.2014.01300
Papadatou-Pastou M (2018) Handedness and cognitive ability: using meta-analysis to make sense of the data. Prog Brain Res 238:179–206. https://doi.org/10.1016/bs.pbr.2018.06.008
Papadatou-Pastou M, Ntolka E, Schmitz J, Martin M, Munafò MR, Ocklenburg S, Paracchini S (2020) Human handedness: a meta-analysis. Psychol Bull 146(6):481–524
Peters M (1981) Handedness: effect of prolonged practice on between hand performance differences. Neuropsychologia 19(4):587–590. https://doi.org/10.1016/0028-3932(81)90025-7
Pool E-M, Rehme AK, Fink GR, Eickhoff SB, Grefkes C (2014) Handedness and effective connectivity of the motor system. NeuroImage 99(40):451–460. https://doi.org/10.1016/j.neuroimage.2014.05.048
Porac C (2016a) The most compelling research on handedness is mixed a review of laterality: exploring the enigma of left-handedness
Porac C (2016b) Laterality. Exploring the enigma of left-handedness. Elsevier Science, Amsterdam. Online verfügbar unter http://www.sciencedirect.com/science/book/9780128012390
Porac C, Coren S (1981) Lateral preferences and human behavior. Springer, New York
Prichard E, Propper RE, Christman SD (2013) Degree of handedness, but not direction, is a systematic predictor of cognitive performance. Front Psychol 4:9. https://doi.org/10.3389/fpsyg.2013.00009
Quinn K, Geffen G (1986) The development of tactile transfer of information. Neuropsychologia 24(6):793–804
Raymond M, Pontier D (2004) Is there geographical variation in human handedness? Laterality 9(1):35–51. https://doi.org/10.1080/13576500244000274
Rigal RA (1992) Which handedness: preference or performance? Percept Mot Skills 75(3):851–866. https://doi.org/10.2466/pms.1992.75.3.851
Rönnqvist L, Domellöf E (2006) Quantitative assessment of right and left reaching movements in infants: a longitudinal study from 6 to 36 months. Dev Psychobiol 48(6):444–459. https://doi.org/10.1002/dev.20160
Sacrey L-AR, Arnold B, Whishaw IQ, Gonzalez CLR (2013) Precocious hand use preference in reach-to-eat behavior versus manual construction in 1- to 5-year-old children. Dev Psychobiol 55(8):902–911. https://doi.org/10.1002/dev.21083
Scharoun SM, Bryden PJ (2014) Hand preference, performance abilities, and hand selection in children. Front Psychol 5:82. https://doi.org/10.3389/fpsyg.2014.00082
Schillinger K, Mesoudi A, Lycett SJ (2015) The impact of imitative versus emulative learning mechanisms on artifactual variation: implications for the evolution of material culture. Evol Hum Behav 36(6):446–455
Sivagnanasunderam M, Gonzalez DA, Bryden PJ, Young G, Forsyth A, Roy EA (2015) Handedness throughout the lifespan: cross-sectional view on sex differences as asymmetries change. Front Psychol 5:1556
Sovák M (1962) Lateralität & Sprache. Wissenschaftliche Zeitschrift Martin-Luther Universität 11:1695–1702
Sovak M (1974) Measuring of lateral preference earlier and now. Stud Psychol 16(3):209
Stilwell JM (1987) The development of manual midline crossing in 2- to 6-year-old children. Am J Occup Ther 41(12):783–789. https://doi.org/10.5014/ajot.41.12.783
Tan LE (1985) Laterality and motor skills in four-year-olds. Child Dev 56(1):119–124
Tapley SM, Bryden MP (1985) A group test for the assessment of performance between the hands. Neuropsychologia 23(2):215–221. https://doi.org/10.1016/0028-3932(85)90105-8
Triggs WJ, Calvanio R, Levine M, Heaton RK, Heilman KM (2000) Predicting hand preference with performance on motor tasks. Cortex 36(5):679–689. https://doi.org/10.1016/S0010-9452(08)70545-8

Uomini NT (2009) The prehistory of handedness: archaeological data and comparative ethology. J Hum Evol 57(4):411–419. https://doi.org/10.1016/j.jhevol.2009.02.012
Vaesen K (2012) Cumulative cultural evolution and demography. PLoS One 7(7):e40989
Willems RM, van der Haegen L, Fisher SE, Francks C (2014) On the other hand: including left-handers in cognitive neuroscience and neurogenetics. Nat Rev Neurosci 15(3):193–201. https://doi.org/10.1038/nrn3679
Zickert N, Geuze RH, Riedstra B, Groothuis TGG (2021) Is imitational learning a driving factor for the population bias in human hand preference? J Hum Evol 159:103045

Neural Asymmetries 2

Contents

Surprisingly, the nature of handedness itself has been little looked at using fMRI, the self-evident difference between the two hands being studied surprisingly rarely, despite a general recognition that left-handers are less lateralised than are right-handers. (McManus 2021: 6)

2.1 Introduction

At first glance, the neural support of handedness seems rather obvious since it has been well established for decades that the contralateral motor cortex controls unimanual actions (e.g. Sperry 1968). Recent magnetic resonance imaging (MRI) studies confirm specific asymmetrical brain structures and features related to the difference between left and right motor skill levels. Nevertheless, the implications of the findings remain somewhat ambiguous since it is not clear whether hemispheric asymmetries cause manual asymmetries or whether handedness leads to asymmetrical brain organisation (Andersen and Siebner 2018; Vingerhoets 2019). This question becomes more curious since contralateral cortical control applies to both the dominant and the non-dominant hands. This means that hemispheric asymmetry cannot be equated with hemispheric dominance concerning hand dominance (Tzourio-Mazoyer et al. 2021).

If our aim is to understand children with variable hand use, we need to look at both dexterity and handedness as essential aspects of motor control and manual skill. Neuro-anatomical, physiological structures and processes of handedness as well as dexterity are fundamental to both. In recent years, technological advances have led to significantly more detailed neuroimaging of the brain and consequently to a surge of research focusing on neural asymmetries. From a practice-based approach, we need to know if there are new anatomically-based measures for assessing handedness more reliably. Could such new approaches complement or even replace current behavioural measures?

This chapter investigates a fundamental perspective on handedness looking at neural asym-

E. Kraus, *Beyond Left and Right Handedness*, https://doi.org/10.1007/978-3-031-24389-9_2

metries from three different levels. *Structural asymmetry* refers to the anatomical structures and their neural underpinnings that are associated with handedness. What is the relationship between handedness, neuro-anatomical brain structures and neurophysiological processes? A second level is *functional asymmetry*, where asymmetries, such as sidedness and specific lateralised processes, can be observed. The third level, *manual asymmetry* (referring to lateralised manual activity), focuses on two behavioural asymmetries particularly relevant to a practice-based handedness approach with developing children: midline crossing and bimanual coordination. These three levels of neural asymmetries are fundamental to handedness, its development and establishment, and thus important for our understanding of the phenomenon.

2.2 Structural Asymmetries

Some specific anatomical structures such as the cerebral cortex, corpus callosum, cerebellum and spinal tract have been associated with lateralisation and specialisation, as research findings reveal (Amunts 2010; Kong et al. 2020; Corballis 2010; Germann et al. 2019). These anatomical structures are referred to as *structural asymmetries*. Typically, however, studies investigate structural and functional asymmetries since these are intricately related.

We will now look at some specific neuroanatomical structures that have been shown to be primarily related to handedness: the *primary motor cortex*, *corpus callosum*, *cerebellum* and *corticospinal tract*.

2.2.1 Primary Motor Cortex

Handedness is often seen to be a general indicator of hemispheric lateralisation of the brain and thus frequently assessed in laterality research (Habib and Robichon 2003). It is argued that handedness does not originate in the extremities that execute function (i.e. arms and hands) but from the functional asymmetry of the two hemispheres (Corballis 2003, 2010). Functional asymmetry means that each hemisphere performs separate, opposite or unique functions required to execute a task (Hellige 2010). Very broadly speaking, the left hemisphere is thought to particularly process and control information that is factual, mathematical, sequential, verbal logical and analytical, whilst the right hemisphere deals more with abstract, artistic, imaginative, visual, intuitive and creative information processing and control (e.g. Amunts 2010), such as displayed in Fig. 2.1.

The primary motor cortex is the motor centre of the cerebral cortex—an essential area of the brain concerning motor function, whereby it is always located on the opposite hemisphere that controls the movement of the (♦**contralateral**) extremity (Illert and Kuhtz-Buschbeck 2006). In other words: The left primary motor cortex controls the movements of the right hand, whilst the right primary motor cortex controls the movements of the left hand. The advantage of this hemispheric specialisation is the enablement of complementary processes that do not interfere with each other (Hellige 2010). This allows the leading (dominant) hemisphere to develop and execute more precise and efficient coordination—"predictive control". The assisting (nondominant) hemisphere is responsible for stabilising less efficient but robust control—"impedance modulation" (Przybyla et al. 2013; Yadav and Sainburg 2011, 2014). As a result,

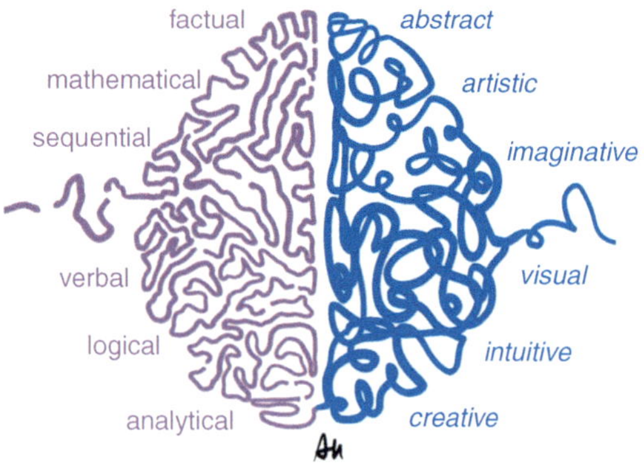

Fig. 2.1 Functional asymmetries of typical functions of the left and right Primary Motor Cortexes. (Illustrated by Amelie Kraus)

motor function is thereby also lateralised, and we are able to perform fluid and coordinated movements. These findings are based on the widely accepted notion that the right hemisphere processes *parallel information*, whilst the left hemisphere specialises in *sequential and serial information* processing (e.g. Todor and Doane 1977). Consequently, some authors argue that the right hand performs better at sequential motor tasks (e.g. Habibi and Chattopadhyay 2021).

Tzourio-Mazoyer and colleagues used finger tapping in left and right hands to investigate specific homotopic brain areas involved (Tzourio-Mazoyer et al. 2021). Both left and right handers showed contralateral activations and deactivation, particularly when the preferred hand was used. Their findings indicate that both handedness groups showed stronger contralateral activity in the cortical and cerebellar motor areas when the right hand was used compared to the left. Moreover, there was a strong deactivation in ipsilateral areas when the dominant hand was used in both groups. The authors conclude that left and right participants perform certain movements faster with their right hand, indicating that the left hand appears to be dominant in some aspects of motor control. The study highlights the complexity of neuro-mechanisms in handedness and indicates that *Left* and *Right Handedness* are not simply a mirror image of one another (Tzourio-Mazoyer et al. 2021).

The different forms of specialisation can be observed in the division of roles between the hands during two-handed actions, the so-called role-differentiated bimanual task (RDBM). The dominant hand typically assumes a more active and leading role, whilst the other hand is engaged in supporting, stabilising and positioning (e.g. Woytowicz et al. 2018). This seems to reflect hemispheric differences, but these differences are also subject to task demands and other environmental influences (Ferre et al. 2020). See also Sect. 2.4.2 for bimanual coordination.

How does lateralisation of the motor cortex take place? The *dynamic dominance's hypothesis* explains this lateralisation process by assuming that the ability to control an extremity is the decisive factor when distinguishing between the dominant and non-dominant arms (Sainburg 2002, 2014). The various hemispheric aspects of specialisation are presumably related to different aspects of sensorimotor function. The preferred hand results from the interaction between neurophysiological asymmetries and action requirements (Przybyla et al. 2013). According to this hypothesis, choosing a hand for an activity depends on which hand is better suited for the required task.

Importantly, the direction and the degree of handedness appear to be separate entities and seem to be encoded independently in the brain (Dassonville et al. 1997). The extent of the activation seems to be related to the degree of handedness since strongly established handers show a more distinct asymmetry of the primary motor cortex during hand movements than individuals with a milder degree of handedness (Dassonville et al. 1997; Pool et al. 2014). Moreover, the hemispheres of left-handed people seem to be somewhat less lateralised and have been found to show different activation patterns compared to those of right handers (Pool et al. 2014; Szaflarski et al. 2002, 2012). See also Chap. 4.

Nevertheless, not all aspects of manual activity are regulated contralaterally. For example, during isolated manual actions (Sadato et al. 1996) or movements with the non-dominant hand (Grabowska et al. 2012), some activated brain regions are ♦**ipsilateral** (same side) to the extremity. It is thus not entirely clear which structures of the cortex are involved in different movement patterns since research findings continue to yield contradictory or insignificant results, despite modern imaging techniques (Ocklenburg et al. 2015). Also, some cortical neurons have been found to have both contralateral and ipsilateral pathways to the extremities, so some of the descending activities as well as the ascending information affect both sides (Kuypers 1982; Michel 2021). The combination of ipsilateral and contralateral pathways and their impact on handedness require further clarification and research, particularly regarding the possible influence this may have on the variability of handedness.

2.2.2 Corpus Callosum

The corpus callosum consists of up to 300 million axons connecting the two hemispheres and transferring information in both directions. For hemispheric specialisation to succeed, the corpus callosum is essential. This brain region, also known as the band of commissural fibres between the cerebral hemispheres, connects the two hemispheres and serves as a "bridge" for exchanging information (Nowicka and Tacikowski 2011). The corpus callosum optimises the functions of the cerebral hemispheres by reducing superfluous information processing. For example, when an activity is selectively activated in the opposite hemisphere, this same activity is inhibited and thus prevented in the other hemisphere (Nowicka and Tacikowski 2011; Schnitzler et al. 1996). More specifically, it has been found that the corpus callosum supports manual preference, particularly by inhibitory modulation of the ipsilateral motor cortex (e.g. Budisavljevic et al. 2021).

Numerous studies investigated handedness in relation to the corpus callosum. For the purpose of this book, we will look at three aspects: studies investigating the relationship between callosal size and handedness, those investigating the function of the corpus callosum and those exploring the role and development of the corpus callosum in bimanual cooperation.

Callosal Size and Handedness

Several studies compared the size of the corpus callosum across different handedness groups, and some found that the corpus callosum is significantly larger in left and "mixed" handers (e.g. Cowell and Gurd 2018; Habib et al. 1991). In the 1980s, Witelson had also found a larger corpus callosum in individuals that were "mixed" handed compared to consistent right handers. She concluded that more efficient callosal connectivity was associated with a lower degree of handedness (Witelson 1989). Based on these findings, Witelson and Nowakowski postulated that the degree of functional hemispheric asymmetry is determined by the loss of callosal axons during postnatal development (Witelson and Nowakowski 1991). This would mean that little axon loss promotes a larger corpus callosum and more variable hand use, and vice versa.

Luders and colleagues also found evidence for a relationship between the size of the corpus callosum and the degree of handedness. According to them, the larger the "bridge" between the hemisphere, the lesser the degree of handedness (and the greater the variability of hand use) in both left- and right-handed individuals (Luders et al. 2010). This supports the suggestion that a strong lateralisation of the brain requires less interhemispheric communication and a smaller corpus callosum (ibid.). However, brain size correlates with the size of the corpus callosum (Jäncke et al. 1997), so this might be a confounding variable that has not been explicitly controlled. Furthermore, Westerhausen and colleagues did not find a larger corpus callosum and mixed handedness (Westerhausen et al. 2004), nor could Luders and colleagues find differences between the callosal size and handedness groups (Luders et al. 2003). Moreover, the research focus has usually been on the relationship between handedness *direction* and corpus callosum. Corballis argues that the *degree* of handedness concerning callosal size might be more revealing (Corballis 2009).

More recently, Westerhausen and Papadatou-Pastou conducted a meta-analysis to evaluate the association between the corpus callosum and handedness. They excluded all studies where handedness was used as a controlled variable (Westerhausen and Papadatou-Pastou 2022). A total of 24 data sets were included. The authors also failed to find support for the often-cited association between a higher interhemispheric connectivity and inconsistent or mixed handedness, as was proposed by Witelson and others earlier (Witelson 1989). Westerhausen and Papadatou-Pastou recommended that large-scale studies on the corpus callosum and handedness be conducted more specifically on brain size effects, sex differences and performance measures (Westerhausen and Papadatou-Pastou 2022). It is also likely that once again, the highly heterogenous and opaque group of "mixed"-handed individuals would influence the outcome of the studies.

Function of Corpus Callosum

It is widely documented in the literature that bimanual cooperation of the hands is dependent on a well-functioning corpus callosum (Fagard and Corroyer 2003; Fling et al. 2011). However, how exactly the interhemispheric communication affects the development of functional hemispheric asymmetries remains controversial. It appears to have both excitatory and inhibitory functions (see van der Knaap and van der Ham 2011 for review). At birth, the corpus callosum is underdeveloped, and bimanual coordination only emerges when the corpus callosum is well functioning. Ferre and colleagues suggest that its development should be a focus in developmental studies since it can be seen as a predictor of manual lateralisation and bimanual coordination (Ferre et al. 2020).

When investigating the function of the corpus callosum in development, Sacco and team assessed hand preference of 1-year-old children with and without a corpus callosum ($N = 24$). It was found that there was no difference between the groups in hand preference in unimanual tasks. However, during bimanual tasks, the hand use of children without a corpus callosum differed from their typically developed counterparts (Sacco et al. 2006). The authors conclude that agenesis (i.e. the complete absence) of the corpus callosum may impair the establishment of a more differentiated bimanual development.

Several functional magnetic resonance imaging studies investigated the relationship between interhemispheric functional connectivity and temporal correlation between physiological signals. Interestingly, the interhemispheric functional connectivity may be intact even without the corpus callosum. Rolland and colleagues investigated 22 patients where the corpus callosum had been surgically removed because of medically refractory epilepsy. The interhemispheric functional connectivity was significantly less after the operation, particularly in the multimodal associated areas in the parietal and frontal lobes (Roland et al. 2017). In the longitudinal follow-up, there was no evidence of recovery. Partial and complete callosotomy revealed that callosal as well as extra-colossal anatomical connections play a role (ibid.). These findings suggest that the corpus callosum is not solely responsible for interhemispheric communication, even though it seems necessary for role-differentiated movement.

Corpus Callosum and Bimanual Role Differentiation

The callosal bridge enables complex role-differentiated bimanual manipulation (Babik 2014). ♦ **Role-differentiated bimanual movement/manipulation (RDBM)** refers to bimanual actions in which one hand (usually the ♦**dominant** hand) performs precise movements, and the other hand (usually the non-dominant one) stabilises or adaptively supports the movement (Michel et al. 2013). An example of a role-differentiated action is unscrewing the lid of a tube: the non-dominant hand would hold the tube, whilst the dominant hand would perform the screwing movement.

Babik suggests that early deficiencies in the role-differentiated bimanual manipulation may be due to a delay in the development of the corpus callosum affecting underlying interhemispheric communication (Babik 2014). On this basis, the developmental pattern of role-differentiated bimanual abilities could be used as an indicator for functions of the corpus callosum and hemispheric specialisation (ibid.). Ferre and colleagues explain the relationship between bimanual cooperation and corpus callosum: If interhemispheric communication is suboptimal, bimanual actions are more complex and thus difficult to learn. This may lead to the avoidance of fine motor and bimanual activities, which in turn are necessary to develop and maintain the corpus callosum and impede a child's development (Ferre et al. 2020).

During child development, it appears that there are individual aspects, such as the relative rather than absolute division of labour between the hemispheres, which inform the action programming or type of information processing

(Michel 2021). At the same time, since the corpus callosum structurally and functionally connects the two hemispheres, each hemisphere can access and potentially process all information required to learn a skill.

> *It is likely that handedness reduces the decision time for the initiation of unimanual tasks (putting food in mouth, throwing or swinging a stick) and for the selection of the different actions in role-differentiated bimanual manipulations (RDBM). During RDBM, the preference efficiently dictates the sequence of the actions of each hand, and the practice of manual actions improves their skill of execution.* (Michel 2021: 9)

Thus, to understand the specialisation process between the hemispheres, the development of the colossal functioning needs to be considered in developmental studies (Michel 2021).

2.2.3 Cerebellum

The cerebellum plays a vital role in planning, executing and controlling movement and motor action. It is involved in spatiotemporal coordination, fine-tuning movements, motor learning, stabilising postural aspects, and balance (Illert and Kuhtz-Buschbeck 2006). Some authors argue that there is evidence that the cerebellum is also important for the development of handedness (Musalek 2015; Tichy and Belacek 2009) and that hand preference correlates with a strong cortical asymmetry (Volkmann et al. 1998a). Similar results were obtained in a study with 8- to 10-year-old children investigating the relationship between cerebellar dominance and hand performance (Musalek 2015).

The cerebellum also controls muscle tone. Studies have shown that the non-dominant arm is usually more relaxed and has a lower muscle tone than the dominant arm (Tichy and Belacek 2009), indicating that the cerebellum lateralised asymmetrically. However, the exact role of the cerebellum in the formation of handedness is unclear and requires further research (e.g. Germann et al. 2019; Kavaklioglu et al. 2017; Rosch et al. 2010).

2.2.4 Corticospinal Tract

Handedness and manual dexterity are usually linked to the contralateral primary motor cortex, the origin of the corticospinal tract. It is the main pathway for voluntary movement, with the majority of axons crossing over at the pyramidal decussation (Nathan et al. 1990). Looking at the ontogenesis of handedness, some findings question the assumption that the brain constitutes the sole structural origin of handedness. For example, it has been found that a preferred hand for thumb sucking is already evident in foetuses even before brain maturation (Hepper et al. 1991, 1998, 2005; Hepper 2013). Furthermore, a more recent study on gene activities in the spinal cord of embryos suggests that first manual asymmetries may be formed before the spinal cord even connects with the brain (Ocklenburg et al. 2017). However, it is not clear whether these early lateralisation processes lead to a particular laterality/sidedness and hand preference.

Figure 2.2 summarises the main functions of the four neural structures that have been shown to be involved in handedness formation, illustrating the typical asymmetry seen in right handers. Whilst cortical control is also located in the contralateral hemisphere in left handers (i.e. the right hemisphere), many left handers also display similar asymmetries in other areas such as language, and they are thus not the mirror image of right handers (see Chap. 4).

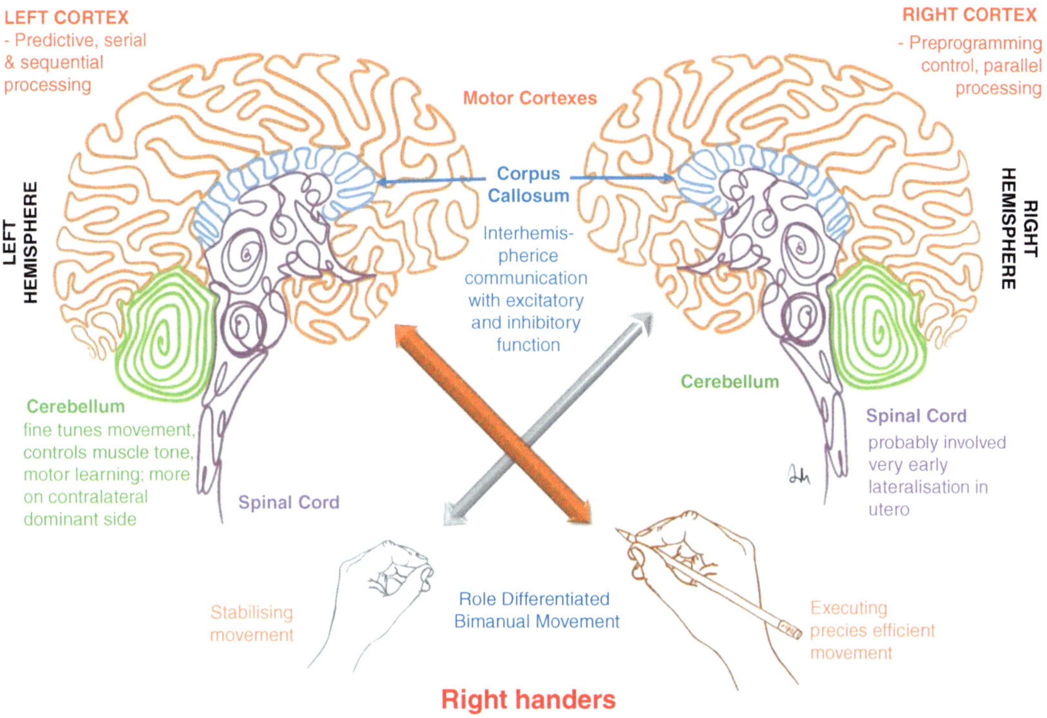

Fig. 2.2 Cortexes, corpus callosum, cerebellum and spinal cord involved in handedness formation using right handers as an example. (Illustrated by Amelie Kraus)

2.3 Functional Asymmetries

This section will look at laterality/sidedness in terms of functional asymmetry. It is widely documented that the preferred and more proficient hand does not necessarily correlate with other preferred modalities such as eyes or ears. However, footedness generally concords with handedness (Porac 2016). Crossed dominance[1] is not uncommon, e.g. a right-handed person may prefer to look through a keyhole with his/her left eye. In fact, about 50% of the normal population seems to exhibit such cross sidedness (ibid.). Porac investigated the four lateral preferences in terms of consistency. She found that only 4% of subjects were uniformly left sided and 46% uniformly right sided for the hand, foot, eye and ear (ibid.). Since footedness correlates most highly with handedness, it receives particular attention.

[1]When a person's handedness does not correspond to the laterality of foot, eye or ear, the term "crossed dominance" is frequently used.

2.3.1 Footedness

Unlike handedness, footedness does not seem to be influenced substantially by social and cultural factors and may provide valuable information on the development and underlying genetic architecture of lateral motor biases (Packheiser et al. 2020). Porac investigated the relationship between footedness and handedness. She found that 91% of right handers show right-sided footedness, of which 83% is consistent, compared to 61% of left handers and their footedness (Porac 2016). Thus, we could expect that most right handers use the right foot for actions such as kicking a ball or picking up a small object with their toes. However, this would not necessarily apply to left handers (ibid.). A meta-analysis on footedness by Packheiser and team using four different classification systems across 164 studies (N = 145,135 individuals) also showed a significant difference between left and right handers. In particular, they found that only 3.2% of right handers were left footed, whilst 39.9% of left handers were not left footed (Packheiser et al. 2020).

Practitioners such as occupational therapists often use footedness to assess handedness, probably based on the premise that there is a correlation between handedness and footedness, observed particularly in right handers. However, there are several problems with this approach.

Firstly, as we have seen, the correlation appears to be significantly high only in *right handers* and may thus not accurately identify left handers.

Secondly, research generally appears to be a lack of differentiation between footedness and leggedness. It is well known that *proximal* muscles are less lateralised than *distal* muscles. Distal muscles are controlled almost exclusively by the contralateral hemisphere, whereas proximal muscles have both contralateral and ipsilateral pathways (e.g. Geschwind and Galaburda 1985; Rigal 1992). This means that this could influence the consistency of gross leg movements such as kicking, and it indicates that the measures used to assess footedness, similar to handedness, are dependent on the task.

Thirdly, repeated observations in occupational therapy practice show that there is often a discrepancy between the leg with the better *standing balance* and the one preferred for *kicking*. So, using standing balance as a measure of footedness may yield very different results. Fourthly, should a child also engage in sports such as football *training*, the focus is likely to be on training both legs to be equally good at kicking, thereby also reducing the asymmetry between them. This consideration complies with a study by Saccoa and colleagues, who investigated the relationship between footedness and handedness with 2236 young Italian sportspersons. They found a significantly lower association between the two variables compared to other studies (Saccoa et al. 2018).

In research, too, there have been attempts to obtain more specific results indicating a clearer correlation between footedness and handedness, also in left handers. For example, the following principle was incorporated: the more demanding an action, the more lateralised the response. Musalek, for example, found that in right handers, tapping with the foot ("foot tapping") correlates highly with handedness (hand preference) but not with foot performances such as the one-leg stand (Musalek 2015). He thus concluded that fine motor foot tapping could also be used to measure handedness. However, it is unclear if this would apply to left handers to the same extent.

From a practice-based perspective, we can conclude that more specific research is warranted in this area, with a focus on left handers. More complex, fine movement patterns involving distal musculature of the foot are most likely to correlate with handedness, particularly if these actions are not influenced by practice and training. More specific footedness tasks could possibly be useful as an additional "neutral" measure of handedness.

2.3.2 Sensory Dominance

When one sensory modality, be it eye or ear, is used more frequently and receives preferential processing, it is referred to as sensory dominance: eyedness and earedness. Whilst the correlation between handedness and either eyedness or earedness has not been strong, it has been shown that when the two sensory modalities are linked, a more stable association between the sensory and motor modalities is seen in right handers (Yang et al. 2021). This preferential link appears independent of task demands and complexity but varies greatly between individuals. For example, Porac found that 66% of right handers display a dominant right eye, compared to 57% of left handers being left eyed, and that 60% of people generally show a right-ear and 40% a left-ear preference. The overall correlation to a corresponding handedness is 63% (Porac 2016).

Research has also focused on other asymmetries in terms of visual and auditory perceptual processing, somatosensory body representation (Hach and Schütz-Bosbach 2014) and lateralisation of emotion processing (Brancucci et al.

2009). Possibly, such laterality features could expand our understanding of handedness, but to date, we lack insight into possible relationships for the same reasons: lack of uniform definitions and measures. Overall, the correlation of lateral asymmetries of eyedness, earedness and movement-related asymmetries (e.g. body rotations) with hand preference seems to vary greatly.

In conventional clinical practice, occupational therapists often tend to use sensory asymmetries as a measure of handedness. This is probably based on the assumption that laterality and handedness are one construct. This may lead to therapists concluding that a child is left handed because s/he? kicks the ball with the left foot or shows a preference for the right eye. It is therefore important to clearly differentiate between laterality and handedness, since there appear to be different lateralisation processes underpinning handedness and laterality/sidedness.

2.3.3 Language and Handedness

In the nineteenth century, Broca and Wernicke found that in most people (left and right handers), the language centre is situated in the left hemisphere of the cerebral cortex (see Rutten 2022 for review). Since then, the hemispheric specialisation of language and manual skills have been linked. However, the relationship between handedness and language is neither simple nor straightforward (Corballis 2003). For example, according to Christman, 96% of right-handed people have the speech centre located in their left hemisphere compared to 70% of left handers (Christman 2012). In addition, Knecht found that of the 30% of left handers with a right dominant cerebral speech centre, 15% showed activations in both hemispheres (Knecht 2000). Similarly, it has been shown that, on average, left handers are less lateralised of language (see (Bruckert et al. 2021; Häberling et al. 2016; Vingerhoets 2019). Chapter 4 will detail the differences between left and right handers.

There is growing evidence that the relationship between language and handedness is multifactorial and develops over time. Nelson and colleagues found that hand preference *consistency* in role-differentiated bimanual movement (RDBM) tasks in early childhood is associated with language skill development since language measure outcomes are related to the hand preference trajectories (Nelson et al. 2017). In addition, the earlier a right-hand preference appeared, the higher the language assessment score compared to children with late right or late left trajectories (ibid.). Similarly, it was found that toddlers who used their right hand consistently during RDBM showed greater receptive and expressive language skills at the age of 5 compared to left and moderate handers (Gonzalez et al. 2020). Other developmental studies focusing on mixed handedness as a risk factor for developmental language in later childhood did not find sufficient evidence for this (Pritchard et al. 2019; Roland et al. 2017).

The complex relationship between language and handedness becomes more pertinent when developmental studies use a *multifactorial* approach (e.g. Sommer 2010). In addition, there is a need for repeated testing over time in *longitudinal studies* with multiple test points to accommodate the typical fluctuations in hand use as well as language (Gonzalez et al. 2020). Based on our current knowledge, handedness appears to be a *dynamic developmental phenomenon* rather than a trait used to focus on predicting later language outcomes or vice versa.

2.4 Manual Asymmetries

In addition to the neuro-anatomical structures of handedness, certain neurophysiological processes associated with manual asymmetries during the execution of movement and actions are also relevant to our understanding of handedness and handedness formation.[2] I focus on two neurophysiological phenomena closely related to

[2] In this book, the term ↖**handedness formation** refers to the entire process of handedness establishment, including all its influences and individual predispositions, which create and constitute a certain handedness. ↖**Handedness development** is considered to be part of handedness formation, but refers only to the first 6 years of life.

handedness and particularly relevant to a practice-based approach. They are crossing the body midline as a more complex form of hand preference and bimanual cooperation as a form of more complex proficiency (compared to unimanual performance).

A definition of these two manual asymmetries is warranted to understand the terminology.

In this book, the phenomenon of ♦**crossing the body midline** refers to the spontaneous reaching of one hand into the opposite or ♦**contralateral** space in relation to the vertical upper body midline. This occurs, for example, when a person picks up an object with the right hand when the object is placed on the left side. To "successfully" cross over, the impulse to move ♦**ipsilaterally** (on the same side) must be inhibited (Bishop 1990).

We perform most tasks in our everyday life with both hands, which can be termed as bimanual actions or activities, where asymmetries in hand use are particularly evident. For the effective and efficient execution of bimanual tasks, our hands have to cooperate with each other, referred to as ♦**bimanual cooperation** or ♦**bimanual coordination**. More specifically, our hands have to assume different roles: usually, one hand leads or performs the action, and the other stabilises or assists, whether this is whilst opening the lid of a jar, adjusting the paper when cutting with scissors or playing the piano. As mentioned under Sect. 2.2.2, this is referred to as ♦**role-differentiated bimanual movement (RDBM).**

2.4.1 Crossing the Body Midline

The ability to cross the body midline, or contralateral reaching, is thought to be an indication of neurological maturity, particularly involving the corpus callosum. It reflects the extent of lateralisation and specialisation of the two cerebral hemispheres (Surburg 1999). Furthermore, crossing the midline is considered to be a typical milestone in the sensory-motor development of children (Ayres 2013; Kephart 1977). Consequently, avoidance of crossing over indicates developmental delay (Michell and Wood 1999). Accordingly, tests for crossing the body midline are included in some developmental tests (Scharoun and Bryden 2014, 2015; Ayres 1972, 2013).

The reason for contralateral reaching seems to be rooted in the brain's strife to maximise its efficiency in an action or movement to achieve the highest possible desired outcome at the lowest possible effort (Shadmehr et al. 2016). This maximisation of utility makes it likely that several potential motor plans are encoded simultaneously, and the brain's sensorimotor region selects the most efficient motor plan or chooses the hand that can perform the action best. The establishment of handedness ensures a predetermined (dominant) hand, which decreases the reaction time (see van Helvert et al. 2021).

Moreover, motor planning actions seem to involve ipsilateral or contralateral reaching as part of the movement sequence that are task dependent. For example, if the task demand is low, the hand closest to the object to be taken or manipulated will often be used on the same side (ipsilateral). On the other hand, if the task demand is high, such as using a tool, the dominant hand will usually reach contralaterally to pick it up and use it since this is more time efficient (e.g. Xiao et al. 2019). Contralateral reaching is also related to hand preference: in established handers, the dominant hand will spontaneously cross the middle of the body more frequently and further than the non-dominant hand (Bryden et al. 2000; Brown et al. 2006; Bryden and Roy 2006; Kraus 2006), as can be seen in Fig. 2.3.

Crossing over with the dominant hand has been found to be more pronounced in right handers: left handers cross their body midline less often whilst using their non-dominant right hand more frequently (Gabbard et al. 2001; Kraus 2006). Regardless, crossing the midline has been used to assess the degree of hand preference (Bishop et al. 1996). Since left handers are often less pronounced in their handedness (lower degree), the differences in results may be attributed to this variability.

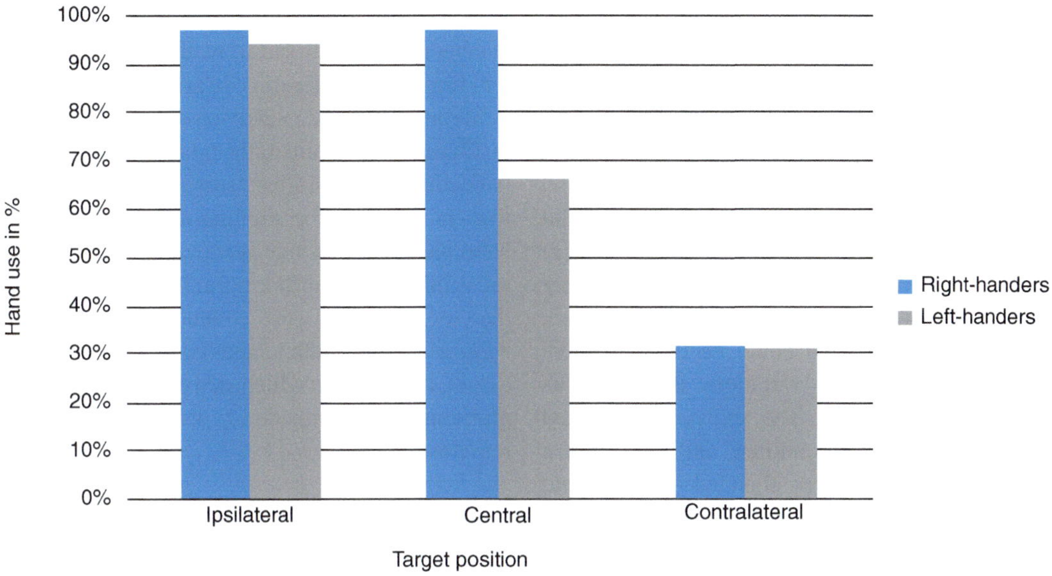

Fig. 2.3 Ipsilateral, central and contralateral hand use in left and right handers (own presentation based on the data of Bryden et al. 2000)

In the 1970s, it was proposed that crossing the body midline is a necessary prerequisite for the development of hand preference (Ayres and Rasokat 1979; Provine and Westerman 1979). More recently, Scharoun and Bryden found that crossing over exhibits a similar developmental pattern to handedness (Scharoun and Bryden 2014). The ability to cross the body midline is already evident in early childhood, intensifying during later childhood and then decreasing somewhat with age. Thus, infants begin crossing over at the age of 18–20 weeks in the course of exploring their environment (Liederman 1983; Provine and Westerman 1979). However, this crossing over involves trunk rotation (i.e. the crossing over the body occurs at abdominal rather than chest level) and may not be identical to crossing the upper body midline. Indeed, infants and young children tend to avoid contralateral reaching at the "upper" level (Brown et al. 2006). Overall, the ability to cross over increases steadily between 2 and 6 years (Stilwell 1987), or between 3 and 8 years (Schofield 1976), and crossing over with either hand is also common (Scharoun and Bryden 2014). Once development is completed, adults show a clear, albeit reduced, tendency to cross the midline more often with their dominant hand (Brown et al. 2006; Kraus 2006). This indicates that the development of midline crossing is not linear. Scharoun and Bryden also found evidence that preferential contralateral reaching decreases with age (Scharoun and Bryden 2014). Brown and colleagues propose the following explanation for non-linear development (Brown et al. 2006):

- 4-year-old children tend to avoid crossing over because their motor skills are still developing, and they are exploring their environment with both hands.
- 10-year-old children use their preferred hand, regardless of where they move it in space, which could indicate temporary overregulation of the dominant hand.
- Adolescents and adults have reached a stage where both hands are capable of high motor functions and are used effectively with little effort, resulting in the non-dominant hand being used more frequently, thereby decreasing contralateral movements with the dominant hand.

This non-linear development appears similar to the findings of Scharoun and Bryden on the development of consistent hand preference (Scharoun and Bryden 2014; see Sect. 1.3.2).

In addition, there is evidence that the environment (in terms of distance) and task demand (related to the object being a tool) influence hand use when crossing over. For example, in a study with 4- to 9-year-old children, the hand picking up blocks was observed and documented. Although an age trend could be demonstrated, there were significant variations in the results (Cermak et al. 1980). The study was repeated with 5- to 7-year-old children, and the *distance* between the blocks was changed (Atwood and Cermak 1986). Since only a few of the younger children reached contralaterally, it was concluded that a greater distance to the test objects makes crossing over more difficult (ibid.). Similarly, the type of action (pointing or picking up and manipulating) and the nature of the item (an arbitrary object or an instrument to perform a certain function) appear to influence crossing the midline. An increased number of contralateral actions with the dominant hand was observed when a *tool* was picked up compared to a simple object (Bryden et al. 2011) and when the object was actually used (Hill and Khanem 2009). Therefore, it has been suggested that whilst hand use is initially controlled by hand preference, it is also influenced by the position of the object and the complexity of the task (Brown et al. 2006).

Visual feedback, too, appears to influence reaching to the opposite side. For example, blindfolded subjects mainly used their dominant hand ipsilaterally and in the centre, but on the contralateral side, they used their non-dominant hand, thereby avoiding crossing the body midline (Gabbard et al. 2001). However, other researchers consider the impact of visual feedback during ipsilateral reaching to be less important, focusing instead on other influencing factors such as motor control during reaching (Carey et al. 1996). The greater the motor control, the more frequent the performance with that hand. As the dominant is usually more proficient and crosses the body midline more frequently than the non-dominant hand, midline crossing has been recommended to be used as an indicator for hand preference (Carlier et al. 2006; Scharoun and Bryden 2014).

Overall, the nature of the relationship between handedness and midline crossing remains tentative. Is crossing the midline a prerequisite for hand preference or vice versa, or is there a reciprocal influence? Furthermore, it should be noted that most studies were conducted with people *without* motoric deficiencies or deficits. To what extent and during which activities such motor problems may impede a person's hand use remains unclear.

2.4.2 Bimanual Cooperation and Coordination[3]

Bimanual coordination is considered to be a behavioural indicator of interhemispheric communication (e.g. Michel 2021). Whilst most of the motor and sensory innervations of the upper limb are controlled by the contralateral cerebral hemisphere, some cortical neurons have both contralateral and ipsilateral tracts. This means that during bimanual coordinated movement, the two hemispheres process and control not only contralateral ascending and descending pathways of the two sides but also ipsilateral ones (ibid.). Michel concluded that understanding the intermanual transfer of haptic experience and bimanual coordination mechanisms is fundamental for comprehending interhemispheric communication (ibid.).

We will take a closer look at research targeting the development of bimanual cooperation, mirror movements, bimanual coupling, bimanual cooperation and vision since these are most interesting and relevant for a practice-based approach to handedness.

[3] In this section, the terms bimanual cooperation and bimanual coordination will be used interchangeably, since there is no clear distinction in the literature. In the context of the book, however, the term ♦**bimanual cooperation** will be used consistently.

Development of Bimanual Coordination

To better understand bimanual movement and coordination, looking at its development in infants and toddlers indicates swift and vivid changes in motor skills, with great variability within and between children. Research in this area has resulted in a dynamical system approach responsible for motor development rather than specific structures (see Brakke and Pacheco 2019).

Children show greater variability in bimanual performance than adults, especially with their non-dominant hands (Kuhtz-Buschbeck et al. 1999). Rather than interpreting this as an immature behaviour, it has been proposed to be an instability necessary for the emergence of new behaviour.

In particular, practising motor behaviour can be seen as a problem-solving exercise, and it has been investigated to understand its contribution to skill acquisition over time. Furthermore, Brakke and colleagues proposed a conceptual model that incorporates maturational information, experiences, task properties and task constraint, as well as perceptual variability affecting motor behaviour (Brakke and Pacheco 2019).

Numerous findings link the development of bimanual coordination with the maturation of neuro-anatomical structures such as the corpus callosum (Fagard et al. 2001). However, the imminent influence of factors such as experience, age range, context and experience of tasks becomes increasingly apparent over time (Brakke and Pacheco 2019). For example, whin the first 2 years of life, infants develop a relatively stable but flexible role differentiation between the hands, starting with simple tasks such as holding an object with one hand and manipulating or exploring it actively with the other hand (e.g. Babik 2014). Also, between 12 and 15 months, toddlers imitate manual movement, corresponding to their cortical development and an emerging neural system coupling perception and action (Yoo et al. 2016). More specifically, the development of bimanual coordination can be seen from the results of a RDBM study by Nelson and team with 3-year-old children (N = 64). 7.8% of children were found to have a left-hand preference, 76.6% showed a right-hand preference and 15.6% showed no preference for RDBM (Nelson et al. 2019). In comparison, in adults (N = 1051), 4.1% demonstrated a left-hand preference for RDBM, 61.2% showed a right-hand preference and 34.7% showed no preference for RDBM (Gonzalez and Nelson 2021).

Mirror Movements

The demands of bimanual coordination are significantly increased when both hands perform different movements (Swinnen and Wenderoth 2004). Humans have a natural tendency to synchronise the motor performance of their hands, thus preferring to do the same action on both sides. The phenomenon when the arms or hands mirror and thereby synchronise each other's movement is also referred to as "mirror movement" (Cattaert et al. 1999). ⧫**Mirror movements** are a normal phenomenon in the motor learning process (Leinen et al. 2016), as can be seen in children during their first 5 years of life (Fagard and Corroyer 2003). If movements are not mirrored actively, they may still be observed as associated movements. In particular, children and older adults tend to generate more involuntary simultaneous muscle activation with the non-performing side of the body when moving intentionally with the opposite side (Addamo et al. 2009; Leinen et al. 2016).

Interestingly, the tendency for involuntary mirror movement appears to be particularly observable in strongly established left and right handers (i.e. with a high degree of handedness). In comparison, less lateralised individuals (i.e. with a low degree of handedness) do not seem to be much affected by an increased coordination effort (Kourtis et al. 2014). This seems to indicate that the extent of bimanual cooperation depends rather on the degree and direction of handedness (ibid.): a mild degree of handedness correlates with an increase in brain activity during bimanual movements, which in turn enhances the ability to plan and organise bimanual movements (ibid.).

Bimanual Coupling and Decoupling

Spatial and temporal independence between the hands during bimanual activities is also referred to as "bimanual coupling" (Crites and Gorman 2017). ♦**Bimanual coupling** was investigated in more detail in 413 3- to 10-year-old children to examine the extent to which the hands can act independently of each other. In 3- and 5-year-old children, there was a strong tendency for both hands to want to perform the same movement, therefore "interfering" with each other ("immature coupling"). However, this tendency decreased in children between 5 and 7 years, and 7- to 9-year-olds were gradually able to use their hands independently and fluently (van Grunsven et al. 2009). The authors conclude that this development of bimanual coordination is due to the specific distribution of tasks (i.e. role differentiation) between the hands and forms the basis for complex tasks such as fluent writing (ibid.).

Also investigating bimanual coupling, Janssen and colleagues conducted several studies looking at simultaneous grasps and the tendency to avoid a so-called uncomfortable end posture (Janssen et al. 2009, 2011). They concluded that the ability to motor plan is specialised in the left hemisphere, independent of the direction of handedness. Hughes and colleagues conducted a similar experiment, examining motor planning and execution during bimanual grasping and placing tasks. They did not find differences between the hands in the gross postures between the left and right hands and attributed this to the different task demands. However, the authors observed a shorter object transport time with the left hand for both left and right handers. This is in accordance with research on manual asymmetries suggesting that hemispheric advantages during motor action observed in unimanual tasks are not necessarily related to the direction of handedness (Hughes et al. 2011).

It is generally assumed that unimanual actions must be individually decoupled and controlled to allow independent movements on both sides. In the 1970s, the hypothesis was put forward that role complementarity is a necessary prerequisite for the development of hand preference (Bresson et al. 1977). The process of "uncoupling" and the decrease in mirror movements seem to overlap with the extent of myelination, i.e. the complete corpus callosum development (Chicoine et al. 2000). Therefore, the maturation of the corpus callosum is thought to play an essential role in the formation of bimanual cooperation (Leinen et al. 2016; van Grunsven et al. 2009).

Bimanual Motor Learning

There is evidence that both hands benefit from each other when they act simultaneously but in different ways: in right handers, the left hand "learns" about movement direction and patterns from the right hand, and the right hand "learns" about controlling positioning from the left hand (Kagerer 2015). These results indicate that different information is exchanged between the hemispheres during simultaneous bimanual movement. Interestingly, it has been observed that people who initially practice a motor task with their non-dominant hand learn faster compared to those who first practice with their dominant one. This is particularly the case with actions that require spatial accuracy (Senff and Weigelt 2011; Stolze 2012). If the task to be learned requires strength and precision, it seems more effective to start training with the dominant hand (Stolze 2012). Moreover, proprioception (i.e. the awareness of the position and movement of the body) seems to be better developed in the non-dominant hand in right handers, presumably to facilitate more accurate positions when assisting and stabilising (Adamo and Martin 2009; Goble and Brown 2010). This could also influence the asymmetry between the hands when learning and performing bimanual motor tasks.

Vision seems an even stronger factor than proprioception influencing the learning and execution of bimanual tasks. During simultaneous bimanual movements, Krager found that *visual feedback monitoring* of one hand positively affects the performance of the other hand, suggesting that there is crossmodal information sharing between the hemisphere to complement each hand's function (Kagerer 2015). The underlying mechanisms of concurrent bimanual movement have received much research attention. There have been two contrasting theories on handedness supporting mechanically coupled bilateral movements: (1) complementary dominance, where each hemisphere specialises in specific motor control aspects (Woytowicz et al. 2018), and (2) global dominance, where the contralateral hemisphere to the extremity specialises in all aspects of motor control (Volkmann et al. 1998). Woytosict and colleagues found support for the complementary dominance hypothesis, where each cerebral hemisphere specialises for dynamic control mechanisms and impedance during bilateral interactions (Woytowicz et al. 2017, 2018).

Using *visual copying* when learning a bimanual task also appears to influence the learning process. A study by Zickert and colleagues investigated the influence of learning a bimanual task (complex knotting) from someone with the same handedness compared to someone with discordant handedness. It was found that the more complex and unfamiliar the bimanual task with greater role differentiation between the hands, the more important the concordant handedness when visually copying the task during skill acquisition (Zickert et al. 2021).

In addition to lateralised influencing factors such as proprioception, visual feedback and visual learning, the *degree* of handedness (often referred to as consistency) affects the manual asymmetry in bimanual motor learning. Oswald and Bo investigated 56 adults using an in-phase and out-of-phase tapping task leading with the left or right hand (Oswald and Bo 2019). A bimanual advantage was only evident in subjects with a degree handedness. The authors conclude that the so-called bimanual advantage may thus depend on the degree of handedness as well as its direction. Another influencing factor, *speed*, has been found by Panzer and colleagues, who tested "limb dominance" and showed that the speed of limb movement influences manual asymmetry in bimanual coordination tasks in both left and right handers (Panzer et al. 2021).

Overall, the above studies confirm the intertwined and complex development of bimanual cooperation and show that the development of role-differentiated bimanual manipulation may be a *requirement* for the final developmental stages of handedness.

2.5 Concluding Remarks

The aim of this chapter has been to look at relevant neural structural, functional and manual asymmetry concerning the origins of handedness to see what contribution research in this area could make to a practice-based approach to handedness. For *structural asymmetries*, we can conclude that several neurophysiological structures and processes are associated with the neuroanatomical origins of handedness. Indeed, the neural foundations of handedness remain somewhat indefinable. The state-of-the-art methodologies of MRI research allow us to gain specific insights into the structural and functional foundations and reveal a reciprocal relationship between handedness and neural traits. However, whilst many interesting findings in this area increase the knowledge base of handedness, the neural research focus tends to be isolated on micro aspects, like pieces of a very large puzzle that are still being sorted. In addition, the complexity of handedness as a multifactorial and multidimensional phenomenon also transpires at the neural level. Together with the well-known problem of inconsistent definitions, categorisation and measures, this likely contributes to the contradictory results. Accordingly, Tzourio-Mazoyer and colleagues suggest that future research should combine developmental trajectories of dexterity and handedness with behavioural and neural processes whilst also integrating information on hand function and hand use in longitudinal developmental studies mapping brain maturation (Tzourio-Mazoyer et al. 2021). Such a multifactorial approach might also look include specific variants, such as the hemisphere dominant for language in a sufficient number of left-handed individuals, which may also account for some of the high variability in left handers.

Whilst findings at the structural asymmetry level do not directly impact a practice-based approach, some findings at the functional asymmetry (e.g. footedness) and manual asymmetry levels provide practitioners with useful implications. Laterality of modalities, such as footedness, should be treated as a separate phenomenon from handedness. Handedness can be seen as the most lateralised and specialised form of laterality and is its most complex form, and it serves as a foundation for complex manual activities that are incomparable to lateralised actions such as kicking a ball or looking through a lens with the preferred modality. Nevertheless, footedness, in particular, could be used as an additional supporting measure when assessing unclear handedness in children; other sensory laterality measures, such as eyedness and earedness, should not be used since the correlation to handedness is too weak.

For midline crossing as a *manual asymmetry*, it is important for practitioners to note that contralateral reaching tests used to measure hand preference may not differentiate the two constructs accurately. Developmentally delayed children who avoid midline crossing may show a clear hand preference in midline but will not display this preference when engaging in a contralateral reaching task. Interestingly, children with atypical handedness establishment have also been observed in occupational therapy to engage in contralateral reaching with either hand, thereby not displaying a crossing avoidance (on the contrary) but certainly showing "mixed" handedness (Kraus 2019). The differences between left- and right-handed individuals and the fact that crossing over appears closely related to the degree of handedness add to the complexity of the relationship between handedness and midline crossing. For a practice-based approach, we can conclude that on the one hand, contralateral reaching appears to be a key aspect of hand preference, whilst on the other hand, it is also a separate and distinct phenomenon.

Also, practitioners working with atypically developed children should look at bimanual coordination skills in relation to handedness establishment and division of roles between the hands. It is likely that unestablished handedness impedes bimanual coordination development and/or vice versa. Therefore, understanding the development of bimanual coordination and the bimanual coupling tendency is useful. In addition, considering the influencing factors of proprioception, visual feedback, visual learning, degree of handedness and speed of the activity is imperative since they all impact bimanual performance. These research findings thus serve as a helpful knowledge base when treating children with problems in this area.

Overall, we need to see how these structural, functional and manual asymmetries are related to other behavioural measures and features of handedness. This way, we can deepen our understanding of handedness as a multidimensional phenomenon and the related factors that influence it. The following chapter will explore some of these factors that co-determine handedness in a practice-based approach.

References

Adamo DE, Martin BJ (2009) Position sense asymmetry. Exp Brain Res 192(1):87–95. https://doi.org/10.1007/s00221-008-1560-0

Addamo PK, Farrow M, Hoy KE, Bradshaw JL, Georgiou-Karistianis N (2009) The influence of task characteristics on younger and older adult motor overflow. Q J Exp Psychol 62(2):239–247. https://doi.org/10.1080/17470210802269217

Amunts K (2010) Structural indices of asymmetry. In: The two halves of the brain, pp 145–176

Andersen KW, Siebner HR (2018) Mapping dexterity and handedness: recent insights and future challenges. Curr Opin Behav Sci 20:123–129

Atwood RM, Cermak SA (1986) Crossing the midline as a function of distance from midline. Am J Occup Ther 40(10):685–690. https://doi.org/10.5014/ajot.40.10.685

Ayres AJ (1972) Sensory integration and learning disorders. Western Psychological Services, Los Angeles

Ayres AJ (2013) Bausteine der kindlichen Entwicklung. Sensorische Integration verstehen & anwenden ; das Original in der modernen Neuauflage ; überarbeitet & erweitert durch das Pediatric Therapy Network. 5., überarb. & erw. Aufl. Springer, Berlin

Ayres AJ, Rasokat C (1979) Lernstörungen. Sensorisch-integrative Dysfunktionen Springer, Heidelberg; Stiftung Rehabilitation (Rehabilitation & prävention, 6)

Babik I (2014) Development of handedness for role-differentiated bimanual manipulation of objects in relation to the development of hand-use preferences for acquisition. Dissertation. The University of North Carolina at Greensboro, Greensboro

Bishop DVM (1990) Handedness and developmental disorders. Mac Keith Press; J.B. Lippincott, Oxford, Philadelphia (Clinics in developmental medicine, 110)

Bishop DV, Ross VA, Daniels MS, Bright P (1996) The measurement of hand preference: a validation study comparing three groups of right-handers. Br J Psychol 87(Pt 2):269–285. https://doi.org/10.1111/j.2044-8295.1996.tb02590.x

Brakke K, Pacheco MM (2019) The development of bimanual coordination across toddlerhood. Monogr Soc Res Child Dev 84(2):7–147. https://doi.org/10.1111/mono.12405

Brancucci A, Lucci G, Mazzatenta A, Tommasi L (2009) Asymmetries of the human social brain in the visual, auditory and chemical modalities. Phil Trans R Soc B 364(1519):895–914. https://doi.org/10.1098/rstb.2008.0279

Bresson F, Maury L, Pieraut-Le Bonniec G, de Schonen S (1977) Organization and lateralization of reaching in infants: an instance of asymmetric functions in hands collaboration. Neuropsychologia 15(2):311–320. https://doi.org/10.1016/0028-3932(77)90040-9

Brown S, Roy E, Rohr L, Bryden P (2006) Using hand performance measures to predict handedness. Laterality 11(1):1–14. https://doi.org/10.1080/1357650054200000440

Bruckert L, Thompson PA, Watkins KE, Bishop DVM, Woodhead ZVJ (2021) Investigating the effects of handedness on the consistency of lateralization for speech production and semantic processing tasks using functional transcranial Doppler sonography. Laterality 26(6):680–705. https://doi.org/10.1080/1357650X.2021.1898416

Bryden PJ, Roy EA (2006) Preferential reaching across regions of hemispace in adults and children. Dev Psychobiol 48(2):121–132. https://doi.org/10.1002/dev.20120

Bryden PJ, Pryde KM, Roy EA (2000) A performance measure of the degree of hand preference. Brain Cogn 44(3):402–414. https://doi.org/10.1006/brcg.1999.1201

Bryden PJ, Mayer M, Roy EA (2011) Influences of task complexity, object location, and object type on hand selection in reaching in left and right-handed children and adults. Dev Psychobiol 53(1):47–58. https://doi.org/10.1002/dev.20486

Budisavljevic S, Castiello U, Begliomini C (2021) Handedness and White matter networks. Neuroscientist 27(1):88–103. https://doi.org/10.1177/1073858420937657

Carey DP, Hargreaves EL, Goodale MA (1996) Reaching to ipsilateral or contralateral targets: within-hemisphere visuomotor processing cannot explain hemispatial differences in motor control. Exp Brain Res 112(3):496–504. https://doi.org/10.1007/BF00227955

Carlier M, Doyen A-L, Lamard C (2006) Midline crossing: developmental trend from 3 to 10 years of age in a preferential card-reaching task. Brain Cogn 61(3):255–261. https://doi.org/10.1016/j.bandc.2006.01.007

Cattaert D, Semjen A, Summers JJ (1999) Simulating a neural cross-talk model for between-hand interference during bimanual circle drawing. Biol Cybern 81(4):343–358

Cermak SA, Quintero EJ, Cohen PM (1980) Developmental age trends in crossing the body midline in normal children. Am J Occup Ther 34(5):313–319. https://doi.org/10.5014/ajot.34.5.313

Chicoine A-J, Proteau L, Lassonde M (2000) Absence of interhemispheric transfer of unilateral visuomotor learning in young children and individuals with agenesis of the corpus callosum. Dev Neuropsychol 18(1):73–94. https://doi.org/10.1207/S15326942DN1801_5

Christman SD (2012) Handedness. In: Ramachandran VS (Hg.) Encyclopedia of human behavior. Elsevier Academic Press, Amsterdam, pp 290–296

Corballis MC (2003) From mouth to hand: gesture, speech, and the evolution of right-handedness. Behav Brain Sci 26(2):199–208; discussion 208-60. https://doi.org/10.1017/s0140525x03000062

Corballis MC (2009) The evolution and genetics of cerebral asymmetry. Philos Trans R Soc B 364(1519):867–879

Corballis MC (Hg.) (2010) Handedness and cerebral asymmetry. An evolutionary perspective. MIT Press, Cambridge

Cowell P, Gurd J (2018) Handedness and the corpus callosum: a review and further analyses of discordant twins. Neuroscience 388:57–68

Crites M, Gorman JC (Hg.) (2017) Bimanual coupling and the intermanual speed advantage. Proceedings of the human factors and ergonomics society annual meeting 61(1)

Dassonville P, Zhu XH, Uurbil K, Kim SG, Ashe J (1997) Functional activation in motor cortex reflects the direction and the degree of handedness. Proc Natl Acad Sci U S A 94(25):14015–14018. https://doi.org/10.1073/pnas.94.25.14015

Fagard J, Corroyer D (2003) Using a continuous index of laterality to determine how laterality is related to interhemispheric transfer and bimanual coordination in children. Dev Psychobiol 43(1):44–56. https://doi.org/10.1002/dev.10117

Fagard J, Hardy-Léger I, Kervella C, Marks A (2001) Changes in interhemispheric transfer rate and the development of bimanual coordination during childhood. J Exp Child Psychol 80(1):1–22. https://doi.org/10.1006/jecp.2000.2623

Ferre CL, Babik I, Michel GF (2020) A perspective on the development of hemispheric specialization, infant handedness, and cerebral palsy. Cortex 127:208–220. https://doi.org/10.1016/j.cortex.2020.02.017

Fling BW, Walsh CM, Bangert AS, Reuter-Lorenz PA, Welsh RC, Seidler RD (2011) Differential callosal contributions to bimanual control in young and older adults. J Cogn Neurosci 23(9):2171–2185

Gabbard C, Helbig CR, Gentry V (2001) Lateralized effects on reaching by children. Dev Neuropsychol 19(1):41–51. https://doi.org/10.1207/S15326942DN1901_4

Germann J, Petrides M, Chakravarty MM (2019) Hand preference and local asymmetry in cerebral cortex, basal ganglia, and cerebellar white matter. Brain Struct Funct 224(8):2899–2905. https://doi.org/10.1007/s00429-019-01941-6

Geschwind N, Galaburda AM (1985) Cerebral lateralization. Biological mechanisms, associations, and pathology. II A hypothesis and a program for research. Arch Neurol 42(6):521–552

Goble DJ, Brown SH (2010) Upper limb asymmetries in the perception of proprioceptively determined dynamic position sense. J Exp Psychol Hum Percept Perform 36(3):768–775

Gonzalez SL, Nelson EL (2021) Factor analysis of the home handedness questionnaire: unimanual and role differentiated bimanual manipulation as separate dimensions of handedness. Appl Neuropsychol Adult 28(2):173–184

Gonzalez SL, Campbell JM, Marcinowski EC, Michel GF, Coxe S, Nelson EL (2020) Preschool language ability is predicted by toddler hand preference trajectories. Dev Psychol 56(4):699

Grabowska A, Gut M, Binder M, Forsberg L, Rymarczyk K, Urbanik A (2012) Switching handedness: fMRI study of hand motor control in right-handers, left-handers and converted left-handers. Acta Neurobiol Exp 72(4):439–451

Häberling IS, Corballis PM, Corballis MC (2016) Language, gesture, and handedness: evidence for independent lateralized networks. Cortex 82:72–85

Habib M, Robichon F (2003) Structural correlates of brain asymmetry: studies in left-handed and dyslexic individuals. In: The asymmetrical brain, pp 681–716

Habib M, Gayraud D, Oliva A, Regis J, Salamon G, Khalil R (1991) Effects of handedness and sex on the morphology of the corpus callosum: a study with brain magnetic resonance imaging. Brain Cogn 16(1):41–61

Habibi P, Chattopadhyay D (2021) The impact of handedness on user performance in touchless input. Int J Hum Comp Stud 149:102600

Hach S, Schütz-Bosbach S (2014) In (or outside of) your neck of the woods: laterality in spatial body representation. Front Psychol 5:123. https://doi.org/10.3389/fpsyg.2014.00123

Hellige JB (2010) Hemispheric specialisation: language, space and sexual differentiation. In: Koob GF, Le Moal M, Thompson RF (Hg.) Encyclopedia of behavioral neuroscience. Elsevier Science, Burlington, pp 21–26

Hepper PG (2013) The developmental origins of laterality: fetal handedness. Dev Psychobiol 55(6):588–595. https://doi.org/10.1002/dev.21119

Hepper PG, Shahidullah S, White R (1991) Handedness in the human fetus. Neuropsychologia 29(11):1107–1111. https://doi.org/10.1016/0028-3932(91)90080-r

Hepper PG, McCartney GR, Shannon EA (1998) Lateralised behaviour in first trimester human foetuses. Neuropsychologia 36(6):531–534. https://doi.org/10.1016/s0028-3932(97)00156-5

Hepper PG, Wells DL, Lynch C (2005) Prenatal thumb sucking is related to postnatal handedness. Neuropsychologia 43(3):313–315. https://doi.org/10.1016/j.neuropsychologia.2004.08.009

Hill EL, Khanem F (2009) The development of hand preference in children: the effect of task demands and links with manual dexterity. Brain Cogn 71(2):99–107. https://doi.org/10.1016/j.bandc.2009.04.006

Hughes CML, Reißig P, Seegelke C (2011) Motor planning and execution in left-and right-handed individuals during a bimanual grasping and placing task. Acta Psychol 138(1):111–118

Illert M, Kuhtz-Buschbeck JP (2006) Motorisches system. In: Neuro-& Sinnesphysiologie. Springer, pp 94–130

Jäncke L, Staiger JF, Schlaug G, Huang Y, Steinmetz H (1997) The relationship between corpus callosum size and forebrain volume. Cereb Cortex 7(1):48–56

Janssen L, Beuting M, Meulenbroek R, Steenbergen B (2009) Combined effects of planning and execution constraints on bimanual task performance. Exp Brain Res 192(1):61–73

Janssen L, Meulenbroek RGJ, Steenbergen B (2011) Behavioral evidence for left-hemisphere specialization of motor planning. Exp Brain Res 209(1):65–72

Kagerer FA (2015) Control of discrete bimanual movements: how each hand benefits from the other. Neurosci Lett 584(Pt 7):33–38. https://doi.org/10.1016/j.neulet.2014.10.002

Kavaklioglu T, Guadalupe T, Zwiers M, Marquand AF, Onnink M, Shumskaya E et al (2017) Structural asymmetries of the human cerebellum in relation to cerebral cortical asymmetries and handedness. Brain Struct Funct 222(4):1611–1623. https://doi.org/10.1007/s00429-016-1295-9

Kephart NC (1977) Das lernbehinderte Kind im Unterricht. Ernst Reinhart Verl, München

Knecht S (2000) Handedness and hemispheric language dominance in healthy humans. Brain 123(12):2512–2518. https://doi.org/10.1093/brain/123.12.2512

Kong X-Z, Postema MC, Guadalupe T, de Kovel C, Boedhoe PSW, Hoogman M et al (2020) Mapping brain asymmetry in health and disease through the ENIGMA consortium. Hum Brain Mapp 43(1):167–181

Kourtis D, de Saedeleer L, Vingerhoets G (2014) Handedness consistency influences bimanual coordination: a behavioural and electrophysiological investigation. Neuropsychologia 58:81–87. https://doi.org/10.1016/j.neuropsychologia.2014.04.002

Kraus E (2006) Ist das Überkreuzen der Körpermittellinie ein Indikator für die Handpräferenz bei Kindern? Ergoscience 1(3):100–109. https://doi.org/10.1055/s-2006-927098

Kraus E (2019) Mögliche Ursachen eines wechselnden Handgebrauchs. In: Zwischen Links-& Rechtshändigkeit. Springer, pp 69–110

Kuhtz-Buschbeck JP, Boczek-Funcke A, Illert M, Joehnk K, Stolze H (1999) Prehension movements and motor development in children. Exp Brain Res 128(1):65–68

Kuypers HGJM (1982) A new look at the organization of the motor system. Prog Brain Res 57:381–403

Leinen P, Vieluf S, Kennedy D, Aschersleben G, Shea CH, Panzer S (2016) Life span changes: performing a continuous 1:2 bimanual coordination task. Hum Mov Sci 46(3):209–220. https://doi.org/10.1016/j.humov.2016.01.004

Liederman J (1983) Mechanisms underlying instability in the development of hand preference. In: Young G, Corter CM, Segalowitz SJ, Trehub SE (Hg.) Manual specialization and the developing brain: an overview: Academic New York, pp 71–90

Luders E, Rex DE, Narr KL, Woods RP, Jancke L, Thompson PM et al (2003) Relationships between sulcal asymmetries and corpus callosum size: gender and handedness effects. Cereb Cortex 13(10):1084–1093

Luders E, Cherbuin N, Thompson PM, Gutman B, Anstey KJ, Sachdev P, Toga AW (2010) When more is less: associations between corpus callosum size and handedness lateralization. NeuroImage 52(1):43–49. https://doi.org/10.1016/j.neuroimage.2010.04.016

McManus C (2019) Half a century of handedness research: Myths, truths; fictions, facts; backwards, but mostly forwards. Brain Neurosci Adv 3, 2398212818820513.

Michel GF (2021) Handedness development: a model for investigating the development of hemispheric specialization and interhemispheric coordination. Symmetry 13(6):992

Michel GF, Nelson EL, Babik I, Campbell JM, Marcinowski EC (2013) Multiple trajectories in the developmental psychobiology of human handedness. Adv Child Dev Behav 45:227–260

Michell D, Wood N (1999) An investigation of midline crossing in three-year-old children. Physiotherapy 85(11):607–615. https://doi.org/10.1016/S0031-9406(05)66041-5

Musalek M (2015) Skilled performance tests and their use in diagnosing handedness and footedness at children of lower school age 8–10. Front Psychol 5(998):641. https://doi.org/10.3389/fpsyg.2014.01513

Nathan PW, Smith MC, Deacon P (1990) The corticospinal tracts in man: course and location of fibres at different segmental levels. Brain 113(2):303–324

Nelson EL, Gonzalez SL, Coxe S, Campbell JM, Marcinowski EC, Michel GF (2017) Toddler hand preference trajectories predict 3-year language outcome. Dev Psychobiol 59(7):876–887. https://doi.org/10.1002/dev.21560

Nelson EL, Gonzalez SL, El-Asmar JM, Ziade MF, Abu-Rustum RS (2019) The home handedness questionnaire: pilot data from preschoolers. Laterality 24(4):482–503. https://doi.org/10.1080/1357650X.2018.1543313

Nowicka A, Tacikowski P (2011) Transcallosal transfer of information and functional asymmetry of the human brain. Laterality 16(1):35–74. https://doi.org/10.1080/13576500903154231

Ocklenburg S, Garland A, Ströckens F, Uber Reinert A (2015) Investigating the neural architecture of handedness. Front Psychol 6(820):216. https://doi.org/10.3389/fpsyg.2015.00148

Ocklenburg S, Schmitz J, Moinfar Z, Moser D, Klose R, Lor S et al (2017) Epigenetic regulation of lateralized fetal spinal gene expression underlies hemispheric asymmetries. eLife 6:e22784. https://doi.org/10.7554/eLife.22784

Oswald K, Bo J (2019) Impact of handedness consistency on bimanual and unimanual continuous movements. J Motor Behav 51(2):161–170. https://doi.org/10.1080/00222895.2018.1443906

Packheiser J, Schmitz J, Berretz G, Carey DP, Paracchini S, Papadatou-Pastou M, Ocklenburg S (2020) Four meta-analyses across 164 studies on atypical footedness prevalence and its relation to handedness. Sci Rep 10(1):14501. https://doi.org/10.1038/s41598-020-71478-w

Panzer S, Kennedy D, Leinen P, Pfeifer C, Shea C (2021) Bimanual coordination associated with left- and right-hand dominance: testing the limb assignment and limb dominance hypothesis. Exp Brain Res 239(5):1595–1605. https://doi.org/10.1007/s00221-021-06082-z

Pool E-M, Rehme AK, Fink GR, Eickhoff SB, Grefkes C (2014) Handedness and effective connectivity of the motor system. NeuroImage 99:451–460

Porac C (2016) Laterality. Exploring the enigma of left-handedness. Elsevier Science, Amsterdam. http://www.sciencedirect.com/science/book/9780128012390

Pritchard VE, Malone SA, Burgoyne K, Heron-Delaney M, Bishop DVM, Hulme C (2019) Stage 2 registered report: there is no appreciable relationship between strength of hand preference and language ability in 6- to 7-year-old children. Wellcome Open Res 4:81. https://doi.org/10.12688/wellcomeopenres.15254.1

Provine RR, Westerman JA (1979) Crossing the midline: limits of early eye-hand behavior. Child Dev 50(2):437–441

Przybyla A, Coelho CJ, Akpinar S, Kirazci S, Sainburg RL (2013) Sensorimotor performance asymmetries predict hand selection. Neuroscience 228(Pt. 2):349–360. https://doi.org/10.1016/j.neuroscience.2012.10.046

Rigal RA (1992) Which handedness: preference or performance? Percept Mot Skills 75(3):851–866. https://doi.org/10.2466/pms.1992.75.3.851

Roland JL, Snyder AZ, Hacker CD, Mitra A, Shimony JS, Limbrick DD et al (2017) On the role of the corpus callosum in interhemispheric functional connectivity in humans. Proc Natl Acad Sci U S A 114(50):13278–13283

Rosch RE, Ronan L, Cherkas L, Gurd JM (2010) Cerebellar asymmetry in a pair of monozygotic handedness-discordant twins. J Anat 217(1):38–47

Rutten G-J (2022) Broca-Wernicke theories: a historical perspective. Handb Clin Neurol 185:25–34

Sacco S, Moutard M-L, Fagard J (2006) Agenesis of the corpus callosum and the establishment of handedness. Dev Psychobiol 48(6):472–481. https://doi.org/10.1002/dev.20162

Saccoa C, Michele D, Rocco, Semprini G, Merni F, Soffritti G (2018) Joint assessment of handedness

and footedness through latent class factor analysis. Laterality 23(6):643–663
Sadato N, Campbell G, Ibáñez V, Deiber M, Hallett M (1996) Complexity affects regional cerebral blood flow change during sequential finger movements. J Neurosci 16(8):2691–2700
Sainburg R (2002) Evidence for a dynamic-dominance hypothesis of handedness. Exp Brain Res 142(2):241–258. https://doi.org/10.1007/s00221-001-0913-8
Sainburg RL (2014) Convergent models of handedness and brain lateralization. Front Psychol 5(92):97. https://doi.org/10.3389/fpsyg.2014.01092
Scharoun SM, Bryden PJ (2014) Hand preference, performance abilities, and hand selection in children. Front Psychol 5:82. https://doi.org/10.3389/fpsyg.2014.00082
Scharoun SM, Bryden PJ (2015) Is strength of handedness reliable over repeated testing? An examination of typical development and autism spectrum disorder. Front Psychol 6:17
Schnitzler A, Kessler KR, Benecke R (1996) Transcallosally mediated inhibition of interneurons within human primary motor cortex. Exp Brain Res 112(3):381–391. https://doi.org/10.1007/BF00227944
Schofield WN (1976) Do children find movements which cross the body midline difficult? Q J Exp Psychol 28(4):571–582. https://doi.org/10.1080/14640747608400584
Senff O, Weigelt M (2011) Sequential effects after practice with the dominant and non-dominant hand on the acquisition of a sliding task in schoolchildren. Laterality 16(2):227–239. https://doi.org/10.1080/13576500903549414
Shadmehr R, Huang HJ, Ahmed AA (2016) A representation of effort in decision-making and motor control. Curr Biol 26(14):1929–1934
Sommer IEC (2010) 10 sex differences in handedness, brain asymmetry, and language lateralization. In: The two halves of the brain, pp 287
Sperry RW (1968) Hemisphere deconnection and unity in conscious awareness. Am Psychol 28:723–733
Stilwell JM (1987) The development of manual midline crossing in 2- to 6-year-old children. Am J Occup Ther 41(12):783–789. https://doi.org/10.5014/ajot.41.12.783
Stolze H (2012) Brain lateralisation and motor learning: selective effects of dominant and non-dominant hand practice on the early acquisition of throwing skills. Laterality 17(1):18–37. https://doi.org/10.1080/1357650X.2010.524222
Surburg PR (1999) Midline-crossing inhibition: an indicator of developmental delay. Laterality 4(4):333–343. https://doi.org/10.1080/713754347
Swinnen SP, Wenderoth N (2004) Two hands, one brain: cognitive neuroscience of bimanual skill. Trends Cogn Sci 8(1):18–25. https://doi.org/10.1016/j.tics.2003.10.017
Szaflarski JP, Binder JR, Possing ET, McKiernan KA, Ward BD, Hammeke TA (2002) Language lateralization in left-handed and ambidextrous people. Neurology 59(2):238–244. https://doi.org/10.1212/WNL.59.2.238
Szaflarski JP, Rajagopal A, Altaye M, Byars AW, Jacola L, Schmithorst VJ et al (2012) Left-handedness and language lateralization in children. Brain Res 1433(1129–39):85–97. https://doi.org/10.1016/j.brainres.2011.11.026
Tichy J, Belacek J (2009) Laterality in children: cerebellar dominance, handedness, footedness and hair whorl. Acta Nerv Super Rediviva 51(1–2):9–20
Todor JI, Doane T (1977) Handedness classification: preference versus proficiency. Percept Mot Skills 45(3 Pt 2):1041–1042. https://doi.org/10.2466/pms.1977.45.3f.1041
Tzourio-Mazoyer N, Labache L, Zago L, Hesling I, Mazoyer B (2021) Neural support of manual preference revealed by BOLD variations during right and left finger-tapping in a sample of 287 healthy adults balanced for handedness. Laterality 26(4):398–420
van der Knaap LJ, van der Ham IJM (2011) How does the corpus callosum mediate interhemispheric transfer? A review. Behav Brain Res 223(1):211–221
van Grunsven W, Vuylsteke-Wauters M, Njiokiktjien C, Vranken M (2009) Ontogenesis of laterality in 3- to 10-yr.-old children: increased unimanual Independence grounded on improved bimanual motor function. Percept Motor Skills 109(1):3–29. https://doi.org/10.2466/pms.109.1.3-29
van Helvert MJL, Wijdenes LO, Geerligs L, Medendorp WP (2021) Beta-band desynchronization reflects uncertainty in effector selection during motor planning. bioRxiv
Vingerhoets G (2019) Phenotypes in hemispheric functional segregation? Perspectives and challenges. Elsevier (30)
Volkmann J, Schnitzler A, Witte OW, Freund H-J (1998) Handedness and asymmetry of hand representation in human motor cortex. J Neurophysiol 79(4):2149–2154
Westerhausen R, Papadatou-Pastou M (2022) Handedness and midsagittal corpus callosum morphology: a meta-analytic evaluation. Brain Struct Funct 227(2):545–559. https://doi.org/10.1007/s00429-021-02431-4
Westerhausen R, Kreuder F, Dos Santos Sequeira S, Walter C, Woerner W, Wittling RA et al (2004) Effects of handedness and gender on macro-and microstructure of the corpus callosum and its subregions: a combined high-resolution and diffusion-tensor MRI study. Brain Res Cogn Brain Res 21(3):418–426
Witelson SF (1989) Hand and sex differences in the isthmus and genu of the human corpus callosum. Brain 112(3):799–835. https://doi.org/10.1093/brain/112.3.799
Witelson SF, Nowakowski RS (1991) Left out axons make men right: a hypothesis for the origin of handedness and functional asymmetry. Neuropsychologia 29(4):327–333. https://doi.org/10.1016/0028-3932(91)90046-b
Woytowicz EJ, Rietschel JC, Goodman RN, Conroy SS, Sorkin JD, Whitall J, Waller SMC (2017) Determining levels of upper extremity movement impairment by applying a cluster analysis to the Fugl-Meyer assess-

ment of the upper extremity in chronic stroke. Arch Phys Med Rehabil 98(3):456–462

Woytowicz EJ, Westlake KP, Whitall J, Sainburg RL (2018) Handedness results from complementary hemispheric dominance, not global hemispheric dominance: evidence from mechanically coupled bilateral movements. J Neurophysiol 120(2):729–740

Xiao X, Hu H, Li L, Li L (2019) Comparison of dominant hand to non-dominant hand in conduction of reaching task from 3D kinematic data: trade-off between successful rate and movement efficiency. Math Biosci Eng 16(3):1611–1624

Yadav V, Sainburg RL (2011) Motor lateralization is characterized by a serial hybrid control scheme. Neuroscience 196(2):153–167. https://doi.org/10.1016/j.neuroscience.2011.08.039

Yadav V, Sainburg RL (2014) Limb dominance results from asymmetries in predictive and impedance control mechanisms. PLoS One 9(4):e93892. https://doi.org/10.1371/journal.pone.0093892

Yang Y, Weiss PH, Fink GR, Chen Q (2021) Hand preference for the visual and auditory modalities in humans. Sci Rep 11(1):7868. https://doi.org/10.1038/s41598-021-87396-4

Yoo KH, Cannon EN, Thorpe SG, Fox NA (2016) Desynchronization in EEG during perception of means-end actions and relations with infants' grasping skill. Br J Dev Psychol 34(1):24–37

Zickert N, Geuze RH, Riedstra B, Groothuis TGG (2021) Is imitational learning a driving factor for the population bias in human hand preference? J Hum Evol 159:103045

3 Co-determinants of Handedness

Contents

Multiple handedness measures collected in large samples are likely to lead to novel breakthroughs with the increased level of digitisation and online testing. These types of data sets are becoming more likely and extremely exciting possibilities. For now, one of the key advances in the field is a new appreciation for the complexity that underlies handedness, a trait apparently very simple at both behavioral and molecular level. (Paracchini 2021: 9)

3.1 Introduction

The evolutionary, developmental and neural asymmetry research perspectives on handedness help us better understand the origins, processes and structures of handedness. However, a practice-based approach needs to understand those factors that influence and co-determine handedness as part of an assessment and its interpretation. In other words, what observable and behavioural influences or co-determinants for handedness can be identified when children present with atypical handedness, particularly when the writing hand is not clear? These handedness determinants are critical to understanding different manifestations of handedness and thus to developing a *Handedness Typology* (see Chap. 10).

In this chapter, we explore determining factors and look at a more behavioural research perspective on handedness. Research findings that are relevant to a practice-based approach to handedness are presented. In this chapter, these findings are divided into four clusters which I propose to be multivariate ⧫**co-determinants** of multidimensional handedness. The first cluster

E. Kraus, *Beyond Left and Right Handedness*, https://doi.org/10.1007/978-3-031-24389-9_3

deals with research findings around *inheritance and genetics*, the second with *developmental factors*, the third with *environmental influences* and the fourth with motor-sensory impact or *pathological factors* affecting the dominant hand.

3.2 Inheritance of Handedness and Motor Abilities

In this section, we look at the inheritance and genetic basis for both handedness and motor abilities, including motor planning.

3.2.1 Inheritance of Handedness

A variety of research findings suggest that handedness is at least partially heritable. These studies have often focused on explaining possible inheritable reasons for *Left Handedness*. Different approaches have been used, ranging from analysing *distributions of Left Handedness* to *twin studies, familial Left Handedness, genetic theories, molecular gene studies* and *polygenetic predisposition*.

Distributions of *Left Handedness*

Children of left-handed parents have been found to be more often left handed than children of right-handed parents (McKeever 2000; McManus 1991). Also, Carter-Salzman found that adopted children show more agreement with the handedness of their biological parents than with their adoptive ones (Carter-Saltzman 1980).

Twin Studies

The results of studies on identical twins have been the subject of much debate. If handedness is indeed heritable, one would expect that all uniovular twins should also have the same direction of handedness, but this is not the case. For example, identical and fraternal twins have a 75–80% match in their handedness (Sicotte et al. 1999). Moreover, based on a study of more than 25,000 people from twin families, researchers calculated that only about 25% of handedness is heritable (Medland et al. 2004, 2009; Kong et al. 2018). This would mean that genetic factors account for only a quarter of the influences that form *Left* or *Right Handedness*.

Familial *Left Handedness*

A more indirect background measure of the inheritability of handedness is based on the so-called familial sinistrality (*Left Handedness*) in the immediate and extended family. It has been found that about 30% of all people have a left-handed family member and that there is a relationship between the incidence of *Left Handedness* and left-handed family members (Porac 2016).

Genetic Theories

Until we know more about the genetic basis of handedness, its incidence is frequently explained by various genetic theories, such as the *Right-Shift Theory* (Annett 1985) and the *Dextral Chance Model* (McManus 1985). Both theories explain the data from twins and family studies as well as the relationship between cerebral language dominance and handedness, by incorporating a random component, some genetic material expressing a basic tendency towards *Right Handedness*. Annett refers to this as the right-shift factor and postulates that in its absence, the direction of handedness is subject to a 50–50 chance of being left or right handed. The two theories differ in relation to the handedness phenotypes, whereby McManus proposes two discrete handedness categories (McManus 1985, 2007), left and right, and Annett a continuum (Annett 1985). Figure 3.1 illustrates Annett's theory, based on two moderate right handers whose offspring has about a 12% chance of becoming left handed.

Molecular Genetics

Based on a review of recent findings of molecular genetics studies, Paracchini concluded that using different *types* of handedness measures could be beneficial for genetic research on handedness, particularly in the light that handwriting is typically used as a single indicator of handedness (Paracchini 2021). However, this does not consider the distinct dimensions of handedness,

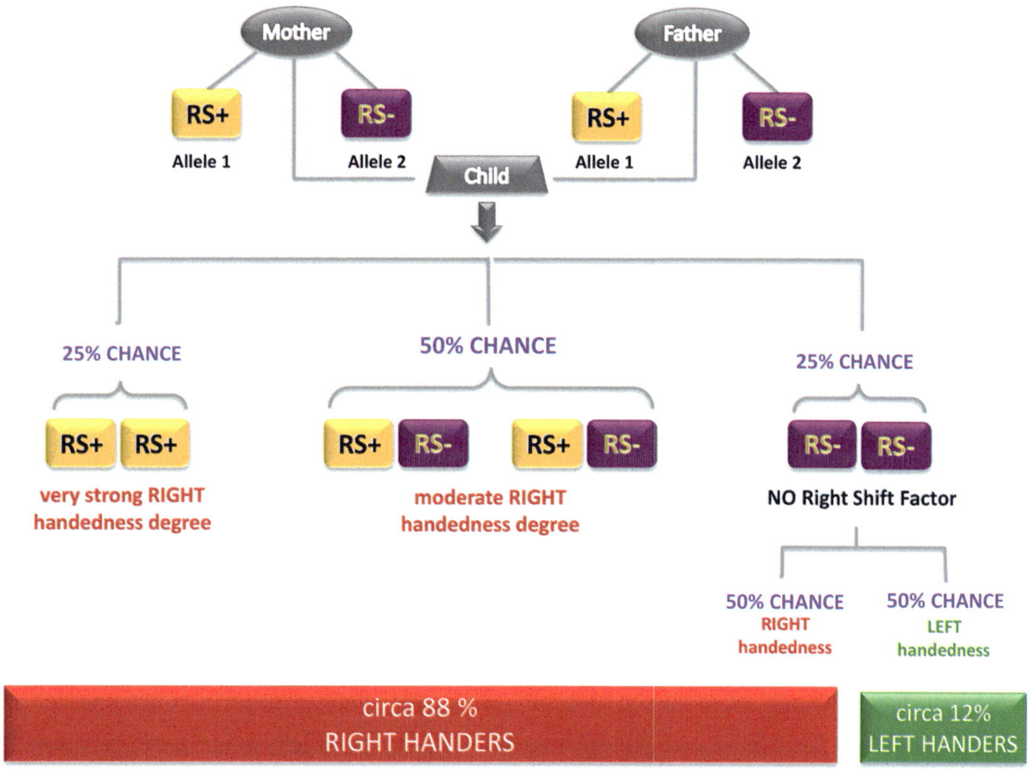

Fig. 3.1 Illustrating Annett's Right-Shift Theory. *RS* inherited right-shift factor

which might relate to the genetic information more specifically, particularly if there are categorical measures of hand preference.

Polygenetic Predisposition

Although there is some substantiation of different genes or alleles that may influence the inheritance of handedness, such as the androgen receptor gene (Arning et al. 2015), there is no evidence to date that a "handedness gene" exists. Instead, at least 40 gene loci (sites in the genome) have been found that seem to participate in the development of handedness (McManus et al. 2013). In addition, it is debated whether the direction and the degree of handedness are two separate phenotypes that are also subject to different genetic factors (Ocklenburg et al. 2014). Against this background, it is generally concluded that handedness is a polygenetic phenomenon and that other non-genetic factors also play a significant role (Porac 2016). However, some researchers such as Kovel and Francks, who conducted a genome-wide analysis of hand preference in the UK with over 331,000 subjects, found no major genetic link. Furthermore, they did not find an association between genes associated with visceral laterality and hand preference (de Kovel and Francks 2019).

3.2.2 Inheritance of Motor Abilities

Handedness is comprised of hand preference and hand proficiency. Exploring the hereditary and genetic base of handedness should thus include the inheritance of motor abilities in general. It can be assumed that a certain predisposition to motor coordination is inherited since children whose parents were highly coordinated also tend to be motorically gifted (Vasileva and Georgiev 2017). Furthermore, Klissouras and colleagues researching the potential in athletes state that "genetic influence is so ubiquitous and persuasive that we ask not what is heritable but what is not heritable" (Klissouras et al. 2007: 35) since nature and nurture cannot be separated. Their complex reciprocal interrelationship is most pertinent during training since training produces results within the genotype variability range, but they are still subject to innate individual abilities (ibid).

3.3 Development of Motor Abilities

In the previous chapter, we looked at the development of handedness. The general focus here is the development of a preferred hand, which generally becomes the more proficient hand with practice. However, there are important factors critical to a practice-based approach that influence hand proficiency. Practitioners need to understand the foundations and prerequisites for motor abilities and motor planning when working with developmentally delayed children and how these relate to handedness.

3.3.1 Foundations for Motor Skills

Specific prerequisites influence manual proficiency. For example, movement needs to be controlled, and sensory consequences of this control need to be predicted. This has been related to manual asymmetry: the dominant hand shows greater ability to *control movement* rather than to predict it (Mathew et al. 2019). Another aspect significantly influencing motor control is *visual and proprioceptive monitoring*. Goble and Brown found that visual feedback was particularly used with the preferred hand, whilst the non-preferred hand relied more on proprioception (Goble and Brown 2007, 2008, 2010). Interestingly, visual monitoring may not always be helpful. It has been shown that visual feedback can also interfere with a learning process (Saunders and Knill 2004) or decrease motor efficiency (Mayer et al. 2018).

From a developmental perspective, we see that typically developing infants use spontaneous self-generated movement accompanied by *tactile, proprioceptive, kinaesthetic and vestibular* input. These form the basis for later emerging motor skills. This input is proposed to create topological representations in the spinal cord and brain and shape the primary sensory and motor pathways (Ferre et al. 2020).

Another influencing factor in the development of proficiency is the type of musculature involved in an action. ♦**Proximal** (close to the body core such as shoulder muscles) and ♦**distal** (further away from the body core such as finger muscles) musculature is controlled differently, which affects the extent of asymmetry. Spinal motor neurons innervate the distal fingers, hand and wrist with more monosynaptic cortico-motoneuronal projections from the motor and premotor regions of the brain, compared to the motor neurons innervating the proximal elbow and shoulder (Rathelot and Strick 2006; Kuypers 1982). As a result, distal movement patterns tend to be more lateralised than proximal ones.

3.3.2 Motor Planning

Motor planning is the process where action outcomes and goals are predicted and motor behaviours are organised to meet specific action goals. In particular, bimanual coordination, proximal and distal movement control and motor planning affect motor abilities and support efficient movement. See also Chap. 2 for bimanual coordination.

The early anticipatory grasp adjustment is probably one of the most rudimentary motor planning abilities (Rosenbaum et al. 2012), whereby complexity increases with age. In addition, goal adjustment in sequential actions becomes more refined (Chen et al. 2010) and responds to increased task complexity, which in turn requires more time to plan, establish and execute an action (Krajenbrink et al. 2020). By school-going age, motor planning in sequential goal-directed manual movements appears fairly well established (ibid.).

A study focusing on the kinematic movement registration in children with autism spectrum disorders (ASD) found that children with ASD demonstrate less functional anticipatory strategies, probably linked to a reduced motor planning ability and causing difficulties with everyday actions (Bäckström et al. 2021). Similarly, when motor planning abilities between children with ASD and typically developed children were compared, Rodgers and colleagues found that the difference depended on the interaction of both task complexity and age (Rodgers et al. 2019). Children with ASD showed less smooth movements and were less proficient in motor planning tasks, particularly at the end of sequential movement patterns (i.e. the fitting phase). In addition, they showed higher individual variability and neurodevelopmental comorbidities, making them a more heterogenous group (Bäckström et al. 2021). Cognitive abilities may also influence motor planning and control (Ansuini et al. 2018), although findings are inconsistent (Cavallo et al. 2018). Moreover, the sensorimotor impairments typical to children with ASD may also be influenced by deficits in motor memory systems (Neely et al. 2019). Since children with ASD tend to have motor planning problems, research specifying the aspects of these problems is helpful to practitioners working with these children.

If we link motor planning skills to handedness, the question arises if motor planning of dominant hand actions would differ from non-dominant hand actions in right and left handers. This research question was investigated by Janssen and colleagues (Janssen et al. 2011). They found support for a left hemispheric dominance in task performance for motor planning at a behavioural level. In particular, learning motor sequences seem to take place most effectively before and during motor action (Ariani and Diedrichsen 2019). These researchers also found several influences affecting sequential movement, including the ability to select and plan multiple sequence elements that needed to be executed.

3.4 Environmental Influences

Since genetics are thought to explain about 25% of the handedness direction (Medland et al. 2009), there must be further influencing factors. Environmental factors and their influence on handedness comprise a large body of knowledge, and they make up the third co-determinant of handedness. For clinical practice, background information on conditions around birth and other influencing factors in the early years is usually integrated into the assessment process to contextualise and understand developmental processes, including handedness. These influences are also important when dealing with developmental disorders or delays, where certain risk factors have been identified (de Moura et al. 2010). In this section, we will look at circumstances around birth influencing early development, particularly at developmental risk factors, as well as at the more general influence of a rightward-biassed environment.

3.4.1 Pre-, Peri- and Postnatal Circumstances

There is evidence that handedness (or at least laterality) seems to develop very early in life. However, this lateralisation process is also influenced by several different factors (Schaafsma et al. 2009). Moreover, it is unclear whether these prenatal preferences can already be interpreted as a manifestation of early handedness, or whether the asymmetries in the womb influence the development and formation of handedness. From birth onwards, handedness develops over various phases (see Chap. 2), which are also intricately linked to environmental influences and opportunities for practice. Therefore, the environmental perspective is critical in our quest to understand the determinants of handedness. We can roughly divide early environmental influences on handedness into those before, at and after birth. For each of these developmental stages, different assumptions or theoretical postulates will be outlined briefly.

Environmental Influences Before Birth

Looking at ***distributions***, it has been found that foetuses show signs of manual asymmetry already in the womb. For example, most embryos prefer their right thumb for sucking and move their right arm more often than their left (Hepper et al. 1991), and their head is tilted more to the right side (Ververs et al. 1994). It has also been shown that the preference for thumb sucking during the last trimester of pregnancy corresponds to the subsequent handedness of a child (Hepper et al. 2005). Parma and colleagues argue that using standard ultrasonography for assessing human handedness should be implemented more in research, as they found a high correlation between foetus reaching to the mouth, the eyes or the uterus wall (Parma et al. 2017).

There have indeed been several attempts to explain these observed early asymmetries in utero. ***Previc's vestibular-monoaminergic theory*** assumes that handedness and cerebral lateralisation are influenced by early asymmetric development of equilibrium (Previc 1991). Previc's theory is based on the observed correlation between the foetal position (i.e. an inclination to the left or right side) during the last trimester of pregnancy. In addition, it considers abnormalities and the higher number of mixed and left handers[1] than assumed to be present in the general population (Previc 1996). He furthermore postulated that intrauterine position leads to asymmetric prenatal auditory and vestibular experiences and influences developmental processes accordingly (Previc 1991). More recent studies with imaging techniques have also shown that the vestibular system is predominantly activated in the contralateral region of the brain, indicating possible differences in this regard between left- and right-handed individuals (Dietrich 2003; Janzen et al. 2008; Schmidt et al. 2013). Since the vestibular system forms early in child development, these asymmetries could have a causal influence on handedness (Dietrich 2003). These are interesting findings for occupational therapists working with a sensory integration approach, which includes vestibular processing.

The idea that the hormone ***testosterone*** in utero may also affect the development and formation of handedness has also attracted research attention. There are two opposing theories explaining the effects of testosterone. The so-called *Geschwind-Behan-Galaburda model* establishes a connection between an increased prenatal testosterone level and *Left Handedness* (Geschwind and Galaburda 1985). The *Witelson theory*, on the other hand, is based on a correlation between low prenatal testosterone levels and *Left Handedness* (Witelson and Nowakowski 1991). Subsequent studies into the relationship between this hormone and handedness tend to support the Witelson theory (e.g. Medland et al. 2005; Vuoksimaa et al. 2010). The research findings on the relationship between testosterone and handedness remain in need of further clarification (see also Beaton et al. 2011; Papadatou-Pastou et al. 2017; Pfannkuche et al. 2009). Furthermore, it is unclear if this hormonal influence is essential in the developmental process of handedness.

There are many further studies on factors influencing handedness before birth, in particular, resulting in more left-handed children. These include research looking at the ***mother's mental ill-health*** (Rodriguez and Waldenström 2008) and ***increased mother's age*** at the birth of their child (Bailey and McKeever 2004; Coren 1992); ***smoking during pregnancy*** (Bakan 1991; Rodriguez and Waldenström 2008); and ***seasons around birth*** (Jones and Martin 2008; Fagard et al. 2021). All these multifactorial influences could be considered collectively when documenting a child's medical history. However, their usefulness to a practice-based approach is questionable since their impact is relatively vague and may lead practitioners to erroneous conclusions.

Environmental Influences at Birth

The impact of ***preterm birth***, (i.e. children born before the 37th week of pregnancy), on handedness has been the subject of many studies, and this is most often also related to ***low birth weight***. Domellöf and colleagues conducted a meta-analysis involving close to 2000 preterm infants and more than 8.000 control infants in studies published between 1980 and 2010. They found twice as many preterm left- and/or mixed-handed children as full-term children (Domellöf et al. 2011). Ross and team found that 63% of preterm infants

[1] Previc referred to mixed and left handers as "non-right handers".

showed *Right Handedness*, compared with 80% of normal births in 4-year-olds (Ross et al. 1987). Moreover, preterm birth can have several consequences on brain development and can also lead to motor disorders such as cerebral palsy or developmental coordination disorder (DCD), affecting motor function (Williams et al. 2010). Also, weaker fine motor skills were associated with preterm children (van Heerwaarde et al. 2020).

Importantly, not all studies found a relationship between ***birth stress*** and *Left Handedness*. Tan and colleagues conducted a study of over 900 subjects. They investigated hand preference using a 14-item questionnaire and information about conditions around birth. There was no evidence supporting birth stress as the main cause of *Left Handedness* (Tan and Nettleton 1980).

Environmental Influences After Birth

Two well-documented environmental influences on handedness development after birth include ***breastfeeding*** (e.g. Denny 2012; Hujoel 2019) and ***cradling*** (e.g. Donnot et al. 2008; Todd and Banerjee 2016; Schaafsma et al. 2009). In addition, the general rightward bias of physical and social-cultural influences is likely to considerably impact handedness development (see Sect. 3.4.2). For a practice-based approach, the results of breastfeeding and cradle studies remain inconclusive, and the direct impact of these factors on handedness development remains unspecific.

Early brain damage before, at or after birth has been associated with increased mixed and *Left Handedness*, especially among boys. Interestingly, this was not related to other developmental milestones such as language or cognitive deficits in school performance (Saigal et al. 1992; Satz 1972). This indicates that an increase in mixed or *Left Handedness* is not necessarily an indicator of developmental delay or vice versa.

3.4.2 Sociocultural and Physical Influences with a Rightward Bias

Over the last centuries of recorded history, religious and cultural perspectives, values as well as the use of language have shaped our perception of *Left* and *Right Handedness*. Very often, the right is viewed as positive or strong, whilst the left is portrayed as something negative or weak (see Christman 2012). This is reflected in major *religions*, such as Christianity, Judaism, Islam and Buddhism, the right side is reserved for the "good" and "correct". For example, the Bible refers to the right side of God as reserved for the "righteous", whilst sinners are assigned to the left side on Judgement Day. An example of a *cultural practice* is shaking hands with the "right" hand when greeting. Children are taught this practice frequently by referring to shaking hands with the "good", "nice" or "better" hand. Similarly, many *languages* use "left" to denote something negative or degrading. For example, in English, there are phrases such as "having two left feet" that insinuate clumsiness, as contrasted to "being right" or "righteous", where positive attributes are implied (see Porac 2016; Christman 2012 for reviews).

The strong right-biassed environment is widely seen as leading to repeated imitation and learning of culturally relevant tasks with the right hand. As such, a cluster of research has shown that environmental factors, particularly during child development (see Marcori and Okazaki 2020; Merni et al. 2014; Michel et al. 2013; Fagard 2013), strongly influence the direction and degree of handedness. In particular, Campbell and colleagues propose that an infant's *experience* during development may substantially influence the variability of handedness development (Campbell et al. 2018).

In addition, learning effects, imitation of behaviour or cultural pressure due to the predominantly right-orientated physical and sociocultural environment inevitably influence handedness formation (e.g. Janßen 2000). As a result, inherent left handers learn to write with the right non-dominant hand. Writing is not only one of the most complex and demanding human activities, but it is also culturally highly valued across societies and thus particularly prone to conformity.

Furthermore, several authors have argued that societies representing a high degree of conformity or a cultural devaluation of *Left Handedness* produce increased numbers of ♦**converted**

(switched) left handers, particularly since handwriting is a culturally highly valued activity (DeAgostini et al. 1997; Dahmen and Fagard 2005; Kushner 2013). Until the turn of the last century, switching *Left Handedness* was a common practice in the Western world, strongly endorsed and recommended by scientists, educators, priests and physicians of the time, and is often subject to social and cultural discrimination (see Kushner 2017 for review).

A historical example is Germany, where *Left Handedness* was considered deviant and undesirable under the Nazi regime, and thus suppressed (Siebner et al. 2002; Dobel 2006). These negative attitudes prevailed well into the 1970s with deliberate handedness conversions commonly attempted to prevent left-handed writing in schools, sometimes with harsh measures (e.g. by hitting the fingers—Ocklenburg and Gunturkun 2017). Also, in North America, a study from the 1950s shows that particularly left-handed fathers insisted that their children use their right hands. A common argument was that left handers experience disadvantages in the right-handed world, which the child should be spared (Falek 1959). More details on *Converted Left Handedness* are discussed in Chap. 4.

There is evidence that the sociocultural pressures to convert handedness have decreased over the last decades. Indeed, a study based on large data sets of Canadians and Americans indicates that handedness conversion has decreased over time (Porac 1996).

However, even if the situation in the labour market and negative attitudes towards *Left Handedness* have decreased over the years, they still prevail. Typically, handedness conversions occur at home within families where pressure towards *Right Handedness* is exerted. Certain factors such as the parents' educational level, occupation and income may also influence the tendency to switch left handers (Porac 2016). Meyer suspects that switching the writing hand still occurs today but often in a more hidden or subtle manner. These discrete conversions are based on *sociocultural* influences, such as offering rewards, exerting moral pressure or making negative comments when a person is using the left hand for more complex tasks (Sattler and Klußmann 2014; Meyer 2007). The *physical* environment also affects hand use, for example, when parents place objects in their child's right hand or encourage using the right hand during play, eating and brushing teeth (see summary by Porac 2016).

Indeed, it is undeniable that left handers experience difficulties in a right-handed world. Most utensils, tools and facilities (e.g. notebooks, scissors, measuring devices) are designed for right handers (see Zaghloul et al. 2018; Suitner et al. 2017; Masud and Ajmal 2012; Sattler 2000a, b). The impact of these environmental factors on handedness might be difficult to measure and individualistic but should not be underestimated.

Studies on switched/converted left handers most often support the first variant: switched left handers write with the right hand but continue to perform all or most other tasks with the left hand (Klöppel et al. 2007). It is, however, likely that the subjects in this study had an inherently high degree of *Left Handedness*. Had these left handers been less explicit, it would have been more likely that their hand use would have been more variable. This will be discussed in more detail in Chap. 4.

3.5 Pathological Handedness

As discussed earlier, ♦**pathological handedness** is based on repeated observations that premature infants' asymmetric brain injury presumably impacts the dominant motor cortex before, at or after birth (Ross et al. 1992). As a result, the inherently non-dominant hand engages in more reaching and manipulation tasks, thereby developing superior motor skills compared to the inherently dominant hand and becoming more proficient over time. Figures 3.2 and 3.3 illustrate how a pathological impact can change the direction of ♦**handedness formation**.

Bishop calculated a possible distribution of left and right pathological handedness, conserva-

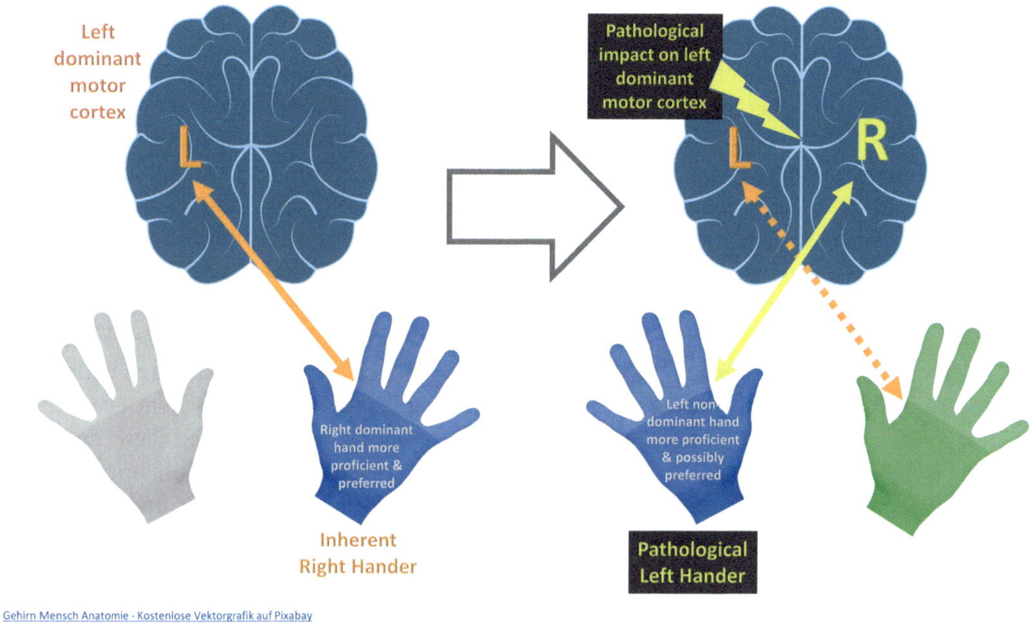

Fig. 3.2 Early pathological impact resulting in *pathological Left Handedness*

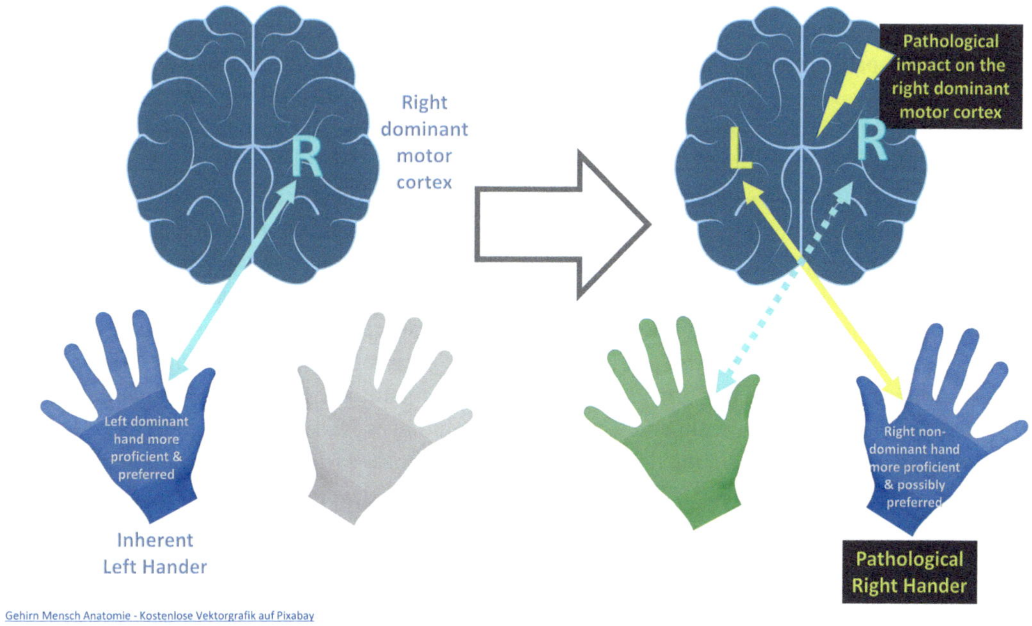

Fig. 3.3 Early pathological impact resulting in *pathological Right Handedness*

tively assuming that 90% of people are right handed (with a left cortical dominance) and 10% are left handed (with right cortical dominance). In addition, she based her calculations on an average of 5% of births incurring pre-, peri- or postnatal complications causing a pathological impact, presumed to be equally distributed between the hemispheres (Bishop 1990).

In other words, of these assumed distributions, the 5% are divided as follows:

- 2.25% will become ***pathological left handers*** because of the impact on their left dominant cortex, with motor deficiencies, particularly on their right side.
- 2.3% will remain ***right handers*** because of the impact on their right dominant cortex, with motor deficiencies, particularly on the left side.
- 0.25% will become ***pathological right handers*** because of the impact on their right dominant cortex, with motor deficiencies, particularly on the left side.
- 0.2% will remain ***left handers*** because of the impact on their left dominant cortex, with motor deficiencies, particularly on the right side.

Pathological Right Handedness is much rarer simply because there is a considerably lower incidence of left handedness than right handedness in the general population. Other authors investigated and confirmed *pathological Right Handedness* (Kim et al. 2001; Coren 1990). However, it is difficult to determine the exact number of pathological handers, particularly since no comprehensive and uniform assessment is used to determine pathological handedness.

Some authors have extended the discourse on the existence of pathological handedness, proposing that one hemisphere is more likely to be affected than the other. For example, when investigating children with hemiplegia, it has been proposed that the left hemisphere may be more susceptible to damage at birth since it is somewhat less developed compared to the right hemisphere at birth (Goodman 1994; Uvebrant 1988). It is argued that there are anatomical reasons for this, such as reduced blood supply to the left hemisphere compared to the right (Perlmutter et al. 1987). If the left hemisphere initially indeed matures more slowly than the right hemisphere, it may be affected more severely by, for example, oxygen deprivation. This, in turn, can lead to intracranial focal lesions and intracranial haemorrhages (Schuhmacher et al. 1988). Such a hypothesis would also support the significantly larger number of pathological left handers. However, it does not explain why some studies have found more left-sided hemiplegic children with mainly right hemispheric damage (Cioni et al. 1999). Influencing factors explaining these discrepancies may be related to differentiating between the severity and type of the brain insult and looking at the handedness measures used. Section 6.5 explores typical manifestations of pathological handedness in more detail.

3.6 Developmental Delay and Disorders

♦**Developmental delay** is defined in the context of this book as a milder form of ♦**developmental disorders** where certain milestones are delayed, but the child is functioning age-appropriately in other areas[2] (World Health Organisation 2016). In most cases, language development, visuospatial and movement coordination are affected. As a rule, the delay or deficiency is defined from the earliest possible point of recognition. As many of these children grow older, these delays often diminish progressively, although some deficits may remain into adulthood (Noterdaeme and Hutzelmeyer-Nickels 2010).

There are early risk factors typically associated with developmental delay and/or other clinical conditions, including infection of the

[2] According to the World Health Organization International Classification of Diseases, the ICD-10-WHO version 2016 (F80-F89), developmental disorders have the following common features: onset occurs invariably in infancy or childhood; a developmental restriction or delay of functions is closely related to the biological maturation of the central nervous system; and there is a steady progression without remissions and recurrences.

mother during pregnancy or anoxia of the infant at birth. The impact of these risk factors may affect development generally and/or specifically affect the development of handedness. For example, suppose the motor cortex of the inherently dominant hand is affected. In that case, the infant will grow up with a dominant arm and hand with motor dysfunction compared to the (relatively) unaffected non-dominant side. Children with hemiplegic cerebral palsy (CP) would be an extreme example of asymmetric development and motor dysfunction due to pathological conditions around birth (Ferre et al. 2020).

In addition to pathological birth factors, research has shown that other conditions may also cause an individual to change the direction of handedness and result in a significantly weaker dominant side. These include brain tumours (Crawford 2013), epilepsy (Dellatolas et al. 1993), premature birth (Domellöf et al. 2011) and early childhood meningitis (Ramadhani et al. 2006).

In the 1970s and 1980s, some research findings proposed that *Left Handedness* is per se disorder related (Bakan et al. 1973), or at least partially (Satz et al. 1985; Soper and Satz 1984). Since then, the notion that *Right Handedness* is the norm and *Left Handedness* to deviate from this norm due to pathological influences or impacts has been widely disputed, based on a differentiation between different groups of left handers. In particular, Annett distinguishes between familial left handers ("natural sinistrality") and so-called ♦***pathological Left Handedness***[3] (see Sects. 3.5 and 4.4), showing that familial left handers performed similarly to right handers on all motor, cognitive and behavioural levels (Annett 1994).

In this section, we will look at developmental disorders and developmental delays, with a particular focus on midline crossing, a typical indicator of developmental delay related to manual lateralisation and specialisation. Importantly, the distinction between developmental delay and atypical handedness is often diffuse, and the two variables appear to overlap. Many developmentally delayed children are *also* delayed in their handedness development, and pathological handers may also be developmentally delayed in other areas.

3.6.1 Motor-Based Developmental Disorders

In the context of a practice-based approach to handedness, those problems related to *motor-based developmental disorders* at the cortical "control level" rather than the skeletal-muscle level are often referred to as developmental coordination disorders[4]. They typically present in occupational therapy and will thus be the focus in this book. These children may have problems with body image and spatial perception, or experience difficulties in planning, coordinating, executing or controlling movement sequences (Krombholz 2005, 2008).

The development of handedness is considered to be a developmental milestone in sensory-motor development (Cermak et al. 1980; Stilwell 1987—see also Sect. 1.3). A large number of studies have investigated motor development concerning handedness, although the findings are somewhat ambiguous. We will focus on two aspects that are most relevant to a practice-based approach to handedness and decisively influencing a child's development: *sensory-motor abilities* and *crossing of the body midline, which is seen as an indicator of developmental delay*.

[3]Pathological *Left* and *Right Handedness* refers to inherently left and right handers where the motor abilities of dominant side are significantly weaker, probably due to pre-, peri- or postnatal impact, causing a shift in the direction of handedness.

[4]Developmental coordination disorder (DCD), also known as dyspraxia, is a condition affecting physical coordination. It causes a child to perform less well than expected in daily activities for their age and appear to move clumsily.

3.6.2 Sensory-Motor Abilities and Handedness

Mori and colleagues investigated hand preference and visual-motor skills in 5- to 6-year-old children (Mori et al. 2006). The children repeated the performance of six activities (writing, drawing, eating with a spoon/chopstick, cutting, throwing and brushing teeth). Mori's research team divided the children into two groups: those with "consistent" and those with "inconsistent" hand use. Consistent children showed superior performance in the visual-motor tasks compared to inconsistent children. The authors concluded that interhemispheric communication, which integrates information from proprioceptors, was more efficient in clearly established left and right handers than in mixed handers.

Using similar preference items for their assessment and relating hand preference to coordination disorders, Goez and Zelnik found similar results. They investigated the relationship between left, right and mixed hand preference concerning coordination disorders in children aged 6–17 (Goez and Zelnik 2008). Hand preference was assessed based on three activities: writing, throwing a ball and holding a spoon. Children who wrote with either hand were classified as mixed handed ("ambidextrous"). The analysis shows that left-handed and mixed-handed children with coordination disorders were overrepresented compared to the incidence in the normal population, with 30% left handers and 13% mixed handers.

Bruckner and colleagues examined hand preference in 4- to 5-year-old children with the HAPT 4–6,[5] which also measures consistency within an activity by repeating each item three times, and found differences between boys and girls. They then compared the consistency with a tracing task. Girls with "consistent" hand preference performed better at tracing than girls with inconsistent hand preference. Children with sub-average tracing performance were more often inconsistent in their hand use, with the boys being more inconsistent with hand use than the girls (Bruckner et al. 2011b).

However, not all research supports the relationship between decreased lateralisation and motor problems. For example, Gabbard' research team did not find any difference between the three groups (left, right and mixed handed) in 4- to 6-year-old children, based on a finger tapping test and three preference items (writing, throwing a ball and stacking dice) (Gabbard et al. 1995). However, since the assessment involved proficiency, the results are not sufficiently comparable with the other two studies that used preference as a measure.

Similarly, Krombholz failed to find a correlation between left or mixed handedness, and deficits in motor abilities (Krombholz 2008). Proficiency was assessed in preschoolers using a dotting test. They were subsequently divided into left-, right- and mixed-handed groups. Fine motor and cognitive tests were conducted at the beginning and end of the kindergarten period. However, 16% of the children changed the direction of their handedness during this period. Compared to the other children with stable handedness, these children showed poorer fine motor and cognitive performances (ibid.). Incidentally, dotting correlates highly with drawing and writing and is thus strongly influenced by a practice effect.

3.6.3 Crossing the Body Midline Avoidance

Several studies used contralateral reaching as a hand preference measure, finding that developmentally delayed children tended to avoid crossing the midline. Bishop, for example, studied 196 twins using the quantification of hand preference task (QHP) involving midline crossing (Bishop 2005). She found that children with a speech disorder were more likely to avoid contralateral reaching, displayed a lower degree of hand preference and performed poorer in proficiency. In a similar study, Hill and Bishop had previously investigated 7- to 11-year-old children, where they compared the data of children with coordination disorders with typically developed chil-

[5] Handpräferenztest, 4–6 years (Bruckner et al. 2011a, b).

dren of the same age as well as younger children (Hill et al. 1998). They found that right-handed children with speech and coordination disorders as well as younger, typically developed children avoided crossing the midline.

However, this tendency was not supported by a study where handedness and crossing the midline were tested in 4-year-olds (Rostoft et al. 2002). Different test procedures were used where contralateral reaching was induced by moving objects, which increased the task demand. Children with motor problems tended to use the right hand. To assess if this phenomenon would be the same for left handers, the study would have to be repeated with a larger number of left-handed subjects.

Bishop also investigated pathological influences on hand preference in children with epilepsy or "mental retardation". Findings revealed no relation to gross motor defects in a secondary analysis of 12,000 children, and there was no association between *Left Handedness* and motor deficit for the preferred hand (Bishop 1984).

Overall, research to date does not conclusively indicate a clear relationship between developmental delay/disorders and handedness groups.

3.7 The Essence of Research Perspectives

Let us look back at the various and diverse research perspectives on handedness so far. It is useful to summarise influencing factors and consider the difference between developmental delay and pathological handedness. This informs my proposal for co-determinants in a practice-based approach.

3.7.1 Summarising Influencing Factors on Handedness Formation

The influencing factors can roughly be divided into internal and external factors. *Internal factors* include the hereditary factors of handedness, motor predisposition (which, in turn, can be influenced by practice) and automation through practice, repetition and multidimensional developmental aspects. *External factors* include birth stress (or stress before, during or after birth), intrauterine influences especially hormones, position of the foetal head before birth, age of the mother, maternal smoking during pregnancy, preterm birth and low birth weight. In addition, after birth, the physical and sociocultural environments play a crucial role in handedness formation. Moreover, trauma or illness at any point in time can affect the development and formation of the preferred and more proficient hand.

These highly complex multidimensional developmental and formation processes are unique and individual for each person. Unfortunately, this individualised complexity is one of the reasons that these multiple factors are seldom taken into account in research. In everyday clinical and educational settings, however, additional information on these factors could help reveal essential aspects of non-typical handedness composition (i.e. how handedness presents at a certain point in time).

3.7.2 Distinguishing Between Developmental Delay and Pathological Handedness

It is difficult to distinguish between developmental delay and pathological handedness since both are the results of early pathological impact and risk factors. At the same time, depending on the location and severity of the lesion, not all developmental delays or disorders result in a change of handedness direction. Whilst similar risk factors may be responsible for cortical damage in both cases, a specific distinction between the two can be helpful, particularly for clinical practice.

Hypothetically, reduced hemispheric and manual lateralisation/specialisation may occur for two reasons in developmental delay/disorders, resulting in *Developmentally Delayed Handedness*. Either both hemispheres are affected by the pathological impact or the hemispheric lateralisation and specialisation processes have not yet taken place sufficiently to demonstrate manual asymmetries. This would mean that neuro-anatomical structures such as the cortexes and the cerebellum are affected bilaterally, resulting in motor abnormalities observed in both hands and both hands performing "equally poorly". Moreover, in my experience, alternating hand use is frequent since such a child tries to perform a task with one hand, struggles to do so and then tries with the other hand.

Conversely, in *pathological handedness*, the contralateral dominant motor cortex is affected (see Sect. 3.6). This can also result in alternating hand use, but it is very likely to result in different swapping patterns. Based on cases in clinical practice, we see two kinds of hand use variability. If the degree of handedness is co-determinant high, the better (non-dominant) hand will be used for tasks requiring greater proficiency, and the dominant less proficient hand will be used for simple low-demand manual tasks. If the handedness degree is low, most tasks might be performed with the non-dominant, more skilled right hand. Instead of the proficiency of *both* hands being equally poor, we would observe a stark difference in the level of motor performance between the hands, with the affected (dominant) hand performing very poorly compared to the unaffected (non-dominant) hand.

To comprehensively differentiate between the two conditions, we need a methodical handedness assessment that considers multifactorial background information and looks at handedness multidimensionally.

3.8 Proposing a Model of Co-determinants of Handedness

For a useful practice-based approach, I propose integrating the various research perspectives in a model consisting of those factors that primarily influence and determine handedness. Based on the literature, four main clusters can be considered co-determinants of handedness relevant to a practice-based approach: *inheritance*, *development*, *environment* and pathological *motor impact* affecting the dominant motor cortexes (see Fig. 3.4).

In my view, the perspectives on evolution and neural asymmetries of handedness, as discussed in Chaps. 1 and 2, are not directly applicable to a practice-based approach, given our current

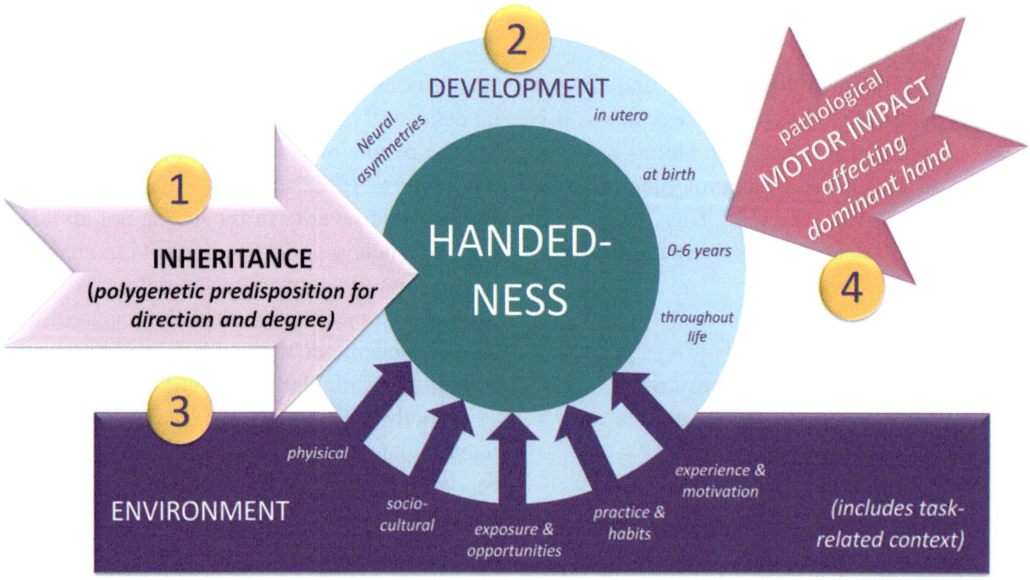

Fig. 3.4 Model for proposing four co-determinants of handedness formation

knowledge in these areas. For this reason, they are not included in the model as co-determinants. The co-determinant *inheritance* refers to the polygenetic predisposition of both the direction and the degree of handedness. The co-determinant *development* is unique in that it is intricately linked to handedness development, pathological motor sensory impact as well as physical and sociocultural environments. The co-determinant *environment* can be divided into a general external environment with physical and sociocultural influences, typically with a rightward bias; and a more task-related situational environment, encompassing exposure and opportunities to practise manual tasks, perceived experiences and motivation to perform them. Finally, the co-determinant pathological *motor impact* particularly determines pathological handedness by affecting the inherently dominant cortex but cannot be clearly separated from the pathological impact on development. In my experience, formulating theses co-determinants of handedness is very useful for practitioners dealing with atypical handedness. They represent a highly complex reciprocal and dynamic process underpinning manual action with the potential to explain the cause of variable hand use. In Chap. 9, we will further explore how these co-determinants inform the multivariate nature of handedness.

3.9 Concluding Remarks

In this chapter, we have taken on three further research perspectives on handedness: genetics or hereditary, factors as well as environmental and pathological factors. *Hereditary factors* have been found to determine only 25% of handedness in individuals, whilst other factors impose major influences, such as the environment or sensory-motor impacts affecting the dominant side. *Environmental influences* based on physical and sociocultural specifics can cause a change in handedness direction (particularly in left handers). In addition, early pathological *motor impact* (pathology) affecting the dominant side can cause the non-dominant hand to gain greater hand proficiency as well as preference. Finally, all of these influences are subject to *development* in terms of dynamically interrelated cascades (see Chap. 2). On this basis, I propose four co-determinants for handedness formation: inheritance, development, environmental and pathological motor-sensory factors. Defining these co-determinants allows practitioners to indirectly draw on research findings in a practice-based approach by providing a specific focus on the background information needed when children present with mixed handedness. With these co-determinants as a knowledge basis for the origins of handedness, we now look at *Left Handedness* in greater detail in the following chapter.

References

Annett M (1985) Left, right, hand, and brain. The right shift theory. L. Erlbaum Associates, London

Annett M (1994) Handedness as a continuous variable with dextral shift: sex, generation, and family handedness in subgroups of left- and right-handers. Behav Genet 24(1):51–63. https://doi.org/10.1007/BF01067928

Ansuini C, Podda J, Battaglia FM, Veneselli E, Becchio C (2018) One hand, two hands, two people: prospective sensorimotor control in children with autism. Dev Cogn Neurosci 29:86–96

Ariani G, Diedrichsen J (2019) Sequence learning is driven by improvements in motor planning. J Neurophysiol 121(6):2088–2100

Arning L, Ocklenburg S, Schulz S, Ness V, Gerding WM, Hengstler JG et al (2015) Handedness and the X chromosome: the role of androgen receptor CAG-repeat length. Sci Rep 5(1):655. https://doi.org/10.1038/srep08325

Bäckström A, Johansson A-M, Rudolfsson T, Rönnqvist L, von Hofsten C, Rosander K, Domellöf E (2021) Motor planning and movement execution during goal-directed sequential manual movements in 6-year-old children with autism spectrum disorder: a kinematic analysis. Res Dev Disabil 115:104014

Bailey L, McKeever W (2004) A large-scale study of handedness and pregnancy/birth risk events: implications for genetic theories of handedness. Laterality 9(2):175–188. https://doi.org/10.1080/13576500342000013

Bakan P (1991) Handedness and maternal smoking during pregnancy. Int J Neurosci 56(1–4):161–168. https://doi.org/10.3109/00207459108985412

Bakan P, Dibb G, Reed P (1973) Handedness and birth stress. Neuropsychologia 11(3):363–366

Beaton AA, Rudling N, Kissling C, Taurines R, Thome J (2011) Digit ratio (2D:4D), salivary testosterone,

and handedness. Laterality 16(2):136–155. https://doi.org/10.1080/13576500903410369
Bishop DV (1984) Using non-preferred hand skill to investigate pathological left-handedness in an unselected population. Dev Med Child Neurol 26(2):214–226. https://doi.org/10.1111/j.1469-8749.1984.tb04434.x
Bishop DV (1990) Handedness, clumsiness and developmental language disorders. Neuropsychologia 28(7):681–690. https://doi.org/10.1016/0028-3932(90)90123-6
Bishop DVM (2005) Handedness and specific language impairment: a study of 6-year-old twins. Dev Psychobiol 46(4):362–369. https://doi.org/10.1002/dev.20062
Bruckner J, Deimann P, Kastner-Koller U (2011a) HAPT 4–6. Handpräferenztest für 4–6-jährige Kinder. Hogrefe, Göttingen
Bruckner J, Kastner-Koller U, Deimann P, Voracek M (2011b) Drawing and handedness of preschoolers: a repeated-measurement approach to hand preference. Percept Mot Skills 112(1):258–266. https://doi.org/10.2466/04.10.PMS.112.1.258-266
Campbell JM, Marcinowski EC, Michel GF (2018) The development of neuromotor skills and hand preference during infancy. Dev Psychobiol 60(2):165–175. https://doi.org/10.1002/dev.21591
Carter-Saltzman L (1980) Biological and sociocultural effects on handedness: comparison between biological and adoptive families. Science 209(4462):1263–1265. https://doi.org/10.1126/science.7403887
Cavallo A, Romeo L, Ansuini C, Podda J, Battaglia F, Veneselli E et al (2018) Prospective motor control obeys to idiosyncratic strategies in autism. Sci Rep 8(1):1–9
Cermak SA, Quintero EJ, Cohen PM (1980) Developmental age trends in crossing the body midline in normal children. Am J Occup Ther 34(5):313–319. https://doi.org/10.5014/ajot.34.5.313
Chen Y, Keen R, Rosander K, von Hofsten C (2010) Task demands affect infants' reaching kinematics. Child Dev 81:1846–1858
Christman SD (2012) Handedness. In: Ramachandran VS (Hg.) Encyclopedia of human behavior. Elsevier Academic Press, Amsterdam, pp 290–296
Cioni G, Sales B, Paolicelli PB, Petacchi E, Scusa MF, Canapicchi R (1999) MRI and clinical characteristics of children with hemiplegic cerebral palsy. Neuropediatrics 30(5):249–255
Coren S (1990) Left-handedness. Behavioural implications and anomalies. Advances in psychology. Elsevier, Burlington
Coren S (1992) The left-hander syndrome. The causes and consequences of left-handedness. Free Press, New York
Crawford J (2013) Childhood brain tumors. Pediatr Rev 34(2):63–78
Dahmen R, Fagard J (2005) The effect of explicit cultural bias on lateral preferences in Tunisia. Cortex 41(6):805–815. https://doi.org/10.1016/s0010-9452(08)70299-5
de Kovel CGF, Francks C (2019) The molecular genetics of hand preference revisited. Sci Rep 9(1):5986. https://doi.org/10.1038/s41598-019-42515-0
de Moura DR, Costa JC, Santos IS, Barros AJD, Matijasevich A, Halpern R et al (2010) Risk factors for suspected developmental delay at age 2 years in a Brazilian birth cohort. Paediatr Perinat Epidemiol 24(3):211–221
DeAgostini M, Khamis AH, Ahui AM, Dellatolas G (1997) Environmental influences in hand preference: an African point of view. Brain Cogn 35(2):151–167. https://doi.org/10.1006/brcg.1997.0935
Dellatolas G, Luciani S, Castresana A, Rémy C, Jallon P, Laplane D, Bancaud J (1993) Pathological left-handedness. Left-handedness correlatives in adult epileptics. Brain 116(Pt 6):1565–1574. https://doi.org/10.1093/brain/116.6.1565
Denny K (2012) Breastfeeding predicts handedness. Laterality 17(3):361–368
Dietrich B (2003) Die Linkshänder in einer rechtsorientierten Gesellschaft: Problembewältigung & Möglichkeiten am Beispiel einer Konzeptentwicklung für eine Linkshänder-Beratungsstelle: diplom. de
Dobel S (2006) Das mach ich mit links. Dobel S (2006). Das mach ich mit links. Artikel vom 13. 08.2006. Stern. https://www.stern.de/panorama/wissen/mensch/linkshaender-das-mach--ich-mit-. In: *Stern*, 13.08.2006. https://www.stern.de/panorama/wissen/mensch/linkshaender-das-mach%2D%2Dich-mit-
Domellöf E, Johansson A-M, Rönnqvist L (2011) Handedness in preterm born children: a systematic review and a meta-analysis. Neuropsychologia 49(9):2299–2310. https://doi.org/10.1016/j.neuropsychologia.2011.04.033
Donnot J, Vauclair J, Bréjard V (2008) Newborn right-holding is related to depressive symptoms in bottle-feeding mothers but not in breastfeeding mothers. Infant Behav Dev 31(3):352–360
Fagard J (2013) The nature and nurture of human infant hand preference. Ann N Y Acad Sci 1288(1):114–123
Fagard J, de Agostini M, Huet V, Granjon L, Heude B (2021) Is handedness at five associated with prenatal factors? Int J Environ Res Public Health 18(7):3529. https://doi.org/10.3390/ijerph18073529
Falek A (1959) Handedness: a family study. Am J Hum Genet 11(1):52
Ferre CL, Babik I, Michel GF (2020) A perspective on the development of hemispheric specialization, infant handedness, and cerebral palsy. Cortex 127:208–220. https://doi.org/10.1016/j.cortex.2020.02.017
Gabbard C, Hart S, Gentry V (1995) A note on trichotomous classification of handedness and fine-motor performance in children. J Genet Psychol 156(1):97–104
Geschwind N, Galaburda AM (1985) Cerebral lateralization. Biological mechanisms, associations, and pathology. II. A hypothesis and a program for research. Arch Neurol 42(6):521–552
Goble DJ, Brown SH (2007) Task-dependent asymmetries in the utilization of proprioceptive feedback for goal-

directed movement. Exp Brain Res 180(4):693–704. https://doi.org/10.1007/s00221-007-0890-7
Goble DJ, Brown SH (2008) Upper limb asymmetries in the matching of proprioceptive versus visual targets. J Neurophysiol 99(6):3063–3074
Goble DJ, Brown SH (2010) Upper limb asymmetries in the perception of proprioceptively determined dynamic position sense. J Exp Psychol Hum Percept Perform 36(3):768–775
Goez H, Zelnik N (2008) Handedness in patients with developmental coordination disorder. J Child Neurol 23(2):151–154. https://doi.org/10.1177/0883073807307978
Goodman R (1994) Childhood hemiplegia: is the side of lesion influenced by a family history of left-handedness? Dev Med Child Neurol 36(5):406–411. https://doi.org/10.1111/j.1469-8749.1994.tb11866.x
Hepper PG, Shahidullah S, White R (1991) Handedness in the human fetus. Neuropsychologia 29(11):1107–1111. https://doi.org/10.1016/0028-3932(91)90080-r
Hepper PG, Wells DL, Lynch C (2005) Prenatal thumb sucking is related to postnatal handedness. Neuropsychologia 43(3):313–315. https://doi.org/10.1016/j.neuropsychologia.2004.08.009
Hill L, Elisabeth, Bishop DVM (1998) A reaching test reveals weak hand preference in specific language impairment and developmental co-ordination disorder. Laterality 3(4):295–310. https://doi.org/10.1080/713754314
Hujoel PP (2019) Breastfeeding and handedness: a systematic review and meta-analysis of individual participant data. Laterality 24(5):582–599. https://doi.org/10.1080/1357650X.2018.1555254
Janßen JP (2000) Foundations of a functional theory of human handedness. Theory Psychol 10(3):375–398. https://doi.org/10.1177/0959354300103004
Janssen L, Meulenbroek RGJ, Steenbergen B (2011) Behavioral evidence for left-hemisphere specialization of motor planning. Exp Brain Res 209(1):65–72
Janzen J, Schlindwein P, Bense S, Bauermann T, Vucurevic G, Stoeter P, Dieterich M (2008) Neural correlates of hemispheric dominance and ipsilaterality within the vestibular system. NeuroImage 42(4):1508–1518. https://doi.org/10.1016/j.neuroimage.2008.06.026
Jones GV, Martin M (2008) Seasonal anisotropy in handedness. Cortex 44(1):8–12
Kim H, Yi S, Son E, Kim J (2001) Evidence for the pathological right-handedness hypothesis. Neuropsychologia 15:510–515
Klissouras V, Geladas N, Koskolou M (2007) Nature prevails over nurture. Int J Sport Psychol 38(1):35–67
Klöppel S, van Eimeren T, Glauche V, Vongerichten A, Münchau A, Frackowiak RSJ et al (2007) The effect of handedness on cortical motor activation during simple bilateral movements. NeuroImage 34(1):274–280
Kong X-Z, Mathias SR, Guadalupe T, ENIGMA Laterality Working Group, Glahn DC, Franke B et al (2018) Mapping cortical brain asymmetry in 17,141 healthy individuals worldwide via the ENIGMA consortium. Proc Natl Acad Sci U S A 115(22):E5154–E5163
Krajenbrink H, Lust J, Wilson P, Steenbergen B (2020) Development of motor planning in children: disentangling elements of the planning process. J Exp Child Psychol 199:104945
Krombholz H (2005) Motorische Entwicklungsstörungen. In: Enzyklopädie der Psychologie 5
Krombholz H (2008) Zusammenhänge zwischen Händigkeit und motorischen und kognitiven Leistungen im Kindesalter. Zeitschrift für Entwicklungspsychologie & Pädagogische Psychologie 40(4):189–199. https://doi.org/10.1026/0049-8637.40.4.189
Kushner HI (2013) Why are there (almost) no left-handers in China? Endeavour 37(2):71–81. https://doi.org/10.1016/j.endeavour.2012.12.003
Kushner HI (2017) On the other hand. Left hand, right brain, mental disorder and history. Johns Hopkins University Press, Baltimore
Kuypers HGJM (1982) A new look at the organization of the motor system. Prog Brain Res 57:381–403
Marcori AJ, Okazaki VHA (2020) A historical, systematic review of handedness origins. Laterality 25(1):87–108. https://doi.org/10.1080/1357650X.2019.1614597
Masud Y, Ajmal MA (2012) Left-handed people in a right-handed world: a phenomenological study. Pak J Social Clin Psychol 10(1):49–60
Mathew J, Sarlegna FR, Bernier P-M, Danion FR (2019) Handedness matters for motor control but not for prediction. Eneuro 6(3)
Mayer S, Schwind V, Schweigert R, Henze N (2018) The effect of offset correction and cursor on mid-air pointing in real and virtual environments. In: Proceedings of the 2018 CHI conference on human factors in computing systems, pp 1–13
McKeever WF (2000) A new family handedness sample with findings consistent with X-linked transmission. Br J Psychol 91(Pt 1):21–39. https://doi.org/10.1348/000712600161655
McManus IC (1985) Handedness, language dominance and aphasia: a genetic model. Psychol Med Monogr Suppl 8:3–40
McManus IC (1991) The inheritance of left-handedness. Ciba Found Symp 162:251–67; discussion 267–81. https://doi.org/10.1002/9780470514160.ch15
McManus IC (2007) The inheritance of left-handedness. In: Ciba Foundation symposium 162-biological asymmetry and handedness: biological asymmetry and handedness: Ciba Foundation symposium 162: Wiley Online Library, pp 251–281
McManus IC, Davison A, Armour JAL (2013) The evolution of human handedness. Ann N Y Acad Sci 1288(1):48
Medland SE, Perelle I, de Monte V, Ehrman L (2004) Effects of culture, sex, and age on the distribution of handedness: an evaluation of the sensitivity of three measures of handedness. Laterality 9(3):287–297. https://doi.org/10.1080/13576500342000040
Medland SE, Duffy DL, Spurdle AB, Wright MJ, Geffen GM, Montgomery GW, Martin NG (2005) Opposite effects of androgen receptor CAG repeat length on

increased risk of left-handedness in males and females. Behav Genet 35(6):735–744. https://doi.org/10.1007/s10519-005-6187-3
Medland SE, Duffy DL, Wright MJ, Geffen GM, Hay DA, Levy F et al (2009) Genetic influences on handedness: data from 25,732 Australian and Dutch twin families. Neuropsychologia 47(2):330–337. https://doi.org/10.1016/j.neuropsychologia.2008.09.005
Merni F, Michele D, Rocco, Soffritti G (2014) Assessment of handedness using latent class factor analysis. Laterality 19(4):405–423. https://doi.org/10.1080/1357650X.2013.845572
Meyer RW (2007) Linkshändig? Ein Ratgeber
Michel GF, Nelson EL, Babik I, Campbell JM, Marcinowski EC (2013) Multiple trajectories in the developmental psychobiology of human handedness. Adv Child Dev Behav 45:227–260
Mori S, Iteya M, Gabbard C (2006) Hand preference consistency and eye-hand coordination in young children during a motor task. Percept Mot Skills 102(1):29–34. https://doi.org/10.2466/pms.102.1.29-34
Neely KA, Mohanty S, Schmitt LM, Wang Z, Sweeney JA, Mosconi MW (2019) Motor memory deficits contribute to motor impairments in autism spectrum disorder. J Autism Dev Disord 49(7):2675–2684
Noterdaeme M, Hutzelmeyer-Nickels A (2010) Early symptoms and recognition of pervasive developmental disorders in Germany. Autism 14(6):575–588
Ocklenburg S, Gunturkun O (2017) The lateralized brain. The neuroscience and evolution of hemispheric asymmetries. Elsevier Science, San Diego
Ocklenburg S, Beste C, Arning L (2014) Handedness genetics: considering the phenotype. Front Psychol 5(9):221. https://doi.org/10.3389/fpsyg.2014.01300
Papadatou-Pastou M, Martin M, Mohr C (2017) Salivary testosterone levels are unrelated to handedness or cerebral lateralization for language. Laterality 22(2):123–156. https://doi.org/10.1080/1357650X.2016.1149485
Paracchini S (2021) Recent advances in handedness genetics. Symmetry 13(10):1792
Parma V, Brasselet R, Zoia S, Bulgheroni M, Castiello U (2017) The origin of human handedness and its role in pre-birth motor control. Sci Rep 7(1):1–9
Perlmutter JS, Powers WJ, Herscovitch P, Fox PT, Raichle ME (1987) Regional asymmetries of cerebral blood flow, blood volume, and oxygen utilization and extraction in normal subjects. J Child Neurol 7(1):64–67. https://doi.org/10.1038/jcbfm.1987.9
Pfannkuche KA, Bouma A, Groothuis TGG (2009) Does testosterone affect lateralization of brain and behaviour? A meta-analysis in humans and other animal species. Phil Trans R Soc B 364(1519):929–942. https://doi.org/10.1098/rstb.2008.0282
Porac C (1996) Attempts to switch the writing hand: relationships to age and side of hand preference. Laterality 1(1):35–44. https://doi.org/10.1080/713754205
Porac C (2016) Laterality. Exploring the enigma of left-handedness. Elsevier Science, Amsterdam. http://www.sciencedirect.com/science/book/9780128012390
Previc FH (1991) A general theory concerning the prenatal origins of cerebral lateralization in humans. Psychol Rev 98(3):299–334. https://doi.org/10.1037/0033-295X.98.3.299
Previc FH (1996) Nonright-handedness, central nervous system and related pathology, and its lateralization: a reformulation and synthesis. Dev Neuropsychol 12(4):443–515. https://doi.org/10.1080/87565649609540663
Ramadhani MK, Koomen I, Grobbee DE, van Donselaar CA, van Marceline Furth A, Uiterwaal CSPM (2006) Increased occurrence of left-handedness after severe childhood bacterial meningitis: support for the pathological left-handedness hypothesis. Neuropsychologia 44(12):2526–2532. https://doi.org/10.1016/j.neuropsychologia.2006.03.026
Rathelot J-A, Strick PL (2006) Muscle representation in the macaque motor cortex: an anatomical perspective. Proc Natl Acad Sci U S A 103(21):8257–8262
Rodgers RA, Travers BG, Mason AH (2019) Bimanual reach to grasp movements in youth with and without autism spectrum disorder. Front Psychol 9:2720
Rodriguez A, Waldenström U (2008) Fetal origins of child non-right-handedness and mental health. J Child Psychol Psychiatry 49(9):967–976. https://doi.org/10.1111/j.1469-7610.2008.01923.x
Rosenbaum DA, Chapman KM, Weigelt M, Weiss DJ, van der Wel R (2012) Cognition, action, and object manipulation. Psychol Bull 138(5):924
Ross G, Lipper EG, Am Auld P (1987) Hand preference of four-year-old children: its relationship to premature birth and neurodevelopmental outcome. Dev Med Child Neurol 29(5):615–622
Ross G, Lipper E, Auld PAM (1992) Hand preference, prematurity and developmental outcome a school age. Neuropsychologia 30(5):483–494
Rostoft MS, Sigmundsson H, Whiting HTA, Ingvaldsen RP (2002) Dynamics of hand preference in 4 year-old children. Behav Brain Res 132(1):59–68. https://doi.org/10.1016/s0166-4328(01)00415-6
Saigal S, Rosenbaum P, Szatmari P, Hoult L (1992) Non-right handedness among ELBW and term children eight years in relation to cognitive function and school performance, pp 425–433
Sattler JB (2000a) Der umgeschulte Linkshänder oder Der Knoten im Gehirn [The switched left-hander or the knot in the brain]
Sattler JB (2000b) Links & Rechts in der Wahrnehmung des Menschen. In: Zur Geschichte der Linkshändigkeit. Auer, Donauwörth
Sattler JB, Klußmann A (2014) Leitlinie Händigkeit. - Bedeutung & Untersuchung /. 002/017 - S1. Unter Mitarbeit von DGAUM. AWMF, zuletzt aktualisiert am 06.2020
Satz P (1972) Pathological left-handedness. An explanatory model. [Place of publication not identified]: Distributed by ERIC Clearinghouse
Satz P, Orsini DL, Saslow E, Henry R (1985) The pathological left-handedness syndrome. Brain Cogn 4(1):27–46

Saunders JA, Knill DC (2004) Visual feedback control of hand movements. J Neurosci 24(13):3223–3234

Schaafsma SM, Riedstra BJ, Pfannkuche KA, Bouma A, Groothuis TGG (2009) Epigenesis of behavioural lateralization in humans and other animals. Philos Trans R Soc B 364(1519):915–927. https://doi.org/10.1098/rstb.2008.0244

Schmidt L, Artinger F, Stumpf O, Kerkhoff G (2013) Differential effects of galvanic vestibular stimulation on arm position sense in right- vs. left-handers. Neuropsychologia 51(5):893–899. https://doi.org/10.1016/j.neuropsychologia.2013.02.013

Schuhmacher RE, Barks JDE, Johnston MV, Down SM, Roloff DW, Barlett RH (1988) Right-sided brain lesions in infants following extracorporeal membrane oxygenation. Pediatrics 82:155–161

Sicotte NL, Woods RP, Mazziotta JC (1999) Handedness in twins: a meta-analysis. Laterality 4(3):265–286. https://doi.org/10.1080/713754339

Siebner HR, Limmer C, Peinemann A, Drzezga A, Bloem BR, Schwaiger M, Conrad B (2002) Long-term consequences of switching handedness: a positron emission tomography study on handwriting in "converted" left-handers. J Neurosci 22(7):2816–2825

Soper HV, Satz P (1984) Pathological left-handedness and ambiguous handedness: a new explanatory model. Neuropsychologia 22(4):511–515. https://doi.org/10.1016/0028-3932(84)90046-0

Stilwell JM (1987) The development of manual midline crossing in 2- to 6-year-old children. Am J Occup Ther 41(12):783–789. https://doi.org/10.5014/ajot.41.12.783

Suitner C, Maass A, Bettinsoli ML, Carraro L, Kumar S (2017) Left-handers' struggle in a rightward wor (l) d: the relation between horizontal spatial bias and effort in directed movements. Laterality 22(1):60–89

Tan LE, Nettleton NC (1980) Left handedness, birth order and birth stress. Cortex 16(3):363–373. https://doi.org/10.1016/s0010-9452(80)80038-4

Todd BK, Banerjee R (2016) Lateralization of infant holding by mothers: a longitudinal evaluation of variations over the first 12 weeks. Laterality 21(1):12–33. https://doi.org/10.1080/1357650X.2015.1059434

Uvebrant P (1988) Hemiplegic cerebral palsy. Aetiology and outcome. Acta Paediatr Scand Suppl 345:1–100. https://doi.org/10.1111/j.1651-2227.1988.tb14939.x

van Heerwaarde AA, van der Kamp LT, van der Aa NE, de Vries LS, Groenendaal F, Jongmans MJ, Dudink J (2020) Non-right-handedness in children born extremely preterm: Relation to early neuroimaging and long-term neurodevelopment. Plos one 15(7):e0235311

Vasileva F, Georgiev G (2017) The heredity of motor engrams in volleyball. Res Phys Educ Sport Health 6(1):57–60

Ververs IA, de Vries JI, van Geijn HP, Hopkins B (1994) Prenatal head position from 12-38 weeks. I. Developmental aspects. Early Human Dev 39(2):83–91. https://doi.org/10.1016/0378-3782(94)90157-0

Vuoksimaa E, Eriksson CJP, Pulkkinen L, Rose RJ, Kaprio J (2010) Decreased prevalence of left-handedness among females with male co-twins: evidence suggesting prenatal testosterone transfer in humans? Psychoneuroendocrinology 35(10):1462–1472. https://doi.org/10.1016/j.psyneuen.2010.04.013

Williams J, Lee KJ, Anderson PJ (2010) Prevalence of motor-skill impairment in preterm children who do not develop cerebral palsy: a systematic review. Dev Med Child Neurol 52(3):232–237. https://doi.org/10.1111/j.1469-8749.2009.03544.x

Witelson SF, Nowakowski RS (1991) Left out axons make men right: a hypothesis for the origin of handedness and functional asymmetry. Neuropsychologia 29(4):327–333. https://doi.org/10.1016/0028-3932(91)90046-b

World Health Organisation (2016) ICD-10 Version. International Statistical Classification of Diseases and Related Health Problems 10th Revision. WHO. https://icd.who.int/browse10/2016/en

Zaghloul MS, Saquib J, Al-Mazrou AR, Saquib N (2018) A qualitative assessment of the impact of handedness among left-handed surgeons in Saudi Arabia. Laterality 23(1):39–50

Left Handedness

4

Contents

Left-handers with inconsistent hand preference write with the left, tap faster with the left, and perform better with the left on the Purdue Pegboard task ... but are stronger in the right hand and throw better with the right hand. In the other two groups, strength and skill activities are laterally congruent. This poses difficulties for theories of handedness. (Peters 1990)

4.1 Introduction

Until the 1970s, it was widely believed that *Left Handedness* was a risk factor for specific neurological conditions and abnormalities (Porac 2016). Over the last decades, research findings have found mixed results. Currently, there is a broad consensus in the literature that ordinary or *familial* (hereditary based) *Left Handedness* does not entail any disadvantage or problems and constitutes a normal variant of handedness (e.g. Kilshaw and Annett 1983; Annett 2004). In contrast, research on *pathological Left Handedness* has documented a range of problems and disorders probably associated with it, based on the research of Satz (Satz 1972; Satz et al. 1985; Soper and Satz 1984). However, large surveys of the general population, such as those using self-reported hand preference, are likely to incorporate familial and pathological left handers in a single group of left handers since researchers often do not differentiate between them. Similarly, the group of right handers are most likely to include *switched* left handers, particularly if writing is one of the measures assessing handedness. In particular, the lack of distinction between familial and *pathological Left Handedness* might also explain why researchers continue to explore associations between *Left Handedness* and medical conditions, problems or abnormalities and often yield contradictory find-

E. Kraus, *Beyond Left and Right Handedness*, https://doi.org/10.1007/978-3-031-24389-9_4

ings to support such correlations. Nevertheless, there is a widely accepted consensus in the literature that left handers are not just the mirror image of right handers.

In this chapter, we explore familial *Left Handedness*, particularly by comparing left handers to right handers, to understand and discuss their differences. I then expand on the discussion of the previous chapter on pathological handedness by focusing on pathological left handers and research investigating the association between *Left Handedness* and medical conditions or disorders. The third part of this chapter deals with research and case studies of converted left handers who have learnt to write with their non-dominant right hand, influenced by the right-biassed physical and sociocultural environments. Finally, based on the literature, my own research and clinical experience, I propose several subgroups of *Left Handedness* and show how these differ from similar subgroups of right handers. Such differentiation is particularly important for practitioners to understand variable hand use.

4.2 Familial *Left Handedness*

The term *familial Left Handedness* has been derived from looking at the so-called familial sinistrality[1], based on the number of left handers in the close and wider family (McKeever and VanDeventer 1977; Satz 1972; Annett 2002). A repeatedly found correlation between left handers and their left-handed family members has been a basis for differentiating "natural" *Left Handedness* as an inherited trait, from pathological handers (Satz 1972). In this book, familial *Left Handedness* is used synonymously with hereditary, naturally occurring *Left Handedness*.

Even though researchers have repeatedly recommended that studies need to differentiate between familial and *pathological Left Handedness* (e.g. Annett 2004 and Satz 1972), many studies do not make such distinctions. Neither do they differentiate between right handers and switched left handers (both classified as right handers). Therefore, there is an inherent flaw in the comparison between left and right handers, which is typically perpetuated in many studies on *Left Handedness*.

This is a constraint affecting almost all handedness research, including this book. Despite these limitations, the general insights on *Left* and *Right Handedness* form a valuable basis for better understanding handedness as a phenomenon.

In particular, several questions arise when we take a practice-based approach to *Left Handedness*. Are there specific *Left-Handedness* features, and if yes, what are they? How do left handers differ from right handers? And what do we need to know about different groups on *Left Handedness*? In this section, we will examine familial *Left Handedness*, particularly by comparing it to (familial) *Right Handedness*.

4.3 Typical Differences Between Left Handers and Right Handers

The difficulties left-handed individuals experience in living in a right-handed world have been addressed by Porac and colleagues who surveyed left handers of all ages (Porac et al. 1998; Porac 2016). Subjects were asked to rate their perceived difficulty adapting to the right-biassed environment on a scale from *1 (very easy)* to *4 (very difficult)*. The authors found unexpectedly that most left handers rated their environmental adaptability at *2—easy*. They proposed that this finding might be related to the greater acceptance of left handers today, and the easy accessibility of left hander items (Porac 2016).

There is a wide variety of research on specific traits of left handers, most often focusing on familial *Left Handedness*. However, these are often clouded with over-simplistic and unsubstantiated statements on *Left Handedness*, particularly regarding social and psychological traits, making them prone to stereotypes and unfounded assumptions. Against this background, Table 4.1 summarises typical differences

[1] In this book, the term sinsitrality referring to *Left Handedness* will not be used because of its negative connotation.

Table 4.1 Comparing typical traits between left and right handers

	Left handers	Right handers
Preference	Left handers usually use the non-dominant right hand more often than right handers (Annett 2004; Bryden et al. 2007; Peters 1996)	Right handers use the non-dominant left hand less often than left handers (Annett 2004; Bryden et al. 2007; Peters 1996)
Proficiency	Left handers show small difference in proficiency between the hands, as the non-dominant right hand is often above average in performance (Bryden et al. 2007)	Right handers show larger differences in proficiency between the hands, as the non-dominant left hand is usually average in performance (Bryden et al. 2007)
Development	Left handers tend to develop handedness later, presumably in part because of their adaptation to the right-biassed environment (McManus et al. 1988; Scharoun and Bryden 2014)	Right-handed people often develop their handedness at an early age, presumably supported by the right-biassed environment (McManus et al. 1988; Scharoun and Bryden 2014)
Classification	Left handers are more heterogenous and can be divided into distinct subgroups (Peters 1990)	Right-handed people are a much more homogeneous group, and such subgroups are not always clearly delineated (Peters 1990)
Movement patterns	Mildly established left-handed people often perform gross motor activities with their right hand (Bryden et al. 2007)	Right-handed people perform most gross and fine motor activities with their right hand (Bryden et al. 2007)
Brain activity	The hemispheres are often less lateralised than those of right-handed people (Szaflarski et al. 2002)	The hemispheres are usually more clearly lateralised in right handers (Szaflarski et al. 2002)
	When left handers use their right hand, there is less left hemisphere activation overall in right handers (Klöppel et al. 2007a)	When right-handed people use their left hand, there is generally more activation of the right hemisphere in left handers (Klöppel et al. 2007a)
Functional brain asymmetry	Left handers' brain asymmetry and hemispheric lateralisation processes tend to be less strong and display a higher variability (Budisavljevic et al. 2021; Szaflarski et al. 2002, 2012)	Right handers generally show a stronger brain asymmetry and stronger hemispheric lateralisation processes (Budisavljevic et al. 2021; Szaflarski et al. 2002, 2012)
Direction of visual tracking and drawing	Visual tracking and drawing tend to be from right to left in left handers (Casasanto and Henetz 2012; Scheirs 1990)	Visual tracking and drawing tend to be left to right in right handers (Casasanto and Henetz 2012; Scheirs 1990)
Motor proficiency	An fMRI study found that left handers showed superior performance in simple tapping tasks with their dominant hand, but in more complex tasks, the inter-hand difference decreased (Verstynen et al. 2005)	An fMRI study found that right handers tap better and faster with their dominant hand in simple and complex tasks. The difference increased with task complexity (Verstynen et al. 2005)
	Inter-hand difference in motor performance tasks is smaller in left handers compared to right handers (for a review, see Tzourio-Mazoyer et al. 2015)	Inter-hand difference in motor performance tasks is larger in right handers compared to left handers (for a review, see Tzourio-Mazoyer et al. 2015)
Bimanual role-differentiated movement (RDBM)	When analysing RDBM data, only relatively few left handers showed a clear left-handed preference in bimanual tasks or movement, suggesting that RDBM is expressed differently in left handers (Gonzalez and Nelson 2021)	Right handers show a clear right-handed preference with a leading right hand during RDBM tasks (Gonzalez and Nelson 2021)

(continued)

Table 4.1 (continued)

	Left handers	Right handers
Spatial abilities	Investigating mental rotation of the hands, five-handedness groups all performed similarly on the left hand stimuli, whilst they were clear differences across the groups for right-hand stimuli. Mixed handers performed more accurately with left-hand stimuli, whilst mixed left handers tended to be more accurate with right-hand stimuli. They also recommend that spatial abilities should be investigated in relation to handedness in future research (Cheng et al. 2020)	Extreme right handers performed better than extreme left handers in general in mental rotation of the hands. The authors conclude that potential cognitive mechanisms might be associated with specific handedness groups (Cheng et al. 2020)
	A spatial bias was investigated in graphomotor tasks. No left placing bias was found in left handers (Faghihi et al. 2019)	A left-placing bias was found in right handers in a graphomotor task (Faghihi et al. 2019)
Language	78% of left handers have language lateralised in the left hemisphere, 15% show little or no lateralisation and 7% are lateralised in the right hemisphere (see Bruckert et al. 2021 for review)	In right handers, language is typically lateralised in the left hemisphere in 90% of right handers, and 10% show little lateralisation (see Bruckert et al. 2021 for review)
Intelligence, sport, music, creativity	Left handers perform better in particular (aspects of) IQ tests than right handers (Jeyalyn and Rajasankar 2016)	Right handers perform worse than left handers in those specific aspects of IQ tests (Jeyalyn and Rajasankar 2016)
Sport and music	There is a significantly higher incidence of left handers in interactive sports, athletics and boxing than in the normal population. Some examples are an elevated number of left handers in ball sports (Jeyalyn and Rajasankar 2016), and left handers show an advantage in sports activities in general (Grouios et al. 2000, 2002)	The incidence of right handers in interactive sports is somewhat lower than in the general population (Grouios et al. 2000, 2002)
Music and art	The ability to compose or improvise and general musical talent were enhanced in left-handed boys (Grouios et al. 2000, 2002). There is also an increased *Left Handedness* among creative artists and architects as compared to the typical population (Preti and Vellante 2007), as well as among architects (Peterson and Lansky 1977)	There was no evidence of general musical talent being enhanced in right-handed boys (Grouios et al. 2000, 2002), or of increased *Right Handedness* among creative artists (Preti and Vellante 2007), as well as among architects (Peterson and Lansky 1977)

between left and right handers with reference to examples from the literature (despite its inherent shortcomings) that may be relevant to a practice-based approach to handedness.

What transpires from these findings, and what has been well documented generally, is that left handers show a **greater variability** of hand use across several handedness dimensions, both neurologically and behaviourally (Bryden 2016; Fagard 2013; Hatta 2007; Hammond 2002). In other words, left handers use their non-dominant right hand much more often and more proficiently than right handers use their non-dominant left hand (Annett 2004; Bryden et al. 2007; Peters 1996). Consequently, differences between the hands (⧫**inter-hand differences (IHDs)**) in both preference and performance in left handers are usually smaller compared to right handers (Bryden et al. 2007).

4.4 *Pathological Left Handedness*

We now turn to the so-called *pathological Left Handedness*, introduced, defined and discussed in Chap. 3 (Sect. 3.5). Pathological left handers are very different to ordinary or familial left handers, who had no early traumatic impact responsible for changing the direction of handedness. However, there is no clear definition of pathological handedness. Some state that only a significant damage to the brain can cause pathological handedness (Annett 1985; McManus and Bryden 1992; Satz et al. 1985; McKeever and VanDeventer 1977; Hécaen and Sauguet 1971). Accordingly, the number of pathological left-handed individuals is relatively small, even though some argue that even minimal damage before, during or after birth can cause *pathological Left Handedness*, increasing its occurrence (Coren 1992).

In clinical practice, very strong manual asymmetries in infancy can be observed. Whilst this may indicate a strong handedness degree, coupled with poor motor control and motor deficits on the other side, it may well be an indicator of pathological handedness. Similar findings have been documented in the literature: the combination of significantly weaker proficiency of the non-preferred (but presumably inherently dominant) hand could be an indicator for early brain damage, leading to either pathological left and right handers (Bishop 1984; Gilbert and Wysocki 1992).

4.4.1 Research on *Pathological Left Handedness* and Disorders

Many studies have associated *Left Handedness* with various disorders. This research is deemed important since a disorder-specific approach to handedness helps to understand the neurobiological mechanisms that underpin the relationship between handedness and disorders (Nastou et al. 2022). According to Nastou and colleagues, these studies can identify handedness as a factor related to specific disorders and reveal conditions where disorders are not associated with *Left Handedness*. Overall, some studies have found evidence for an association between *Left Handedness* and disorders, many more have generated contradictory findings and others have found *Left Handedness* to be a protective factor regarding some conditions. Some of these studies are briefly summarised here. See also Sect. 3.5.

Support for a Correlation Between *Left Handedness* and Conditions

- *Migraine, immune disease and developmental learning disorder*: Geschwind and Bejan found that *Left Handedness* was associated with migraine, immune disease and developmental learning disorder (Geschwind and Behan 1982).

Contradictory and Inconclusive Results

- *Developmental Coordination Disorder (DCD)*: Goez and Zelnik investigated 98 children with DCD and discovered more left handers among them compared to the general population (Goez and Zelnik 2008), as did other authors (Freitas et al. 2014). This finding was confirmed in a systematic review of 36 studies with over 1000 participants. Darvik and colleagues concluded that *Left Handedness* could be seen as a general trait of individuals with DCD (Darvik et al. 2018). Other studies did not find increased levels of *Left Handedness* in children with DCD (e.g. Armitage and Larkin 1993).
- *Attention Deficit Hyperactivity Disorder (ADHD)*: Some found a stronger association between ADHD and *Left Handedness* (Niederhofer 2005), whilst others did not (Biederman et al. 1995; Ghanizadeh 2013).
- *Schizophrenia*: Dragovic and Hammond found that strong *Left Handedness* and mixed handedness were associated with schizophrenia (Dragovic and Hammond 2005). In contrast, Dutton and colleagues followed a similar research question finding a distinct negative correlation and *Left-Handedness* incidence. They concluded that both left handers and schizophrenia might be associated with elevated androgen levels (Dutton et al. 2020).

***Left Handedness* as a Protective Factor**

- *Glioma*: In a large case-control study, Miller and colleagues investigated 1849 people with glioma, a primary malignant brain tumour, and compared them to 1354 healthy individuals in a prospective cohort study. They found an inverse relationship between glioma risk and *Left Handedness*, with left handers being 35% less likely to develop glioma (Miller et al. 2018).

The majority of studies seem to remain inconclusive or contradictory. Once again, some of this disparity can be assigned to the poor comparability across studies due to inconsistent definitions and measures. But more importantly, the lack of differentiating between different groups of *Left Handedness* such as familial *Left Handedness* with various degrees, *converted Left Handedness*, *Left Handedness* coexisting with motor disorders, other conditions or *pathological Left Handedness* will inevitably lead to a concoction of left handers with very different attributes and characteristics. It is thus important to define clear subgroups of *Left Handedness*, which will be proposed at the end of the chapter.

4.5 Converted Left Handers

We now turn to the group of left handers who, due to sociocultural pressures inherent in a right-biassed world, learned to write with their right hand (see Chap. 3, Sect. 3.4.2). In this section, we discuss these *converted left handers* who are influenced to perform specific tasks with their right hand, particularly the highly complex activity of handwriting. In addition, the phenomena of *switching repercussions* and *Left-Handedness reversion* (where converted left handers return to writing with their dominant left hand) are discussed.

4.5.1 Influencing Factors on Handedness Conversion

Switched or ♦**converted handedness**[2] typically refers to left-handed persons who have been trained (switched) to their right hand for **writing**[3] because of influences from the physical and sociocultural environments (see Sect. 3.4.2 for details). When this occurs, there is thought to be a conflict between intrinsic preference and external demands that have been shown to result in reduced asymmetrical manual behaviour, which in turn impacts brain activation (Hatta 2007). Furthermore, it has been proposed that handedness conversion may even *cause* neural asymmetries in the brain anatomy. Such asymmetries may indeed develop over the life span since a relationship was found between asymmetries and age (Marcori and Okazaki 2020).

Handwriting with the Non-dominant Hand as the Key Indicator

Since the activity of writing is central to switching handedness, let us look more closely at this process before exploring converted handedness in more detail. Writing is not only an important, if not an essential part of human culture but also a highly complex movement process requiring a remarkably fine-tuned collaboration between the nervous system and the hand and arm muscles. Investigating writing in converted handers is very interesting for handedness research, since writing can be re-learned with the non-dominant hand.

> *If one considers the multitude of components [sic] that the brain uses in planning and execution of the simplest motoric processes, it is astonishing how the comparatively complex process of writing, which involves many centres of the brain [sic], is not only performed but can also be re-learned by the other hand. On this basis, it is understandable why the hand, compared to other parts of the body, is represented by a disproportionate area in the motor cortex.* (Kienle 2011: 7)

Degrees of Handedness

Converted left handers may or may not perform other activities with the right hand, depending on their handedness degree. Incidentally, there are

[2]These terms will be used interchangeably, whereby switching refers mostly to the act of conversion and converted handedness mainly to the state thereof.

[3]In the context of this book and its clinical focus, converted handedness is defined by the act of writing with the non-dominant hand.

also *converted right handers*, who have learnt to write and/or perform other complex activities with their non-dominant left hand. However, this is rare since it requires a concerted effort and motivation to write with the left hand in a right-biassed environment.

Zaghloul and colleagues showed that converted right handers usually switch because of specific interest or in the context of their professional work, taking place mostly in adulthood, such as working with a left-handed surgeon (Zaghloul et al. 2018). In contrast, converted left handers usually switch their writing hand because of externally motivated reasons such as sociocultural factors (e.g. Porac 1996; Porac and Lee Berdel Martin 2007; Sattler 2000). These findings were confirmed more recently by a literature review. Marcori and Okzaki found that converted right handers explained their switching as an experiment with their non-dominant left hand (Marcori and Okazaki 2020).

DeAgostini and colleagues suggest that cultural and environmental factors can alter the inherent ♦**hand dominance** in three ways (DeAgostini et al. 1997). I interpret these categories to correspond with various degrees of handedness.

1. *Switching does not reduce the degree of handedness*: The right non-dominant hand is used *only for writing*, and the dominant left hand continues to be used as the preferred and more proficient hand for other activities. These are likely to be individuals with a *strong degree* of *Left Handedness*.
2. *Switching reduces the degree of handedness*: The right non-dominant hand is used for writing. In addition, other activities are also performed increasingly with the non-dominant right hand. These are likely to be individuals with a *moderate degree* of *Left Handedness*.
3. *Switching results in an overall change in degree and direction*: The right non-dominant hand is used for writing and for many or even most other activities, thereby resembling a right hander. These are likely to be individuals with a *mild degree* of *Left Handedness*.

Some authors have referred to the "successful switching" of a left-handed person as someone who continues to write with the non-dominant right hand. This may occur with or without switching the left hand for other activities (Porac and Buller 1990). For example, Coren estimated that approximately one in ten people will convert their handedness in their lifetime, based on a study looking at "successful" conversions/switching (Coren 1994). He found that 41% of switched left handers continued to write with the right hand, and only 7% of switched right handers continued to write with their left hand (ibid). Similarly, Marcori and colleagues could show that 35% of the switched left handers were "successful" compared to 4% of converted right handers. However, both groups continued to perform several activities with the dominant hand (Marcori et al. 2019). In particular, the authors found a ceiling effect for the capacity to change handedness degree and direction since the reviewed studies did not report complete shifts in behavioural measures (ibid).

Searleman and Porac indeed found that mild-degree left handers were likely to be more "successfully" switched, as they subsequently wrote only with their right hand (Searleman and Porac 2003). In addition to the *degree* of handedness being an influencing factor for "successful" conversion, *lateralised practice* and automation may be other factors playing a significant role in consolidating behavioural and neural asymmetries (Marcori et al. 2019).

However, these studies on switching "success" do not focus on possible ♦**switching repercussions** (see Sect. 4.5.3) or side effects that may result from a conversion, such as motor deficiencies, difficulties in recalling memory or concentration problems, as shown below. If switching repercussions do occur in a converted left hander, it seems paradoxical to refer to this as "successful". Moreover, the relationship between degrees of handedness and possible switching repercussions needs to be researched specifically.

4.5.2 Comparing Converted Left Handers to Non-converted Left Handers

To distinguish the associations made in the literature between *Left Handedness* and specific problems from those related to switching repercussions, I have summarised some of these findings in Table 4.2.

Overall, there appears to be evidence of converted handers encountering more problems than non-converted left handers. In contrast, many of the difficulties non-converted left handers experience seem to be particularly related to the adaptation to a right-biassed environment.

4.5.3 Potential Switching Repercussions

Converting handedness by learning to write with the non-dominant hand has been described as a

Table 4.2 Summary of switching repercussions/symptoms assigned to converted left handers and left handers

Category	Switching repercussion/ symptoms	Evidence of switching repercussions in converted left handers (author(s), year)	Evidence of symptoms in non-converted left handers (author(s), year)
Neural aspects	Neuronal reorganisation	Klöppel et al. (2007b)	
Physical and perception-based aspects	Slowness in writing	Kushner (2017); Steinkopf (2014); Randolph (2007)	Malkhaz et al. (2020); Semenovich (2009)
	Left-right confusion, reversals	Sattler (2000); Soper and Satz (1984); Ansuini et al. (2018); Hildreth (1949); Steinkopf (2014); Randolph (2007)	Malkhaz et al. (2020)
	Difficulty with mental rotation tasks	Cheng et al. (2020)	Malkhaz et al. (2020)
	Disorientation in space	Kushner (2017)	Malkhaz et al. (2020)
	Prone to accidents and injuries	Daniel and Yeo (1991); Hemenway et al. (1994)	Daniel and Yeo (1991)
	Impact on physical well-being	Porac and Searlman (2002); Masud and Ajmal (2012); Denny and O'Sullivan (2007); Sovák (1968)	
	Poor motor coordination	Porac and Searlman (2002); Randolph (2007); Grabowska et al. (2012); Cairney et al. (2008)	Semenovich (2009); Cairney et al. (2008)
Somato-visceral aspects	Bedwetting	Kushner (2017) Sattler (2000)	Malkhaz et al. (2020)
	Nail biting	Kushner (2017)	
	Psychosomatic symptoms	Sattler (2000); Sattler and Klußmann (2014); Sattler (2011)	
Cognition and language	Stuttering	Kushner (2017); Orton and Travis (1929); Foundas et al. (2004); Sattler (2000); Steinkopf (2014); Randolph (2007); Kushner (2012)	Malkhaz et al. (2020); Geschwind and Behan (1982); Dellatolas et al. (1990)
	Memory deficits	Sattler (2000); Steinkopf (2014); Randolph (2007)	Malkhaz et al. (2020); Nikolaeva (2005); Semenovich (2009)
	Slowness in writing	Kushner (2017); Sattler (2000); Steinkopf (2014); Randolph (2007); Grabowska et al. (2012)	Semenovich (2009); Nikolaeva (2005)
	Learning disorders, dyslexia, dysgraphia	Foundas et al. (2004); Johnson and Duke (1935); Sattler (2000); Sovák (1962); Sovak (1974); Porac and Searlman (2002); Sarma (1989); Kotetisvili et al. (2005); Steinkopf (2014); Randolph (2007); Kushner (2012)	Nikolaeva (2005); Semenovich (2009); Cairney et al. (2008)
	Concentration disorders	Hawkyard et al. (2014); Siengthai et al. (2008); Lin and Tsuang (2018)	

Table 4.2 (continued)

Category	Switching repercussion/ symptoms	Evidence of switching repercussions in converted left handers (author(s), year)	Evidence of symptoms in non-converted left handers (author(s), year)
Socio-emotional/ affective	Incidence of fears, anxiety disorders	Malkhaz et al. (2020); Kushner (2017)	
	Prone to psychiatric disorders in general	Sattler (2000); Steinkopf (2014); Randolph (2007)	
	Low frustration tolerance	Sattler and Klußmann (2014)	

significant intrusion into the human brain, as neuroimaging research has confirmed (Sattler 1999; Sattler and Klußmann 2014; Klöppel et al. 2007b; Grabowska et al. 2012; Siebner et al. 2002). Irrespective of the neuro-anatomical and physiological basis, there appears to be behavioural evidence that converting handedness is associated with problems.

Types of Switching Repercussions

Negative consequences of handedness conversion were already documented around the turn of the last century, leading to a much greater acceptance of *Left Handedness* in countries such as the USA, Canada or Australia. In these countries, switching handedness has generally been discouraged from the 1940s onward (Porac and Lee Berdel Martin 2007; Porac 2016). Orton and Travis published a series of articles and books in the late 1920s describing switching repercussions in detail. They demonstrated that half of patients who stuttered were converted left handers. In some historical studies, stuttering stopped when these individuals returned to writing with their left hand (Orton and Travis 1929; Travis 1934). The authors argued that handedness and language are closely related in their hemispheric specialisation processes, concluding that a change in handedness direction could thus result in speech and reading disorders (ibid.).

Some of the current literature on switched left handers focuses more on the nature of sociocultural pressures exerted on left handers, particularly concerning writing with the right hand (see (Porac and Buller 1990). In addition, there is evidence for some typical switching repercussions summarised below:

- *Stuttering* (Orton and Travis 1929; Travis 1934)
- *Learning difficulties* (Rett et al. 1973)
- *Dyslexia and dysgraphia* (Sovák 1962; Sovak 1974)
- *Poor learning* skills/learning difficulties (Sarma 1989; Porac and Searlman 2002)
- *Poor motor coordination* (Porac and Searlman 2002)

In addition, Porac and Searleman found that switched left handers experience *lower physical and psychological well-being* levels than left- and right-handed people. However, the authors relate this finding primarily to the "unsuccessful" switching outcome and speculate that left handers rate themselves lower because they have failed to write with their right hand and, by implication, to adapt to the right-handed environment (Porac and Searleman 2002). Conversely, Sattler deduces that the diminished quality of life often expressed by switched left handers is due to the repercussions of the handedness conversion. These include *low frustration tolerance*, *psychosomatic symptoms* and *aggressive behaviour* (Sattler 2000; Sattler and Klußmann 2014).

Practitioners have also documented observations about switching repercussions within an occupational therapy context. Steinkopf, an experienced teacher specialising in *Left-Handedness* consultations, identifies eight clusters of difficulties: *concentration problems, left-right confusion, blackouts and memory problems, learning disabilities, handwriting production, handwriting legibility, slow physical and mental processing, and language deficits such as stammering* and *word-finding problems* (Steinkopf 2014).

Individual Case Studies on Switching Repercussions

In addition to the cited switching repercussions, individual case studies show that these repercussions appear to have deeper dimensions. For example, Samuel Randolph, a switched left hander, has written his personal account of reverting to his dominant left hand (Randolph 2007). He had always thought of himself as a right hander, until he discovered that he was actually a left hander at the age of 41. He experienced and documented many of the typical conversion repercussions. This is what he writes about his childhood:

> *The growing inner sense of loneliness, humiliation, frustration and hopelessness I felt as I struggled in school are very difficult to convey accurately...Along with the increasing frustration I felt as I fought to overcome submergee [converted hander] deficits came a nagging inner sense that I was deeply flawed. The seeds that would eventually sprout and grow into an ongoing battle with depression began to take root within me.* (Randolph 2007) *(square brackets my inserts).*

Several other individuals have documented similar experiences (e.g. Neumann (2014); Sattler (2000); Kramer (1970); Krombholz (2008)), indicating that reversion processes seem to be linked to complex personality traits and socio-emotional well-being.

Apart from accounts within the general population, specific findings have also been made when looking at individuals with psychiatric disorders. Henninger documented a case with multiple personalities where one was left handed and the other right handed. She concluded that such so-called conditional handedness could be seen as a handedness subtype linked to specific personality characteristics (Henninger 1992). Shimizu and colleagues looked at associations between converted handedness and schizophrenia (Shimizu et al. 1985). Hand preference was assessed in 1774 schizophrenic inpatients, and information on the handed conversion and prevalence of *Left Handedness* was obtained, and data were contrasted to a comparatively large group of normal subjects. Whilst no significant difference was found between the prevalence of left/mixed handedness[4] between the groups, the rate of converted right handers with schizophrenia was higher (ibid.).

Overall, there is a lack of research focusing more specifically on switching repercussions of converted left handers regarding their coping mechanisms and perceptions, degrees of handedness and psychiatric conditions. Furthermore, some authors have argued that converted left handers are likely to be classified in studies as right handers or mixed handers. This may be part of the reason why there are often contradictory and inconsistent findings (Perelle and Ehrman 2005; Vuoksimaa et al. 2009).

Summarising Switching Repercussions for a Practice-Based Approach

In my clinical experience and observations when working with children with switched handedness, many of the above switching repercussions are indeed apparent. It is likely that the discrepancy between the results once again stems from different measures, definitions and classifications of handedness; inconsistent differentiation between pathological and familial left handers; sampling adults rather than developing children; and neglecting various dimensions of handedness and its contextual factors.

For further applied research as well as clinical practice, the most critical primary switching repercussions are not unique to converted handedness but have been identified in specific educational guidelines in Germany (Sattler and Klußmann 2014; Sattler et al. 2014) and summarised below and in Fig. 4.1:

- Memory retention disorders
- Speech disorders such as stuttering
- Attention and concentration problems
- Fine motor difficulties, especially handwriting
- Reading and spelling difficulties
- Visual-spatial and perceptual problems
- Difficulty identifying left and right sides

[4] This group was referred to as "*non-Right handedness*" in the study.

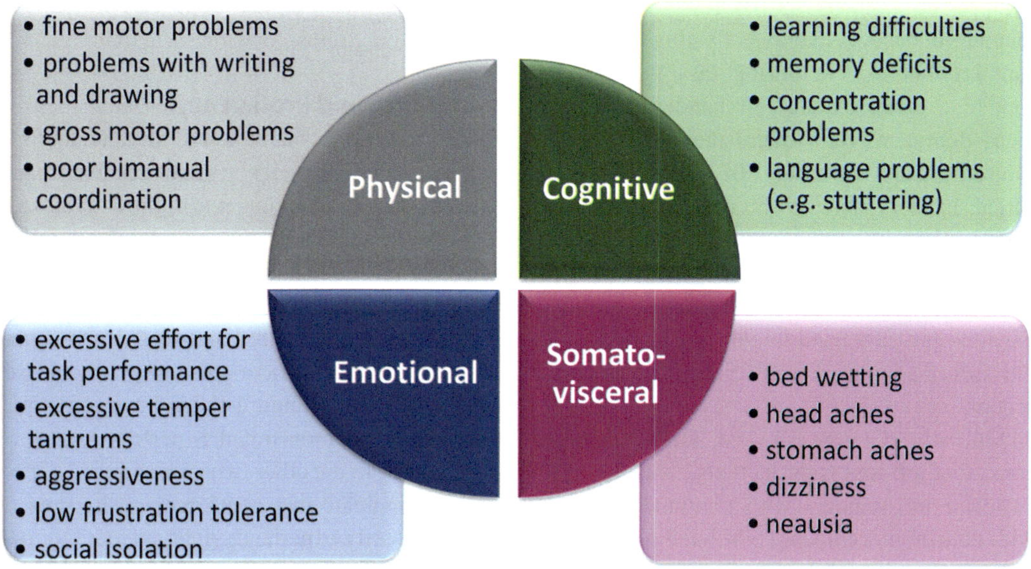

Fig. 4.1 Summarising major conversion repercussions into four clusters: cognitive, somato-visceral, emotional and physical

Secondary repercussions include:

- Withdrawn behaviour, feelings of inferiority
- Inferiority complexes
- Behavioural disorders, including excessive temper tantrums, bed-wetting and nail-biting
- Oppositional and defiant behaviour
- Insecurity
- Overcompensation and disproportionate effort
- Emotional problems

These switching repercussions should be explicitly researched in children with switched handedness, using a comprehensive and well-differentiated handedness assessment as well as background information to capture specific switching characteristics.

4.5.4 Comparing Converted Left Handers to Familial Left Handers and Right Handers

Some researchers investigated the difference between converted and familial left handers and right handers, using both neuroimaging techniques and conventional handedness assessments.

Functional Magnetic Resonance Imaging (fMRI)
Switching repercussions may be extensive in many individuals, but they may also be symptomatic of several other conditions (e.g. in people with ADHD or learning disorders). So, identifying converted handers solely based on these repercussions is problematic. As a guideline for practitioners, it can be assumed that the higher the number of these symptoms co-occuring, the greater the chance that they indicate switching repercussions of a converted (left) hander.

Potentially, advancing technology could significantly contribute to determining switched handedness more reliably. In particular, functional magnetic resonance imaging (fMRI) visualises the brain's anatomical structures and physiological functions (Gerber 2014), thereby allowing us direct insight into its activities. As a result, hypotheses about brain function, including the effect of switched handedness, can be investigated more closely and potentially with greater specificity, particularly to understand the mechanisms of lateralisation and brain plasticity due to environmental influences. Klöppel and colleagues compared ordinary (familial) left handers, converted left handers and right handers

(Klöppel et al. 2007b, 2010). As expected, they found right handers mainly activating their dominant left hemisphere during task performance and, to a lesser extent, left handers activating their dominant right hemisphere since they showed greater variability. In comparison, converted handers showed bilateral activation of both cerebral hemispheres when using the right hand for writing (ibid.). Unfortunately, only the dominant hand was tested—the comparison with the non-dominant hand might have provided further information on the differences between the groups.

Similarly, Grabowska and team compared consistent left and right handers, "successfully" switched left handers who continued to write with their non-dominant right hand and "unsuccessfully" switched left handers who reverted back to left-handed writing (Grabowska et al. 2012). Neuroimaging techniques showed the brain activity of "successfully" retrained left handers to be more similar to that of right handers than that of "unsuccessfully" switched left handers. The authors concluded that converted left-handed people demonstrate changes in plasticity regarding the reorganisation of motor functions, showing a mixture of brain activity patterns typical in left and right handers (ibid.).

Vongerichten investigated the *long-term effects* of switching handedness on brain function based on a tapping task and came to similar conclusions (Vongerichten 2012). She postulated:

> *Attempts at relearning [to write with the right hand] may train the executive areas of the other [non-dominant] hemisphere but not the activity of higher-level motor areas. Instead, relearning actually increases activity in the [right] dominant hemisphere. These results show that left-handers—despite most intensive training—cannot become right-handed* (Vongerichten 2012: 62)

However, research generally does not address the degree of handedness within the group of converted handers. As outlined earlier, some authors propose three variations, ranging from using the switched non-dominant hand only for writing to performing almost other activities with the non-dominant hand (DeAgostini et al. 1997; Llaurens et al. 2009). It seems likely that incorporating a handedness degree variable would yield more differentiated brain activity patterns between the groups.

Preference and Proficiency

Using a self-assessment, Porac investigated both preference and proficiency of switched left handers, familial left handers and right-handed individuals (Porac 2009). For *preference*, subjects rated items requiring high and low skill on a 3-point scale (left–right–mixed). Converted left handers used their right hand significantly more than ordinary left handers. As a *proficiency* task, participants completed a dotting test. Switched left handers demonstrated a performance level comparable to the other two groups (ibid.). These findings indicate that converted left handers do not necessarily experience right-sided motor deficits due to the re-learning to write with the non-dominant hand.

However, this study also failed to consider the degree of handedness. Thus, it is unclear if, and to what extent, the handedness degree may have played a role in being switched in the first place, and how it may impact the research results. In addition, dotting tests are typically used for measuring hand proficiency and correlate highly with handwriting (see also Chap. 6 for assessing handedness). Nevertheless, a dotting task cannot be compared with the highly complex activity of writing. Handwriting involves cognitive, language and affective dimensions in addition to being a highly intricate sensory-motor-based task, and thereby far exceeds the ability needed to make dots as fast as possible. The extent to which these research findings can be transferred to a real-life situation of a switched hander is thus questionable.

4.5.5 Reverting Switched *Left Handedness*

It is possible that converted left handers can return to writing with their dominant left hand. There are documented cases that show that switching repercussions may subsequently decrease or even be reversed. Meng, for example, refers to converted left-handed children who stuttered and showed learning difficulties (Meng 2007). When they returned to writing with the left hand, these problems disappeared, and new competencies emerged.

Individual Case Studies on Reverting Switched *Left Handedness*

There is very little research in this area of ♦**reverting handedness**. However, case studies of reverted left handers enable us to gain more insight into the subsequent changes they experienced, particularly since these are often similar. For example, Randolph describes his reversion experiences as follows:

> *I had somehow managed to trigger a sequence of events that were quickly re-inventing me. All of this came as an exhilarating surprise. Each change and insight was linked to a moment of wonder, the kind we expect to see in children but not in adults. A deeper and more finely detailed sensory awareness was building each day … Because my body and mind were finally being allowed to work as originally intended, the forces of change seemed to run as if they were directed by a hidden master guidance system.* (Randolph 2007: 52–53)

> *On a sensory level … the accelerated development of skill that came in this flood of change included processing enhancements and improved tactile, kinetic, visual and auditory abilities …. On a cognitive level … changes in my thought process took place as a consequence of the improved sensory, memory and mental resources that I enjoyed. In functional terms, I sensed that I was operating in a shifting setting, one that liberated and enhanced cognitive processing. As time passed, I developed enhanced skills and was able to function and move through life much more efficiently.* (Randolph 2007: 56)

Other authors describe similar observations (e.g. Neumann 2014; Sattler 2000; Steinkopf 2014), indicating that handedness appears to be related to more than just sensory-motor abilities, perception, cognitive, language and affective levels, to a strong sense of identity. Working with switched left-handed children and supporting them to revert to their left hand, they and their parents often reported comparable experiences. For example, parents state, "it changed him, he seems to be quite a different child", or a child remarks, "I feel myself now, and it feels like my hand belongs to me". Notably, more research should be conducted in this area, using a multifactorial and multidimensional approach to handedness.

Understanding Brain Plasticity for Handedness Conversion and Reversion

Since there is a lack of research on reverted handedness, let us look at studies investigating neural and behavioural dimensions of brain plasticity typically researched when individuals experimentally learn to write with their non-dominant hand. What allows conversion and reversion of handedness to occur in the first place? It is the phenomenon of the so-called functional plasticity, suggesting that the brain's plasticity as an anatomical and morphological organ is functionally ever-changing (Doyon and Benali 2005; Floyer-Lea and Matthews 2005; Klöppel et al. 2007b; Kienle 2011). Presumably, these processes are also fundamental in reorganising brain activity in switched handers. Pritzel proposes two different processes that may cause functional adaptation in the motor system illustrating brain plasticity (Pritzel 2006). Either the brain has to cope with learning a new task (such as handedness conversion—*my insertion*) or it has to overcome resulting functional limitations after brain damage (or handedness reversion—*my insertion*). In either case, similar neuronal mechanisms seem to be responsible for both processes (ibid.). So, whilst these findings support brain plasticity in handedness conversion and reversion, it is unclear whether the resulting reorganisation is beneficial, a deterrent or indeterminate to the individual.

Research on Training with Non-dominant Hand for Writing

In our quest to better understand the brain's plasticity required for both converting and reverting the dominant hand, we turn to research cases where the non-dominant hand was experimentally trained for writing, or due to amputation rather than environmental influences. Kienle conducted an fMRI study with 19 right-handed typically developed individuals trained to write with their left hand (Kienle 2011). Structural and functional changes in the brain were investigated after the acquisition of writing with the left hand. The results show that the centres for deliberate motor planning were activated in *both* hemispheres of the brain prior to the switching. After the re-learning phase, the activation focus shifted to the *left* hemisphere, which is responsible for motor coordination in routine activities, rather than to the right hemisphere controlling the left motor pathways during writing. In her conclusion, Kienle proposes that writing with the non-dominant hand may cause structural change in the brain and associative connections so that motor information exchange can be optimised between the two hemispheres (ibid.).

Walker and Henneberg also conducted a writing training program with adults over 28 days with their non-dominant hands, using behavioural measures of handwriting (Walker and Henneberg 2007). Whilst the subjects' performance was diverse, writing with the non-dominant hand showed great similarity with that of the dominant hand. Similarly, another study found that, with practice, the non-dominant hand appears to learn to write just as legibly as the preferred hand (Galobardes et al. 1999). Some authors even suggest that with repeated training, there would be no differences in motor aspects such as control, strength or positioning between the hands (Teixeria and Paroli 2000).

Several studies looked at individuals with amputations of the dominant hand or arm and re-learning to write with the non-dominant hand. Results indicate that this can be successfully achieved motorically through practice and repetition. For example, Philip and Frey found that the participants were able to learn to write with their non-dominant left hand but with significantly more effort (Philip and Frey 2014). Similarly, in a programme called "Handwriting for Heroes", veterans with amputation or mutilation of the dominant hand were trained to write with their non-dominant hand. Although good results were achieved, the control group performing the programme with their dominant hand performed better than the veterans (Yancosek 2010).

Practical Implications

Furthermore, Lindemann and Wright argue that handedness may have less to do with an *inherent* disposition than the right-handed environment, repetition, automation and habit (Lindemann and Wright 1998). These findings could well explain why it is possible to convert handedness, but some authors have expressed doubt whether the non-dominant writing hand can, despite repeated training, assume an equal, superior role in function to the dominant hand (Annett 2002; Peters 1981). Also, the investigated writing retraining programmes above were confined to subjects writing a few words repeatedly, based mainly on the motor learning aspect of writing. Conceptual or creative writing would involve quite different cognitive and language processes, as is the case in converted left handers. Such real-life handwriting may result in different writing outcomes.

In summary, these results confirm that handwriting can be automated and performed successfully by the non-dominant hand, even if this means greater effort and possibly related problems. However, transferring these results into everyday life may not be viable, since the experimental wirting programs do not reflect the complexity of writing in real life.

My experience with switched handers in clinical practice supports the notion that the multifaceted and multimodal processes occurring in a fraction of a second during everyday writing do not seem to run as smoothly or efficiently when controlled by the non-dominant motor cortex. In other words, switched handers generally would write better with their dominant hand. When a child learns to write with the non-dominant hand and does not revert, there seem to be different factors influencing whether and to what extent switching repercussions take place. These will be discussed in Chap. 11. So even though the brain's plasticity enables relearning to write with the non-dominant hand, it remains uncertain whether and which switching repercussions may occur in an individual and which factors could facilitate or hinder the process. Clearly, there is a need for further research on converted handedness and switching repercussions.

4.6 Identifying Subgroups of *Left Handedness*

Reviewing the extensive literature on *Left Handedness*, the inconclusive and sometimes contradictory results indicated that many questions remain unanswered. Nevertheless, on four aspects, researchers are generally in agreement:

1. Almost all studies report that there are substantially *more right handers than left handers*, so comparing left handers to right handers

serves as a point of reference (i.e. the two groups are not mirror images of one another).

2. *Left handers differ from right handers* in several ways, even though the literature does not always agree on all differences.
3. Left handers appear to be a more *heterogenous* group than right handers, particularly regarding their high variability and milder degrees of handedness.
4. Distinct subgroups of left handers have been identified, such as *pathological left handers* and *converted left handers*. Whilst counterpart subgroups exist in right handers, these are much rarer.

In addition to the identified subgroups of pathological and converted left handers, it would make sense to include further handedness groups based on the degree of handedness, since there are multiple indications that they differ markedly from one another. Several attempts have been made in this regard by researchers. For example, Bruckert and colleagues propose three distinct groups among left handers (based on a study by Mazoyer and team in 2014, involving 150 left handers): a typically left lateralised group, an ambilateral group with a "weak laterality" and a small atypical group with right lateralisation (Bruckert et al. 2021). The authors further concluded that

> ... *left handers tend to be more variable in laterality than right handers, but also ... that the distribution of laterality across the population is best modelled by multiple subpopulations, rather than one normal distribution. Furthermore, this distribution appears to be different in left and right handers*. (Bruckert et al. 2021: 2)

Whilst left and right handers with a *strong degree* of handedness show very similar patterns of hand use (i.e. perform almost everything with their left or right hand, respectively), most people appear to have a more *moderate degree* of handedness, particularly right handers. In particular, left handers demonstrate a great variability in their hand use not seen in right handers. So proportionally, there are more left handers with a *mild degree* of handedness than right handers. In addition, the group of pathological left handers is significantly larger than pathological right handers as explained in Chap. 3, Sect. 3.5. Similarly, there are many more switched left handers than switched right handers because of the right-biassed environment. These differences between left and right handers as well as the respective subgroups probably stem from a complex combination of genetic predisposition as well as right-biassed physical and sociocultural environments. Figure 4.2 summarises these differences.

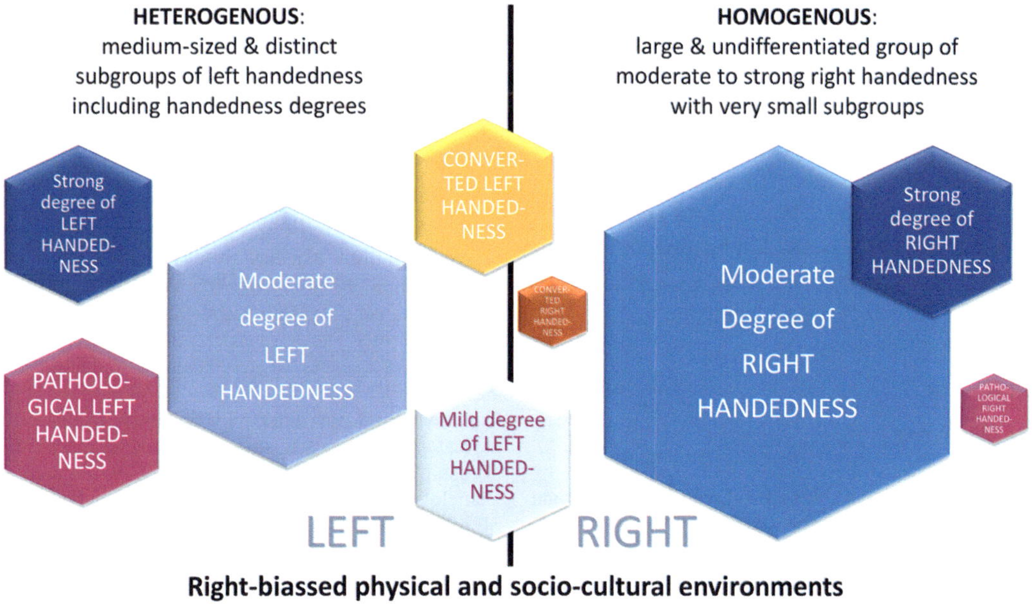

Fig. 4.2 Differences between subgroups in left and right handers

4.7 Concluding Remarks

In this chapter, we looked at a wide range of research studies, which suggest specific traits of left handers, how they differ from right handers, as well as subgroups of pathological left handers and converted left handers. In particular, we gained a better understanding of the conversion and reversion of handedness and its consequences. Since research studies do not consistently measure and categorise *Left Handedness* across studies, defining subgroups of handedness may help to address the challenge of comparing studies. In addition to the already identified subgroups of pathological and converted left handers, the degree of *Left Handedness* is far more variable than in right handedness. Therefore, using handedness degrees as a basis for further handedness subgroups makes sense, since there are multiple indications that they differ. Furthermore, this can help analyse variable hand use in clinical decision-making. The following subgroups for both left and right handers can be identified from the literature: left and right handers with a explicit handedness degree; left and right handers with a moderate degree; left handers with a mild degree (not seen in right handers); converted left and (rarely) converted right handers; and pathological left and (rarely) pathological right handers.

Some of these subgroups will typically use their non-dominant hand more frequently due to their low handedness degree and normal variability, handedness conversion or pathological handedness. In research, individuals in these subgroups will likely be classified as "mixed" handers, forming a highly diverse assemblance of individuals with variable hand use. This inevitably leads to the question on the difference between the so-called mixed handers and left handers or an overlap of proposed subgroups. Chapter 5 will address the phenomenon of mixed handedness.

References

Annett M (1985) Left, right, hand, and brain. The right shift theory. L. Erlbaum Associates, London

Annett M (2002) Handedness and brain asymmetry. The right shift theory. Psychology Press, Hove

Annett M (2004) Hand preference observed in large healthy samples: classification, norms and interpretations of increased non-right-handedness by the right shift theory. Br J Psychol 95(3):339–353. https://doi.org/10.1348/0007126041528130

Ansuini C, Podda J, Battaglia FM, Veneselli E, Becchio C (2018) One hand, two hands, two people: prospective sensorimotor control in children with autism. Dev Cogn Neurosci 29:86–96

Armitage M, Larkin D (1993) Laterality, motor asymmetry and clumsiness in children. Hum Mov Sci 12(1–2):155–177

Biederman J, Wilens T, Mick E, Milberger S, Spencer TJ, Faraone SV (1995) Psychoactive substance use disorders in adults with attention deficit hyperactivity disorder (ADHD): effects of ADHD and psychiatric comorbidity. In: 0002-953X

Bishop DV (1984) Using non-preferred hand skill to investigate pathological left-handedness in an unselected population. Dev Med Child Neurol 26(2):214–226. https://doi.org/10.1111/j.1469-8749.1984.tb04434.x

Bruckert L, Thompson PA, Watkins KE, Bishop DVM, Woodhead ZVJ (2021) Investigating the effects of handedness on the consistency of lateralization for speech production and semantic processing tasks using functional transcranial Doppler sonography. Laterality 26(6):680–705. https://doi.org/10.1080/1357650X.2021.1898416

Bryden PJ (2016) The influence of MP Bryden's work on lateralization of motor skill: is the preferred hand selected for and better at tasks requiring a high degree of skill? Laterality 21(4–6):312–328

Bryden PJ, Roy EA, Rohr LE, Egilo S (2007) Task demands affect manual asymmetries in pegboard performance. Laterality 12(4):364–377. https://doi.org/10.1080/13576500701356244

Budisavljevic S, Castiello U, Begliomini C (2021) Handedness and white matter networks. Neuroscientist 27(1):88–103. https://doi.org/10.1177/1073858420937657

Cairney J, Schmidt LA, Veldhuizen S, Kurdyak P, Hay J, Faught BE (2008) Left-handedness and developmental coordination disorder. Can J Psychiatr 53(10):696–699

Casasanto D, Henetz T (2012) Handedness shapes children's abstract concepts. Cogn Sci 36(2):359–372. https://doi.org/10.1111/j.1551-6709.2011.01199.x

Cheng Y, Hegarty M, Chrastil ER (2020) Telling right from right: the influence of handedness in the mental rotation of hands. Cogn Res Princ Implic 5(1):25. https://doi.org/10.1186/s41235-020-00230-9

Coren S (1992) The left-hander syndrome. The causes and consequences of left-handedness. Free Press, New York

Coren S (1994) Age trends in handedness: evidence for historical changes in social pressure on the writing hand? J Soc Behav Person 9(2):369–376

Daniel WF, Yeo RA (1991) Handedness and accident proneness. Am J Public Health 81(10):1346–1347

Darvik M, Lorås H, Pedersen AV (2018) The prevalence of left-handedness is higher among individuals with

developmental coordination disorder than in the general population. Front Psychol 9:1948
DeAgostini M, Khamis AH, Ahui AM, Dellatolas G (1997) Environmental influences in hand preference: an African point of view. Brain Cogn 35(2):151–167. https://doi.org/10.1006/brcg.1997.0935
Dellatolas G, Annesi I, Jallon P, Chavance M, Lellouch J (1990) An epidemiological reconsideration of the Geschwind-Galaburda theory of cerebral lateralization. Arch Neurol 47(7):778–782. https://doi.org/10.1001/archneur.1990.00530070074013
Denny K, O'Sullivan V (2007) The economic consequences of being left-handed some sinister results. J Hum Resour 42(2):353–374
Doyon J, Benali H (2005) Reorganization and plasticity in the adult brain during learning of motor skills. Curr Opin Neurobiol 15(2):161–167. https://doi.org/10.1016/j.conb.2005.03.004
Dragovic M, Hammond G (2005) Handedness in schizophrenia: a quantitative review of evidence. Acta Psychiatr Scand 111(6):410–419
Dutton E, van der Linden D, Madison G (2020) Why do high IQ societies differ in intellectual achievement? The role of Schizophrenia and left-handedness in per capita scientific publications and Nobel prizes. J Creat Behav 54(4):871–883
Fagard J (2013) The nature and nurture of human infant hand preference. Ann N Y Acad Sci 1288(1):114–123
Faghihi N, Garcia O, Vaid J (2019) Spatial bias in figure placement in representational drawing: associations with handedness and script directionality. Laterality 24(5):614–630
Floyer-Lea A, Matthews PM (2005) Distinguishable brain activation networks for short- and long-term motor skill learning. J Neurophysiol 94(1):512–518. https://doi.org/10.1152/jn.00717.2004
Foundas AL, Bollich AM, Feldman J, Corey DM, Hurley M, Lemen LC, Heilman KM (2004) Aberrant auditory processing and atypical planum temporale in developmental stuttering. Neurology 63(9):1640–1646
Freitas C, Vasconcelos MO, Botelho M (2014) Handedness and developmental coordination disorder in Portuguese children: study with the M-ABC test. Laterality 19(6):655–676
Galobardes B, Bernstein MS, Morabia A (1999) The association between switching hand preference and the declining prevalence of left-handedness with age. Am J Public Health 89(12):1873–1875. https://doi.org/10.2105/ajph.89.12.1873
Gerber N (2014) Transferring industry approaches to resource management for FM in hospitals: a theoretical reflection. Int J Fac Manag 5(2)
Geschwind N, Behan P (1982) Left-handedness: association with immune disease, migraine, and developmental learning disorder. Proc Natl Acad Sci U S A 79(16):5097–5100
Ghanizadeh A (2013) Lack of association of handedness with inattention and hyperactivity symptoms in ADHD. J Atten Disord 17(4):302–307
Gilbert AN, Wysocki CJ (1992) Hand preference and age in the United States. Neuropsychologia 30(7):601–608. https://doi.org/10.1016/0028-3932(92)90065-T
Goez H, Zelnik N (2008) Handedness in patients with developmental coordination disorder. J Child Neurol 23(2):151–154. https://doi.org/10.1177/0883073807307978
Gonzalez SL, Nelson EL (2021) Factor analysis of the home handedness questionnaire: unimanual and role differentiated bimanual manipulation as separate dimensions of handedness. Appl Neuropsychol Adult 28(2):173–184
Grabowska A, Gut M, Binder M, Forsberg L, Rymarczyk K, Urbanik A (2012) Switching handedness: fMRI study of hand motor control in right-handers, left-handers and converted left-handers. Acta Neurobiol Exp 72(4):439–451
Grouios G, Tsorbatzoudis H, Alexandris K, Barkoukis V (2000) Do left-handed competitors have an innate superiority in sports? Percept Motor Skills 90(3_suppl):1273–1282
Grouios G, Tsormpatzoudis C, Alexandris K, Koidou E (2002) Handedness in sport. Aristotle University of Thessaloniki, Thessaloniki
Hammond G (2002) Correlates of human handedness in primary motor cortex: a review and hypothesis. Neurosci Biobehav Rev 26(3):285–292
Hatta T (2007) Handedness and the brain: a review of brain-imaging techniques. Magn Reson Med Sci 6(2):99–112
Hawkyard R, Dempsey I, Arthur-Kelly M (2014) The handwriting experiences of left-handed primary school students in a digital age. Australian data and critique. Aust J Educ 58(2):123–138
Hécaen H, Sauguet J (1971) Cerebral dominance in left-handed subjects. Cortex 7(1):19–48. https://doi.org/10.1016/s0010-9452(71)80020-5
Hemenway D, Azrael DR, Rimm EB, Feskanich D, Willett WC (1994) Risk factors for wrist fracture: effect of age, cigarettes, alcohol, body height, relative weight, and handedness on the risk for distal forearm fractures in men. Am J Epidemiol 140(4):361–367
Henninger P (1992) Conditional handedness: handedness changes in multiple personality disordered subject reflect shift in hemispheric dominance. Conscious Cogn 1(3):265–287
Hildreth G (1949) The development and training of hand dominance; characteristics of handedness. J Genet Psychol 75(2):197–220. https://doi.org/10.1080/08856559.1949.10533517
Jeyalyn S, Rajasankar DS (2016) Correlation between handedness and intelligence among school children. Int J Contem Med Res 3(9):2683–2686
Johnson W, Duke L (1935) Changes in handedness associated with onset or disappearance of stuttering: sixteen cases. J Exp Educ 4(2):112–132
Kienle J (2011) The neuromagnetic equivalents of dynamic effective face perception: Verlag nicht ermittelbar

Kilshaw D, Annett M (1983) Right-and left-hand skill I: effects of age, sex and hand preference showing superior skill in left-handers. Br J Psychol 74(2):253–268
Klöppel S, van Eimeren T, Glauche V, Vongerichten A, Münchau A, Frackowiak RSJ et al (2007a) The effect of handedness on cortical motor activation during simple bilateral movements. NeuroImage 34(1):274–280
Klöppel S, Vongerichten A, van Eimeren T, Frackowiak RSJ, Siebner HR (2007b) Can left-handedness be switched? Insights from an early switch of handwriting. J Neurosci 27(29):7847–7853. https://doi.org/10.1523/JNEUROSCI.1299-07.2007
Klöppel S, Mangin J-F, Vongerichten A, Frackowiak RSJ, Siebner HR (2010) Nurture versus nature: long-term impact of forced right-handedness on structure of pericentral cortex and basal ganglia. J Neurosci 30(9):3271–3275
Kotetisvili B, Salakaia L, Kamkamidze N, Makashvili M, Azmaiparashvili T, Davlianidze G, Kutlia R, Gogia K, Lomidze N (2005) Negative predisposition to the left-handedness of pupils in Georgian schools. In: Georgian Academic Sciences 31
Kramer J (1970) Linkshändigkeit. Arbeiten zur Psychologie, Pädagogik & Heilpädagogik. In: Universität Freiburg/Schweiz, Band 19
Krombholz H (2008) Zusammenhänge zwischen Händigkeit & motorischen & kognitiven Leistungen im Kindesalter. Z Entwicklungspsychol Padagog Psychol 40(4):189–199. https://doi.org/10.1026/0049-8637.40.4.189
Kushner HI (2012) Retraining left-handers and the aetiology of stuttering: the rise and fall of an intriguing theory. Laterality 17(6):673–693
Kushner HI (2017) On the other hand. Left hand, right brain, mental disorder and history. Johns Hopkins University Press, Baltimore
Lin H-L, Tsuang H-C (2018) Handedness and attention deficit/hyperactivity disorder symptoms in college students. Psychiatry Q 89(1):103–110. https://doi.org/10.1007/s11126-017-9517-8
Lindemann PG, Wright CE (1998) Skill acquisition and plans for actions: Learning to write with your other hand. In: 02621504
Llaurens V, Raymond M, Faurie C (2009) Why are some people left-handed? An evolutionary perspective. Philos Trans R Soc B 364(1519):881–894. https://doi.org/10.1098/rstb.2008.0235
Malkhaz M, Elene K, Tamar K, Guram E, Nikoloz A (2020) Left-handers, retrained left-handers and right-handers: a comparative study. World J Adv Res Rev 7(1):41–47. https://doi.org/10.30574/wjarr.2020.7.1.0227
Marcori AJ, Okazaki VHA (2020) A historical, systematic review of handedness origins. Laterality 25(1):87–108. https://doi.org/10.1080/1357650X.2019.1614597
Marcori AJ, Monteiro PHM, Okazaki VHA (2019) Changing handedness: what can we learn from preference shift studies? Neurosci Biobehav Rev 107:313–319
Masud Y, Ajmal MA (2012) Left-handed people in a right-handed world: a phenomenological study. Pak J Soc Clin Psychol 10(1):49–60
McKeever WF, VanDeventer AD (1977) Familial sinistrality and degree of left-handedness. Br J Psychol 68(4):469–471. https://doi.org/10.1111/j.2044-8295.1977.tb01616.x
McManus C, Bryden MP (1992) The genetics of handedness, cerebral dominance and lateralisation
McManus IC, Sik G, Cole DR, Mellon AF, Wong J, Kloss J (1988) The development of handedness in children. Br J Dev Psychol 6(3):257–273. https://doi.org/10.1111/j.2044-835X.1988.tb01099.x
Meng L-F (2007) The rate of handedness conversion and related factors in left-handed children. Laterality 12(2):131–138. https://doi.org/10.1080/13576500601005727
Miller B, Peeri NC, Nabors LB, Creed JH, Thompson ZJ, Rozmeski CM et al (2018) Handedness and the risk of glioma. J Neurooncol 137(3):639–644. https://doi.org/10.1007/s11060-018-2759-y
Nastou E, Ocklenburg S, Papadatou-Pastou M (2022) Handedness in ADHD: meta-analyses. Neuropsychol Rev 32(4):877–892
Neumann M (2014) Natürlich mit Links. Zurück zur Linnkshändigkeit - befreiter leben mit der starken Hand. Ariston, Berlin
Niederhofer H (2005) Serum cholinesterase levels elevated in patients suffering from ADHD. J Atten Disord 9(2):382–383
Nikolaeva EI (2005) Left handed children: diagnostics, training, correction. Detstvo-Press, St. Petersburg
Orton ST, Travis LE (1929) Studies in stuttering: IV. Studies of action currents in stutterers. Arch Neurol Psychiatry 21:61–68
Perelle I, Ehrman L (2005) On the other hand. Behav Genet 35(3):343–350
Peters M (1981) Handedness: effect of prolonged practice on between hand performance differences. Neuropsychologia 19(4):587–590. https://doi.org/10.1016/0028-3932(81)90025-7
Peters M (1990) Subclassification of non-pathological left-handers poses problems for theories of handedness. Neuropsychologia 28(3):279–289. https://doi.org/10.1016/0028-3932(90)90021-f
Peters M (1996) Handedness and performance in left handers. In: Elliott D, Roy EA (Hg.) Manual asymmetries in motor performance. CRC Press, Boca Raton, pp 99–120
Peterson JM, Lansky LM (1977) Left-handedness among architects: partial replication and some new data. Percept Motor Skills 45(3_suppl):1216–1218
Philip BA, Frey SH (2014) Compensatory changes accompanying chronic forced use of the nondominant hand by unilateral amputees. J Neurosci 34(10):3622–3631. https://doi.org/10.1523/JNEUROSCI.3770-13.2014
Porac C (1996) Attempts to switch the writing hand: relationships to age and side of hand preference. Laterality 1(1):35–44. https://doi.org/10.1080/713754205

Porac C (2009) Hand preference and skilled hand performance among individuals with successful rightward conversions of the writing hand. Laterality 14(2):105–121. https://doi.org/10.1080/13576500802299418

Porac C (2016) Laterality. Exploring the enigma of left-handedness. Elsevier Science, Amsterdam. http://www.sciencedirect.com/science/book/9780128012390

Porac C, Buller T (1990) Overt attempts to change hand preference: a study of group and individual characteristics. Can J Psychol 44(4):512–521. https://doi.org/10.1037/h0084268

Porac C, Lee Berdel Martin W (2007) A cross-cultural comparison of pressures to switch left-hand writing: Brazil versus Canada. Laterality 12(3):273–291. https://doi.org/10.1080/13576500701269462

Porac C, Searlman A (2002) The effects of hand preference side and hand preference switch history on measures of psychological and physical well-being and cognitive performance in a sample. Neuropsychologia 40(12):2074–2083

Porac C, Friesen IC, Barnes MP, Gruppuso V (1998) Illness and accidental injury in young and older adult left- and right-handers: implications for genetic theories of hand preference. Dev Neuropsychol 14:157–172

Preti A, Vellante M (2007) Creativity and psychopathology: higher rates of psychosis proneness and nonright-handedness among creative artists compared to same age and gender peers. J Nerv Ment Dis 195(10):837–845

Pritzel M (2006) Händigkeit. In: Karnath HO, Thier P (Hg.) Neuropsychologie. Springer

Randolph SM (2007) Hidden handedness. The emerging story of handedness reversals. Foundation for Handedness Research

Rett A, Kohlmann T, Strauch G (1973) Linkshänder: Analyse einer Minderheit [Left-handers: analysis of a minority]. Jugend & Volk

Sarma PSB (1989) Mixed-handedness and achievement test scores of grade school children. Percept Mot Skills 68(3):839–846. https://doi.org/10.2466/pms.1989.68.3.839

Sattler JB (1999) Linkshänder & umgeschulte Linkshänder in der Ergotherapie. Praxis ergotherapie 12(2):98–110

Sattler JB (2000) Der umgeschulte Linkshänder oder Der Knoten im Gehirn [The switched left-hander or the knot in the brain]

Sattler JB (2011) Der umgeschulte Linkshänder oder der Knoten im Gehirn: Auer

Sattler JB, Klußmann A (2014) Leitlinie Händigkeit. - Bedeutung & Untersuchung/.002/017 - S1. Unter Mitarbeit von DGAUM. AWMF, zuletzt aktualisiert am 06.2020

Sattler JB, Klußmann A, Arnold-Schulz-Gahmen B, Vasterling A, Wagner H, Hartmann B (2014) Händigkeit–Bedeutung & Untersuchung

Satz P (1972) Pathological left-handedness. An explanatory model. [Place of publication not identified]: Distributed by ERIC Clearinghouse

Satz P, Orsini DL, Saslow E, Henry R (1985) The pathological left-handedness syndrome. Brain Cogn 4(1):27–46

Scharoun SM, Bryden PJ (2014) Hand preference, performance abilities, and hand selection in children. Front Psychol 5:82. https://doi.org/10.3389/fpsyg.2014.00082

Scheirs JG (1990) Relationships between the direction of movements and handedness in children. Neuropsychologia 28(7):743–748. https://doi.org/10.1016/0028-3932(90)90130-g

Searleman A, Porac C (2003) Lateral preference profiles and right shift attempt histories of consistent and inconsistent left-handers. Brain Cogn 52(2):175–180

Semenovich AV (2009) Hemispheric organization of mental processes in left-handers. In: Hemispheric interaction (in Russian). Moscow 400, pp 15

Shimizu A, Endo M, Yamaguchi N, Torii H, Isaki K (1985) Hand preference in schizophrenics and handedness conversion in their childhood. Acta Psychiatr Scand 72(3):259–265

Siebner HR, Limmer C, Peinemann A, Drzezga A, Bloem BR, Schwaiger M, Conrad B (2002) Long-term consequences of switching handedness: a positron emission tomography study on handwriting in "converted" left-handers. J Neurosci 22(7):2816–2825

Siengthai B, Kritz-Silverstein D, Barrett-Connor E (2008) Handedness and cognitive function in older men and women: a comparison of methods. J Nutr Health Aging 12(9):641–647

Soper HV, Satz P (1984) Pathological left-handedness and ambiguous handedness: a new explanatory model. Neuropsychologia 22(4):511–515. https://doi.org/10.1016/0028-3932(84)90046-0

Sovák M (1962) Lateralität & Sprache. Wissenschaftliche Zeitschrift Martin-Luther Universität 11:1695–1702

Sovák M (1968) Pädagogische Probleme der lateralität: Verlag Volk u. Gesundheit VEB

Sovak M (1974) Measuring of lateral preference earlier and now. Stud Psychol 16(3):209

Steinkopf F (2014) Schritt für Schritt mit links ins Glück. Jder zweite Mensch ist Linkshänder—meistens weiß er es nur nicht. Left Handers World, Heide

Szaflarski JP, Binder JR, Possing ET, McKiernan KA, Ward BD, Hammeke TA (2002) Language lateralization in left-handed and ambidextrous people. Neurology 59(2):238–244. https://doi.org/10.1212/WNL.59.2.238

Szaflarski JP, Rajagopal A, Altaye M, Byars AW, Jacola L, Schmithorst VJ et al (2012) Left-handedness and language lateralization in children. Brain Res 1433(1129–39):85–97. https://doi.org/10.1016/j.brainres.2011.11.026

Teixeria LA, Paroli R (2000) Lateral asymmetries in motor actions: preference versus training. Moritz 6(1):18

Travis LE (1934) Stuttering and the concept of handedness

Tzourio-Mazoyer N, Petit L, Zago L, Crivello F, Vinuesa N, Joliot M et al (2015) Between-hand difference in ipsilateral deactivation is associated with hand lateral-

ization: fMRI mapping of 284 volunteers balanced for handedness. Front Hum Neurosci 9:5
Verstynen T, Diedrichsen J, Albert N, Aparicio P, Ivry RB (2005) Ipsilateral motor cortex activity during unimanual hand movements relates to task complexity. J Neurophysiol 93(3):1209–1222
Vongerichten A (2012) Angeborene & anerzogene funktionelle Korrelate von Händigkeit im motorischen Kortex. Eine fMRT Studie
Vuoksimaa E, Koskenvuo M, Rose RJ, Kaprio J (2009) Origins of handedness: a nationwide study of 30,161 adults. Neuropsychologia 47(5):1294–1301. https://doi.org/10.1016/j.neuropsychologia.2009.01.007
Walker L, Henneberg M (2007) Writing with the nondominant hand: cross-handedness trainability in adult individuals. Laterality 12(2):121–130. https://doi.org/10.1080/13576500600989665
Yancosek KE (2010) Injury-induced hand dominance transfer. University of Kentucky Libraries, Lexington
Zaghloul MS, Saquib J, Al-Mazrou AR, Saquib N (2018) A qualitative assessment of the impact of handedness among left-handed surgeons in Saudi Arabia. Laterality 23(1):39–50

Mixed Handedness

5

Contents

There may be three distinct populations of individuals: a 'typical' left lateralised population; a smaller 'ambilateral' population with weak laterality; and a small 'atypical' population with right lateralisation. Interestingly, the 'atypical' group were all left handed. This finding lends support to the idea that left handers tend to be more variable in laterality than right handers, but also suggests that the distribution of laterality across the population is best modelled by multiple subpopulations, rather than one normal distribution. Furthermore, this distribution appears to be different in left and right handers. (Bruckert et al. 2021: 2)

5.1 Introduction

Over the last decade, researchers have increasingly concluded that the *degree* rather than the direction of handedness is particularly associated with disorders. Indeed, there appears to be some evidence that the so-called inconsistent or "mixed" hand use is associated with various pathological conditions (e.g. Kastner-Koller et al. 2007; Rodriguez et al. 2010; Somers et al. 2009). Specifically, the *degree* of handedness rather than its *direction* is seen to be a relatively *simple indicator* for specific abilities, predispositions, medical conditions and neurophysiological processes (e.g. Hardie et al. 2016). So similar to some research on *Left Handedness*, there appears to be a quest to identify mixed handedness as a simple indicator for disorders. Whilst this objective is understandable, it is also problematic. As we have seen in the previous chapter, *Left Handedness* research failed to produce unambiguous results in relation to medical conditions and problems, mainly because there is a lack of clear definition

E. Kraus, *Beyond Left and Right Handedness*, https://doi.org/10.1007/978-3-031-24389-9_5

and differentiation between subgroups. Do we face the same problems when dealing with mixed handedness? How is it defined, and does it make sense as a category, or is there a need for differentiation?

In this chapter, I first *contextualise* mixed handedness by looking at degrees of handedness and normal variability. I then explore and define *ambidexterity* to differentiate it from mixed handedness and present a pilot study on *analysing the methodology* of some studies on mixed handedness, before looking at a wide variety of *research findings* in the field. This chapter concludes Part I of the book. Drawing on the previous four chapters, I make two proposals: an explanatory *research-orientated model* for a possible reason for the diverse findings by combining degrees of handedness with callosal functioning and a practice-orientated *criteria catalogue* for differentiating mixed handedness for clinical practice.

5.2 Contextualising Mixed Handedness

5.2.1 Defining Mixed Handedness and Related Terms

At first glance, the category of "mixed" handedness seems even more obscure and indistinct, as it appears to comprise all those individuals who do not show consistent hand use. Indeed, there is a wide range of terms used synonymously with mixed handedness for individuals that are not clearly left or right handed, including "inconsistent", "ambiguous", "non-right", "non-left", "confused", "unestablished", "uncertain", "less lateralised", etc. However, since there is no consensus on its definition in the literature, I will use the term "♦**mixed handedness**" as a somewhat artificially fabricated category to include all those handedness groups that are not clearly assigned to being left or right handed and display reduced lateralisation, regardless of the definition, measures or categorisation used.

Furthermore, it is helpful to use consistent terminology for related processes. The term ♦**variable hand use** will be used when referring to an action; ♦**(un)established handedness** when referring to the still uncertain outcome of handedness; ♦**handedness status** referring to the current manifestation or state of handedness; and ♦**handedness formation** concerning the process of establishing handedness over the life span, of which ♦**handedness development** constitutes the early handedness development between birth and 6 years.

5.2.2 Reasons for Normal Handedness Variability

Handedness has been described as typically *variable* across the life span (Corbetta et al. 2006). This inherently means that everybody shows some variability, i.e. uses the non-dominant hand in everyday activities. However, what are the manifestations of such variability? Researchers tend to define an arbitrary cut-off point differentiating mixed handedness from *normal variability*. The diverse determining factors of handedness (e.g. genetic predisposition, motor abilities, individual developmental patterns, experience/practice, physical, social, and cultural environmental influences) seem to contribute to the complexity and variability of handedness. This is expressed particularly in bimanual activities (e.g. Corbetta et al. 2006; Humphrey 1951), since we typically perform most actions and activities in everyday life using both hands. *Bimanual tasks* are usually characterised by role division between the hands, with a leading or more active hand and a stabilising or assisting hand. It has been found (Kagerer 2015) that handedness in bimanual activities shows a higher variability than one-handed activities, as discussed in Sects. 2.4 and 3.3 (e.g. Kuypers 1982; Michel 2021; Kraus 2003, 2019).

Besides normal variability during unimanual and bimanual tasks, there is evidence that the *degree* of handedness is *inherited* (see Collins 1985; Corballis 1997). For example, in studies on the so-called familial sinistrality (FS), participants are classified as *FS+* based on the incidence of *Left Handedness* in the close relatives (e.g. parents, siblings, children) and as *FS−* if there is a family history of *Left Handedness* in more distant relatives such as grandparents, grandchildren, uncles, aunts and cousins (Bryden 1977). Correlations between family sinistrality and mixed ("ambidextrous") handedness have been repeatedly documented, leading researchers to conclude that the FS+ feature might increase interhemispheric interaction and reduce lateralisation (Christman and Butler 2011). *Left handedness* in close family members could thus be a predictive factor for mixed handedness.

Finally, the frequently mentioned and *inconsistent parameters* of capturing handedness may well account for exacerbating or distorting existing variability, making the comparison of respective studies difficult. The diverse cut-off points for *Left* and *Right Handedness* resulting in different handedness categories, the countless test procedures and the inconsistent definition of handedness are obstacles to drawing conclusions within studies and comparing studies on mixed handedness. Despite these inherent shortcomings, the multitude of studies provides us with important tendencies and indications. A particularly contentious area within the field of mixed handedness is the phenomenon and definition of ambidexterity.

5.3 Ambidexterity

Whilst ambidexterity is often used synonymously with mixed handedness, it constitutes a distinct subgroup of mixed handedness within the rationale of this book. Ambidexterity has been of research interest, particularly at the turn of the nineteenth century. Jackson, founder and honorary secretary of the Ambidextral Culture Society at the time, defined ambidexterity as follows:

> *Ambidexterity shall signify that state of expertness, accuracy, and rapidity in which both hands shall be equally skilful, and equally capable of performing every movement and occupation that either of them can be required to engage in—as expert, for example, in writing a letter as in manipulating the keys of the piano.* (Jackson 1905: 109)

Similarly, Hildreth, a frequently cited and historically important researcher, distinguished between a small group of ambidextrous people with a very similar level of proficiency on both sides. There are *ambidextrous* individuals due to good performance in both hands and *ambisinistral* people, those who show a low-value performance on both sides (Hildreth 1949). Other researchers who studied ambidexterity and generally share this definition also conclude that it is a very rare phenomenon (Elneel et al. 2008; Moynihan and Breathnach 1995).

Historically, ambidexterity was thought to be highly desirable by some scientists in the early nineteenth century. This was based on the assumption that training ambidexterity would result in superior performance of the brain. In particular, simultaneous bilateral writing was trained. Lord Baden-Powell describes this as follows:

> *It is hardly possible to lay too much stress upon this bimanual training [of the two hands], or to attach too much importance to the principle ... Moreover, and of equal import to the individual, it is by the movements of these members [hands], that the whole muscular tissues on both sides of the body are exercised, strengthened and perfected.* (Baden-Powell, cited in Jackson 1905: xi—my insertion in square brackets)

However, the idea that ambidexterity would lead to improved brain function and profit society as a whole did not persist since there was a lack of evidence for the benefits of ambidexterity training. On the contrary, by the mid-twentieth century, there was a general consensus that the two hemispheres are not interchangeable but used for different processes and tasks (see Hellige 2010) and that ambidextrous writing would interfere with the inherent specialisation (Peters et al. 2006; Corballis et al. 2008).

Despite the fact that the scientific community distanced itself from promoting ambidexterity over the years, the idea of training ambidexterity to improve movement and mental processes is still quite widespread today. This is also seen in clinical practice, where mixed-handed children may proudly present themselves as ambidextrous or parents declare their admiration for their ambidextrous child. It is thus important to look at current discourses on ambidexterity as a contextual reference when dealing with children in clinical and educational settings. Advertising ambidexterity can be found in various forms, ranging across books, schools and online training programmes. For example, books such as "The Power of Your Other Hand" proclaim that writing and drawing with the non-dominant hand enhance access to the right hemispheric functions like creativity, intuition, feeling and spiritual wisdom (Capacchione 2019). The reader is encouraged to let the left and right hands communicate with each other, so the writing does not take place simultaneously but alternatingly. Using a different approach, Schlaak invites readers to simultaneously engage in two-handedness experiments by writing with both hands (Schlaak 2019).[1] Also, even today, there are schools teaching ambidextrous (simultaneous) writing.[2] In addition, online programmes such as "Ambidexterity Training for Balance, Symmetry, and Brain" instruct that ambidexterity (*The Bioneer*[3]) can be found, or there are forums where visitors are invited to engage with the pros and cons of becoming ambidextrous, like *Quora*.[4]

Broadly speaking, in current literature, ambidexterity is considered to be very rare at approximately 1% of the population (e.g. Vuoksimaa et al. 2009). Moreover, in both the literature and society at large, the term ambidexterity is often used synonymously with all terms describing mixed handedness and laterality. This is not only confusing but also problematic for scientific research. Furthermore, the idea that the equally proficient use of both hands would lead to superior brain function has been disputed. For example, Corballis states on the Scientific American internet site:

> *The two hemispheres of the brain are not interchangeable. These asymmetries probably evolved to allow the two sides of the brain to specialise. To attempt to undo or tamper with this efficient set-up may invite psychological problems.*[5]

I will use the term ♦**ambidexterity** to refer to the rare phenomenon exhibited by individuals with extraordinarily high and equal levels of motor ability on *both* sides. In other words, they are able to perform highly complex tasks such as writing equally well with either hand. In this way, we clearly distinguish the term "ambidexterity" from mixed handedness, assuming that there will be different reasons for variable hand use in the potpourri of mixed handedness. However, based on the literature and my clinical experience, when looking closely at these rare individuals who perform highly complex tasks such as writing equally well with either hand, they still tend to initially start tasks with their left hand. They also report that they have to practise more with their right hand to achieve similar results. There is a lack of research to clearly differentiate between ambidexterity and very mild *Left Handedness*.

5.4 Analysing Research Methodology on Mixed-Handedness Studies

Considering the lack of definition and general confusion around mixed handedness and ambidexterity, it is not surprising that many studies of handedness deal only with clearly established left- or right-handed subjects. Thus, mixed-handed individuals are often excluded from the data collection and analysis, generating findings on right and left handers with moderate to strong degrees of handedness, or exclusively on right handers. Categories in these studies typically range across the following:

[1] In the book, the reader is prompted to first consult their doctor before embarking on the exercises described, alerting to possible symptoms such as headache or dizziness whilst reading, and stating that he/she would not assume any responsibility should the reader's health be damaged (Schlaak 2019).

[2] Indian school where pupils taught to be ambidextrous faces closure | Daily Mail Online

[3] Ambidexterity Training for Balance, Symmetry, and Brain—The Bioneer

[4] What are the pros and cons of becoming ambidextrous?—Quora

[5] Can Training to Become Ambidextrous Improve Brain Function?—Scientific American

- *One category*—right handers only
- *Two categories*—left and right handers with different cut-off points
- *Two categories*—right and "non-right handers", which included all left and mixed handers, whereby the non-right-handed groups would consist of left handers and individuals with low degrees of handedness (Willems et al. 2014)
- *Two categories*—consistent and inconsistent handers, regardless of left or right (i.e. focusing on the degree rather than the direction)
- *Three categories*—right, left and mixed handers with different cut-off points

Apart from the poor comparability between studies, conclusions about handedness are problematic since we know that left and right handers show distinct differences and cannot be representative for all handedness groups. The same applies to the category of mixed handedness. Findings thus remain heterogeneous and opaque, once again, because clear definitions and parameters for categorising individuals with different degrees of handedness are lacking (Porac 2016).

5.4.1 Criteria for Analysing Research Methodologies on Mixed Handedness

Despite these problems, there is a proliferation of studies investigating mixed handedness, yielding results that contribute to our general understanding of the phenomenon. We will look at these studies more closely in terms of their measures, cut-off points and number of categories used to better understand these results. I reviewed 27 studies (see Table 5.2 citing the authors) addressing mixed handedness, using a number of criteria in the form of a checklist presented in Table 5.1.

Table 5.1 Checklist of criteria for research methodologies used in studies on mixed handedness

Categorisation: number of "mixed" groups:	☐ 1 ☐ 2 ☐ 3 ☐ 4 ☐ 5
What is the cut-off point for mixed handedness?	☐ 90% ☐ 80% ☐ 70% ☐ 60% ☐ 50%
Which dimension of handedness was recorded?	☐ Hand preference ☐ Hand performance ☐ Both
How was hand preference recorded?	QUESTIONNAIRE: ☐ Self-assessment ☐ Third-party assessment OBSERVATION-BASED: ☐ Performance ☐ Not at all
How many hand preference items were included?	☐ 1 ☐ 2–3 ☐ 4–5 ☐ 6–8 ☐ 9–10 ☐ 11–15 ☐ 16–20 ☐ 20+
If observation-based, how often was each item performed?	☐ 1x ☐ 2x ☐ 3x ☐ 4x ☐ Not at all/not applicable
Was there a mixture of skilled/unskilled as well as unimanual/bimanual items?	☐ YES ☐ PARTIALLY ☐ NO
Was midline crossing used as a method of assessment?	☐ YES ☐ NO
Which dimension of hand proficiency was recorded?	TRAINED: ☐ Dotting ☐ Tracing ☐ Other UNTRAINED: ☐ Tapping ☐ Pegboard tasks ☐ Hammering ☐ Bimanual circles ☐ Other
What procedures were used in general?	☐ Research-specific ☐ Generally standardised ☐ Standardised for: ○ age groups ○ left and right handed ○ dominant/non-dominant hand
How was proficiency measured?	☐ Speed ☐ Accuracy ☐ Other
What type of proficiency was assessed: unimanual or bimanual motor performance?	☐ Unimanual ☐ Bimanual ☐ Both

(continued)

Table 5.1 (continued)

Were hand preference and proficiency compared in the data analysis?	☐ YES ☐ PARTIALLY ☐ NO
Was background information (that may have influenced the formation of handedness) included in the assessment and analysis?	YES: ☐ *Left Handedness*/mixed handedness in the family ☐ Switched handedness ☐ Trauma to the dominant hand or side ☐ Unilateral head injury/surgery ☐ Risk factors (e.g. stress during childbirth? ☐ NO ☐ Other
What research design was used in the study assessing handedness?	☐ Experimental ☐ Pragmatic ☐ Case studies ☐ Survey ☐ Other
What kind of subjects were included?	☐ Toddlers ☐ Pre-scholars ☐ Primary school children ☐ Youth ☐ Grown-ups ☐ Typically developed individuals ☐ Persons with specific conditions ☐ Atypical/developmentally delayed
What number of subjects and type of recruitment were used?	☐ 1–20 ☐ 21–50 ☐ 61–100 ☐ 101–200 ☐ 201–500 ☐ 501–1000 ☐ 1000+ ☐ similar numbers of left, right and mixed handers ○ YES ○ NO ☐ Groups are of similar size ○ YES ○ NO ☐ Randomised recruitment ○YES ○NO

Fig. 5.1 Number of handedness groups in "mixed"-handedness studies ($N = 27$)

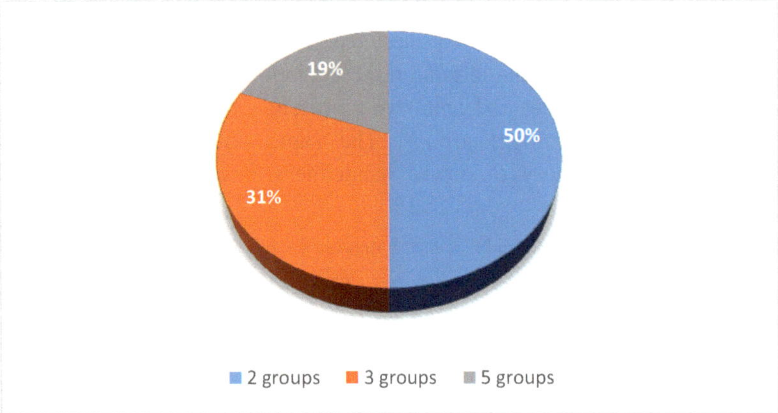

5.4.2 Results of Pilot Study Analysing Methodology of Studies on Mixed Handedness

The results of this pilot study are by no means representative or exhaustive, but they demonstrate tendencies in the methodology of mixed handedness. As shown in Fig. 5.1, 13 of the 27 studies examining mixed handedness defined binary categories comparing right handers with so-called non-right handers (which include left handers). Another eight studies defined three groups, left, right and mixed handers, of which only two specified the mixed-handedness categories in terms of criteria. In five studies, five categories were used: *strongly established left handers, strongly established right handers, left handers, right handers and mixed handers* (consisting of mildly established left and right handers). The binary categories usually consist of right handers and non-right handers. If there are odd numbers of categories, the middle category is usually denoted with a term for mixed handedness. In the case of even-numbered categories, the low-degree categories are often bundled as a mixed category in the data analyses.

In addition to the categories of handedness applied, we need to look at the type of assessment used and whether *preference* and/or *proficiency* were assessed. If it was hand preference, which items were included and how many of them? Were internal consistency and contralateral reaching measured, and was crossing the body midline involved? If *proficiency* was tested, what motor tasks were used (e.g. peg moving, tracing, tapping), and did measurements include accuracy *and* speed or just one of these parameters (see Fig. 6.2 in Chap. 6)? Table 5.2 summarises the number of handedness groups, type of test and

Table 5.2 Summary of relevant findings from 27 studies addressing mixed handedness

	Authors of the studies	Groups	Test	Type	No. of items; internal consistency
1	Glover et al. (2004)	5	Pref	TP-A	6–10; NO
2	Domellöf et al. (2009)	5	Pref	TP-A, S-A, Observation	11+; NO
3	Schiffman et al. (2005)	2	Pref	S-A	11+; NO
4	Oslejskova et al. (2007)	2	Pref	Not specified	Not specified
5	Rodriguez and Waldenström (2008)	3	Pref	TP-A	6–10; NO
6	Cantor et al. (2005)	2	Pref	S-A (EHI)	6–10; NO
7	Forrester et al. (2014)	3	Pref	TP-A, Observation	1–5; NO
8	Floris et al. (2013)	5	Pref	S-A (EHI)	6–10; NO
9	Mulvey et al. (2011)	2	Pref	TP-A	6–10; YES
10	Nicholls et al. (2010)	5	Pref and Prof	S-A	11+; NO
11	Denny and Zhang (2017)	3	Pref and Prof	TP-A	1–5; NO
12	Propper et al. (2004)	2	Pref	S-A (EHI)	6–10; NO
13	Kourtis et al. (2014)	2	Pref	S-A (EHI)	6–10; NO
14	Rodriguez et al. (2010)	3	Pref	TP-A	1–5; NO
15	Bruckner et al. (2011)	2	Pref	TP-A, Observation	11+, YES
16	Preti et al. (2008)	3	Pref	TP-A, S-A, Observation	11+; NO
17	Obel et al. (2003)	2	Pref	TP-A	1–5; NO
18	Vingerhoets and Sarrechia (2009)	3	Pref	S-A (EHI)	11+; NO
19	Davidson and Tremblay (2013)	3	Pref and Prof	S-A (EHI)	6–10; NO
20	Christman (2014)	2	Pref	S-A (EHI)	6–10; NO
21	Christman et al. (2009)	2	Pref	S-A (EHI)	6–10; NO
22	LaVoie et al. (2015)	2	Pref	S-A (EHI)	6–10; NO
23	Dellatolas et al. (1997)	5	Pref	Observation	6–10; NO
24	Fallow and Voyer (2013)	?	Pref	Not specified	11+; NO
25	Isaacs et al. (2006)	3	Pref	S-A (EHI)	6–10; NO
26	Kaploun and Abeare (2010)	2	Pref	S-A (EHI)	11+; NO
27	Newman et al. (2014)	2	Pref	S-A (EHI)	Not specified

Pref hand preference, *Prof* motor proficiency, *S-A* self-assessment, *EHI* Edinburgh Handedness Inventory, *TP-A* third-party assessment, *Observation* observed performance (preference)

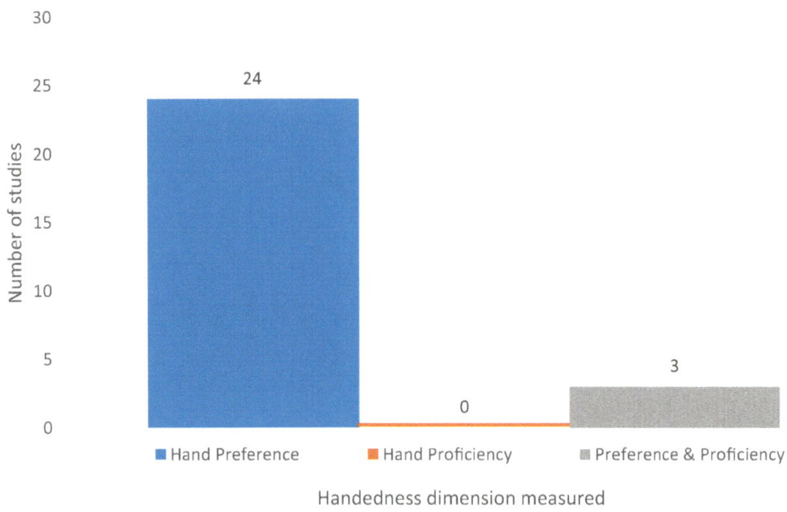

Fig. 5.2 Dimensions of handedness assessed in mixed studies ($N = 27$)

number of test items. Twenty-two studies used questionnaires on hand preference as their handedness measure. Ten of these were based on self-assessment and 12 on third-party assessments. The Edinburgh Handedness Inventory (EHI) was used 12 times. The remaining five studies used performance-based assessment of preference, and only two of these repeated items to measure the internal consistency of an activity.

Finally, it is noteworthy that 24 of the 27 studies used only the dimension of hand preference as a measure for handedness, as illustrated in Fig. 5.2. Different definitions of handedness further compounded this.

Overall, we can conclude from this pilot study that the methodology of many studies investigating mixed handedness tends to focus on the dimension of hand preference based on third-party or self-assessment, with an inclination to use 2–3-handedness categories. These somewhat reductionist methodologies cannot yield differentiated data on mixed handedness that display the multivariate and multidimensional nature of handedness.

Let us now look at the research findings of studies addressing mixed handedness. They can roughly be divided into those that evidence that reduced manual lateralisation is advantageous by finding associations with resources or talents, and others that find mixed handedness to be associated with disadvantages, problems or medical conditions.

5.5 Research Findings on Mixed Handedness

5.5.1 Mixed Handedness as an "Advantage"

The focus on degree, rather than direction, of handedness has emerged over the last years to be a predictor of ***cognitive performance*** (Prichard et al. 2013), particularly concerning the interaction of ***integrated dual processes***. It is postulated that consistent handers find it harder to integrate dual processes, whilst inconsistent (mixed) handers have difficulty separating independent dual processes (see Jasper et al. 2021).

In this regard, there is evidence that less established left and right handers appear to have ***more efficient interhemispheric communication*** (e.g. Davidson and Tremblay 2013). More specifically, the ability to test assumptions on a metacognitive level was investigated in individuals with high and mild degrees of hand proficiency. The mixed handers displayed a greater capacity for metacognition (Niebauer and Garvey 2004). Similar findings were generated by LaVoie and team who showed that right handers with a lower degree of handedness exhibited better ***word stem completions*** and thus presumably greater ***hemispheric interaction*** compared to individuals with high degrees of handedness (LaVoie et al. 2015). These findings are supported by the research of

Luders and colleagues, who showed that mixed (or inconsistent) handedness has been related to a ***larger corpus callosum***. It enables increased interhemispheric communication and integration, as seen when playing instruments that require the integration of right and left hands (e.g. Luders et al. 2010).

The studies examining cognitive flexibility, risk perception and episodic memory revealed correlations between lower degrees of handedness, particularly to right hemispheric processes (Prichard et al. 2013). Others confirmed these results: Greater ***cognitive flexibility*** also in relation to more so-called ***magical ideation*** was also found in mixed handers compared to explicit left and right handers (Badzakova-Trajkov et al. 2011). In terms of memory, mixed handers achieved better results on ***memory tasks*** that require ***interhemispheric communication,*** such as paired associate recall (Lyle and Orsborn 2011; Lyle et al. 2008). Also, they displayed better ***memory*** for the frequency of using one hand or the other in everyday unimanual tasks such as brushing one's teeth (Edlin et al. 2013). Looking more specifically at ***mathematical learning difficulties (MLD),*** Papadatou-Pastou and colleagues conducted a meta-analysis investigating the relationship between handedness and MLD. They did not detect a significant relationship between the two variables, and they concluded that the degree rather than the direction of handedness might yield more specific results (Papadatou-Pastou et al. 2021).

A range of other studies looked at factors such as social and musical abilities as well as motor learning. Denny and Zhang measured hand proficiency on a continuum in 7-, 11- and 16-year-old children and adolescents, together with ***social adaptability***. Whilst they found a correlation between "*non-Right Handedness*" and weak social adaptability in younger subjects, this was not the case in the oldest group: those children with smaller inter-hand differences for proficiency showed a greater social adjustment potential. The authors concluded that the degree rather than the direction of handedness is a significant factor (Denny and Zhang 2017). The competency of ***reading music*** requires high levels of musical ability and sophisticated interhemispheric communication. When correlating the ability to read music with a tapping test used to classify handedness, Kopiez and colleagues found a significantly high correlation between reading music and "*Non-Right Handedness*" (Kopiez and Lee 2006; Kopiez et al. 2006a, b). Finally, in a study, the extent of ***sequential motor learning*** and ***inter-manual transfer*** was researched in relation to degrees of handedness. Less strongly established left handers were better in inter-manual transfer in relation to *sensorimotor adaptation*, whilst less pronounced right handers showed a better inter-manual transfer of *sequential learning*. The results indicate that the involvement of the ipsilateral hemisphere during motor learning influences the extent of inter-manual transfer (Chase and Seidler 2008).

Importantly, many of these studies resulting in findings indicating positive attributes to mixed handers used *proficiency* tests rather than assessing hand preference handedness. This indicates the significance of the *type* of assessment used when assessing handedness (for more detail, see Chap. 6).

5.5.2 Mixed Handedness as a "Disadvantage"

Looking at specific problems rather than conditions, Vingerhoets and Sarrechia concluded that individuals with low degrees of handedness are more likely to have ***left-right confusion*** (Vingerhoets and Sarrechia 2009). Some authors found that mixed (left) handers seem to experience a much higher level of ***social anxiety*** than consistent (strongly established) left and right handers. This was seen especially when the results were combined with familial *Left Handedness* in close family members (Hardie et al. 2016; Yancosek 2010). Persons with low degrees of handedness may also present with ***decreased motor performance***, although not all research results support this proposition (e.g. Gabbard et al. 1993). Using a hand preference (pinboard) test, Gabbard and colleagues found that more consistent preschoolers showed greater

eye-hand coordination than the non-consistent ("ambidextrous") children. The authors concluded that this could be related to the corpus callosum development and the associated interhemispheric communication (ibid.). Based on a square checking task (proficiency), Denny demonstrated that 11-year-old children with the smallest inter-hand differences had the greatest problems in ***verbal, nonverbal*** and ***mathematical ability*** as well as ***reading comprehension*** (Denny 2008). Finally, in Austrian preschool children, a correlation between consistent hand use within an activity and high ***drawing skill*** could be demonstrated only in girls; this was not the case in mixed-handed children (Bruckner et al. 2011).

Focusing on specific medical conditions, a multitude of studies have been conducted, generating evidence for a correlation between mixed handedness and dysfunction or disorders. This has prompted some authors to suggest that these apparent disadvantages may be due to a lack of interhemispheric lateralisation and communication. Table 5.3 summarises some of the studies,

Table 5.3 Summary of literature listing disorders associated with mixed handedness

Condition	Authors and year	Key results and conclusions
Autism	Forrester et al. (2014)	4-year-old boys with autism are less lateralised than typically developed 4-year-old boys
	Floris et al. (2013)	Individuals tend to show right hemispheric lateralisation, but no functional mixed handedness[a]
	Soper and Satz (1984)	Mixed handedness is mainly seen in severely disabled people with autism
	Hauck and Dewey (2001)	Bilateral brain dysfunction is observed, which does not seem to be caused by motor dysfunction
	Markou et al. (2017)	Elevated levels of atypical handedness in individuals with ASD may be attributed to atypical cerebral structures and language lateralisation
Embryo-foetal alcohol syndrome (EFA)	Bookstein et al. (2002)	The corpus callosum is a neuroanatomical focus of foetal alcohol damage, and damage to the corpus callosum before birth persists into adulthood
	Ma et al. (2005)	Investigation of the formation of the corpus callosum found unilateral abnormalities
Prematurity	Marlow et al. (2019)	Although hand lateralisation increases with age, that preterm survivors are more likely to be left or mixed handed at the age of 19 years
Epilepsy	Lewin et al. (1993)	Increased ambidexterity and *Left Handedness* are found in people with epilepsy compared to control groups
	Oslejskova et al. (2007)	Decreased lateralisation and *Right Handedness* are found in 205 10-year-old boys
	Groen et al. (2008)	Low degree of handedness in children with Down syndrome correlates with language deficits
Intellectual disabilities	Papadatou-Pastou and Tomprou (2015)	Elevated levels of atypical handedness were in individuals with intellectual disabilities
Dyslexia	Eglinton and Annett (1994)	Whilst the prevalence of *Left Handedness* was consistent between persons with dyslexia and the control group, the number of mixed handedness doubled in the dyslexic group compared to the control group
ADHD	Rodriguez and Waldenström (2008)	"Ambidexterity" may be an indication of atypical brain laterality and increases the risk of ADHD symptoms in childhood
	Valera et al. (2007)	A meta-analysis of fMRI studies in people with ADHD reveals abnormalities in cerebral asymmetry and interhemispheric signals

Table 5.3 (continued)

Condition	Authors and year	Key results and conclusions
	Nastou et al. (2020)	Based on four meta-analyses, it was found that individuals with ADHD present with a higher incidence of mixed handedness (and not *Left Handedness*) compared to controls
	Peters et al. (2006)	A relationship was found between mixed handedness and increased levels of hyperactivity in a BBC internet study with 255,100 subjects
	Rodriguez et al. (2010)	Mixed-handed children were more likely to present with ADHD symptoms
	Lin and Tsuang (2018)	Mixed-handed individuals showed higher inattentiveness, but not impulsivity, than left and right handers
	Li et al. (2019)	Neuroimaging studies indicate that persons with ADHD display reduced hemispheric asymmetries
Schizophrenia	Dragovic and Hammond (2005)	Atypical hand dominance patterns were significantly greater in subjects with schizophrenia than in control subjects
	Sommer et al. (2001)	The prevalence of mixed and *Left Handedness* ("*non-Right Handedness*") was higher in individuals with Schizophrenia as compared to healthy controls
Antenatal depression	Rodriguez and Waldenström (2008)	Mixed handedness can be a consequence of maternal distress during pregnancy
	Brouwers et al. (2001)	Maternal distress during pregnancy negatively affects child development, including hand formation
Developmental coordination disorder	Goez and Zelnik (2008)	In this study, 13% of the children with DCD were classified as "ambidextrous", resulting in 44% "non-right handers"
	Armitage and Larkin (1993)	Investigating 5–6-year-old children, the authors found 30% to be mixed handed, and 35% in the 8–9-year-old group
	Darvik et al. (2018)	Based on a meta-review, the authors conclude that inconsistent handedness may be more problematic than consistent *Left Handedness* in individuals with DCD
	Lust et al. (2006)	Researchers found 30% of children to have mixed handedness, totalling 40% *non-Right Handedness*

[a] I use the term "mixed handedness" to be consistent with the book's terminology. Authors may have used different terms, such as ambidexterity, ambilaterality and inconsistent handedness.

whereby the distinction between mixed handedness, "*non-Right Handedness*" and "low-degree *Left Handedness*" is not clear and where these have been combined.

5.5.3 Dealing with Contradictory Results of Studies on Mixed Handedness

When we consider these studies with positive and negative attributes or conditions associated with mixed handedness, the results seem contradictory or remain inconclusive. There are four main clusters of possible explanations for this:

1. Depending on what is investigated, the degree of handedness might be advantageous or disadvantageous when performing a specific task, leading to seemingly contradictory results.
2. Using the degree of handedness as a sole indicator for abilities, problems and disorders may be misleading as additional factors are likely to influence and change the outcome.
3. There is a lack of incorporating aspects such as context and task requirements.
4. The diffuse definition and inconsistent categorisation, such as the frequently cited problems of a lack of uniform definition, classification and measurements, may lead to inconclusive results.

More specific research using multidimensional assessments and clearly defined handedness categories and incorporating *multivariate* factors influencing manual performance is required, allowing for the combination and interaction of different variables.

5.6 Proposing an Explanatory Model on Mixed Handedness (D-CC Hypothesis)

To apply a multivariate approach to mixed handedness as an example, the degrees of handedness could be combined with the extent of interhemispheric communication. As discussed in Chap. 2, the corpus callosum in particular is responsible for complex hemispheric interaction (van der Knaap and van der Ham 2011; Cowell and Gurd 2018). Various theories and models attempt to explain underlying neurophysiological processes and reduced lateralisation, such as hemispheric indecisiveness (e.g. Crow et al. 1998) or increased interhemispheric communication, probably due to a larger corpus callosum (e.g. LaVoie et al. 2015). This seems to support an association between *mild degrees of handedness* (mixed handedness) and *interhemispheric interaction*, particularly via the corpus callosum, prompting me to propose an explanatory model in this regard.

Hypothetically, considering the association between *mild degrees of handedness* and *interhemispheric interaction*, there could be (at least) two variations:

- Less lateralised individuals with *mild degrees* of handedness may have *ineffective interhemispheric communication*, which leads to (or coexists with) reduced lateralisation and specialisation of the hemispheres.
- Less lateralised individuals with *mild degrees* of handedness may have a *highly effective interhemispheric interaction* with clear specialisation processes on both sides. This, in turn, may be related to task demands and other contextual factors.

At the level of hemispheric lateralisation, I distinguish between a strong degree (D++) and a mild degree (D−−) of handedness. Since we cannot observe hemispheric processes directly without access to MRI technology, we need to infer them by choosing observable parameters at performance level, as demonstrated by hand preference and proficiency measures. Here we could look at *consistency* within and across unimanual and bimanual tasks[6] in hand preference and proficiency items to behaviourally measure the extent of manual (and indirectly, hemispheric) lateralisation. In addition, I differentiate between a well-functioning and highly effective corpus callosum (CC++) and a suboptimally functioning and less effective one (CC−−) at a **neuro-anatomical level**. Similarly, this could be observed at a behavioural level using simultaneous *bimanual motor tasks*. These require interhemispheric communication and therefore reflect the activity of the corpus callosum. Finally, as a measure, using laterality quotients to quantify both preference and proficiency, *inter-hand differences* (IHD) can be demonstrated.

Using these three measures in relation to degrees of handedness and callosal communication, the combination of these factors, although somewhat reductionist and even over simplistic could hypothetically explain some of the contradictory results found in mixed-handedness research (see Fig. 5.3).

- **D++ CC++** *(top-left quadrant):* If the degree of handedness is strong (D++) and the corpus callosum is efficient (CC++), then it is reasonable to assume that the IHD in the preference tasks is consistent (consistency ↑) as well as high (preference IHD ↑). The hands, however, do not differ significantly with respect to proficiency (proficiency IHD ↑) because the non-dominant hand is also very good. Bimanual coordination would be good since the non-dominant hand works effectively with the non-dominant hand, and there is a clear division of roles (BMK ☺).
- **D−− CC++** *(top-right quadrant):* If the degree of handedness is mild (D−−) and the corpus

[6] We will not differentiate between ♦**internal and external consistency** in the context of this hypothesis and to keep it simple. It would, however, be an important differentiation to make if research were to investigate such a relationship.

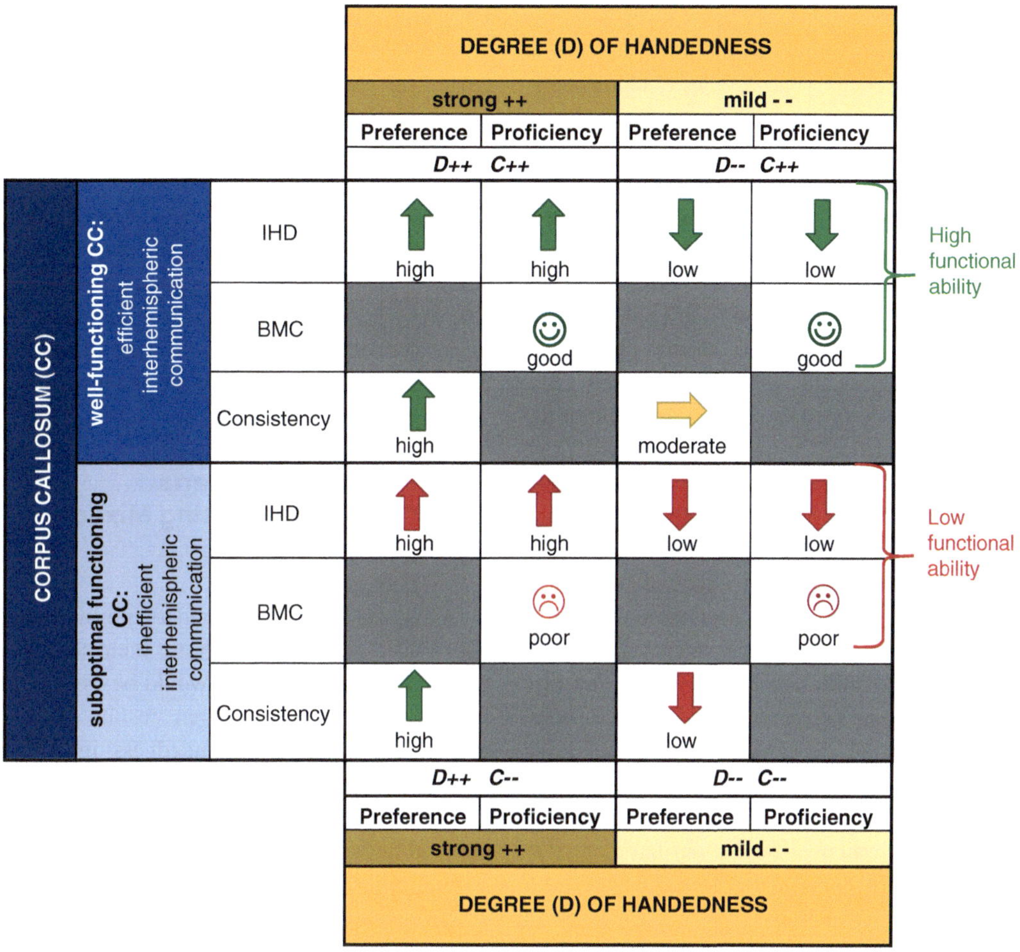

Fig. 5.3 D-CC Hypothesis: Comparison of high and low of degrees of handedness (preference and proficiency) with interhemispheric communication via the corpus callosum. *IHD* inter-hand differences as a behavioural measure for degrees of handedness, *BMC* bimanual cooperation as a behavioural measure for interhemispheric communication, *D* degree

callosum efficient (CC++), the consistency is moderate at best (consistency →); it can be expected that the inter-hand differences will be low (preference IHD ↓, proficiency IHD ↓). Bimanual motor performance would be good (BMK ☺) since both hands are similarly skilled, even though the role division between the hands might not be very consistent.

- **D++ CC−−** *(bottom-left quadrant)*: In the case of a strong degree of handedness (D++) combined with an inefficient corpus callosum (CC−−), the consistency is likely to be high (consistency ↑), as are the inter-hand differences (preference IHD ↑, proficiency IHD ↑) as well as constancy. Bimanual cooperation, however, would be poor (BMK ☹) because, despite good proficiency on each side in unimanual tasks, the hands do not have clear role division and do not work well together.
- **D−− CC−−** *(bottom-right quadrant)*: If the degree of handedness is mild (D−−) and the corpus callosum is inefficient (CC−−), the consistency would be low (consistency ↓) and the inter-hand differences would be small and likely to be poor (preference IHD ↓, proficiency IHD ↓) because of poor lateralisation and interhemispheric communication. Bimanual coordination would be weak, both because proficiency is poor and there is poor division of roles between the hands (BMK ☹), making both hands similarly clumsy.

I hypothesise that different combinations of interhemispheric communication levels (as seen in bimanual cooperation) and degrees of hemispheric lateralisation (as seen in the degree of handedness) may result in a heterogeneous group of mixed handers yielding contradictory results. For example, there are people with good bimanual coordination and large inter-hand differences (strong handedness degree), and there are well-coordinated people with small inter-hand differences (mild handedness degree). Likewise, people with coordination problems could have large or small inter-hand differences. Possibly, the combination of the degree of handedness (representing the extent of hemispheric lateralisation) and bimanual motor performance (representing the efficiency of the corpus callosum) could help us differentiate between different types of mixed handers. Clearly, this D-CC hypothesis would need to be verified.

Other factors, such as environmental influences, inherent motor ability and task demands, are also likely to influence lateralisation and corpus callosal activity. Therefore, background information would also be necessary to contextualise an individual's handedness. For example, some individuals may show variable hand use because they have a moderate handedness degree and are ***converted left handers***. So, they might use their non-dominant right hand for writing but perform many other activities with their dominant left hand (see Sect. 4.5). Another reason for mixed handedness might be ***developmental delay***, retarding also the development of lateralisation and handedness (see Sect. 3.6) since the neurophysiological basis for preferred and more proficient hand use is insufficient. Alternatively, individuals that suffered damages before, at or after birth affecting their inherent dominant hand may develop better proficiency on the non-dominant side (so-called ***pathological handedness***—see Sect. 4.4). However, if the handedness degree is high, they may still use their dominant hand for spontaneous and less demanding actions, thereby also showing variable hand use. Finally, the cause for mixed hand use could simply be a ***low degree*** of handedness, as is apparent particularly in a group of left handers (see Sect. 4.6), or it could indeed be part of the symptomology of certain ***medical conditions***.

Without this contextual information, individuals with fundamentally different causes for their presenting mixed handedness would likely be lumped together in a "mixed" group in research. This background information is critical for a practice-based approach where children frequently present with mixed handedness and the writing hand is not clear. Having a basic understanding of what specific manual behaviours could indicate may be very useful for initial screening. For this purpose, I compiled a set of questions to be used by therapists, educators and other professionals working with younger children, based on a number of criteria to help differentiate between various groups of "mixed" handedness.

5.7 Compiling Criteria for Differentiating Mixed Handedness

As we have seen, mixed handers are individuals with variable hand use who use their non-dominant hand more often than would be expected or considered typical. Research results reveal a broad category of mixed handedness: individuals with differing degrees of handedness, different birth conditions, environmental influences, pathological impact, medical conditions and potential for brain plasticity. So specifically, mixed handedness may include individuals with

- Mild handedness degree
- Converted *Left* and *Right Handedness*
- Developmental delay
- Pathological handedness
- Certain medical conditions or disorders

If we want to investigate mixed handedness in more detail and correlate it to various attributes, characteristics and abilities, we need to differentiate between these different *types* of mixed handedness. Also, more applied research is required to consider all these complex aspects to better understand the variability handedness.

We also need to look at what aspects of handedness are assessed. As we saw in Chap. 1, proficiency and preference have been shown to be different variations of handedness, with hand preference as a J-shaped distribution and proficiency as a bell-shaped distribution (see Fig. 1.2). In regard to mixed handedness, studies have indicated that proficiency measures appear to be more sensitive for this group than preference measures. Williams thus recommends that proficiency rather than preference be used to assess handedness (Williams 1991, 2022). This seems viable since even if mixed handers show little difference in preferred hand use between the hands, they are likely to have a (slightly) better hand.

In everyday life, many parents, teachers, therapists and other professionals are confronted with mixed-handed children but are most often not linked to the scientific community generating relevant insights on handedness. For this purpose, I constructed a summary based on the literature as well as on my own research and clinical experience, in the form of a checklist, posing questions, providing examples and linking this to relevant research findings. This can be a first step in an attempt to differentiate between different forms of mixed handedness (see Table 5.4).

Table 5.4 Proposing criteria for differentiating aspects related to mixed handedness

Criterion	Questions	Example if applicable	Knowledge from research
Consistence	*Is hand use within activities consistent (constant)?*	**YES:** Always paints and cuts with the right, but always throws with left	Inconsistent hand use within the same activity may be indicative of disorders (e.g. Crow et al. 1998)
Degree of handedness	*Is the non-dominant hand used for many activities?*	**YES:** Ball throwing with right and writing with left	Studies come to very different conclusions about the extent to which a low degree of handedness is disadvantageous or advantageous (e.g. Denny and O'Sullivan 2007)
Inheritance, genetic predisposition	*Are there other family members with mixed handedness in the immediate family or extended family circle?*	**YES:** Mother, father or siblings (immediate); or cousin, aunt, uncle, grandparents (extended)	The degree of handedness in individuals with *Left Handedness* in their immediate family tend to be less pronounced. This is also the case with extended family, but to a lesser extent (e.g. Bryden 1987)
	Are there any left-handed people in the immediate or extended family?	**YES:** Mother, father or siblings (close); or cousin, aunt, uncle, grandparents (far)	
Proficiency	*Do both hands perform equally well?* *OR*	**YES:** Ambidextrous: performs highly skilled activities such as drawing and writing equally well with either hand with high proficiency	Very rare. Also associated with disease patterns, but the definition remains inconsistent (e.g. McKeever and VanDeventer 1977)
	Do both hands perform equally poorly?	**YES:** Both hands perform below average in proficiency (tasks requiring speed and accuracy)	Developmentally delayed and motor-deficient individuals show below-average performance on both sides without one hand being significantly better than the other (e.g. Bishop 1990a, b) Diffuse distribution of different components on both sides is a typical feature in developmentally delayed children (e.g. Rodriguez et al. 2010)
	Is one hand performing significantly poorer than the other hand?	**YES:** The "weaker" hand has motor abnormalities; there is evidence of birth stress	Typical of pathological left handers (e.g. Soper and Satz 1984)
	Are certain motor components of motor skills evident on both sides?	**YES:** There are different levels of proprioception, coordination, speed, accuracy, movement fluidity	Diffuse distribution of different components on both sides is a typical feature in developmentally delayed children (e.g. Hauck and Dewey 2001)

(continued)

Table 5.4 (continued)

Criterion	Questions	Example if applicable	Knowledge from research
Preference vs. proficiency	*Is there a mismatch between preference and proficiency?*	**YES:** The one hand is used in many tasks, but proficiency is better on the other hand	This is not uncommon in research, especially for left handers (e.g. Peters 1990)
Crossing the body midline	*Is there an avoidance to cross the body midline*?	**YES:** Picks up items with the left hand on the left side and items on the right side with the right hand	Avoidance of midline crossing is an indication of developmental delay (e.g. Surburg 1999). Usually, individuals cross more with their dominant hand (e.g. Surburg 1999; Carlier et al. 2006)
Converted (switched) handedness	*Is there evidence of converted (switched) handedness in the history/background of the affected individual?*	**YES:** Often, trained activities such as writing and eating are performed with the right hand, and untrained activities are performed with the left hand	Conversion still takes place today and can be more or less "successful" (e.g. Porac 2009)
	Are the typically trained activities performed with the right and the spontaneous activities with the left?	**YES:** Trained activities, such as brushing teeth and writing, are repeatedly demonstrated by others and then practised with the right hand	Switching often affects only certain activities, such as writing, leaving other actions to the left (e.g. Searleman and Porac 2001)
Swapping-hands behaviour	*Is there a particular direction of changing hand use that can be observed?*	**YES:** The left hand starts an activity and then changes it to the right hand (or vice versa)	It could be that the preference is left, but the performance is better on the right (observation from practice) (e.g. Scharoun and Bryden 2014)
	Is the variable hand use related to the task demands and characteristics?	**YES**: Demanding vs. simple actions; practised vs. spontaneous/unpractised activities; trained vs. untrained activities; gross proximal vs. fine distal movements; unimanual vs. bimanual executions	The characteristics of an activity influencing its performance (e.g. (Steenhuis and Bryden 1989). For example, demanding, fine and distal activities are more lateralised (ibid.). Bimanual movements require more complex engagement with the dominant hand (e.g. Fagard and Corroyer 2003)
Disorder or clinical condition	*Is there a developmental disorder or medical condition associated with decreased laterality?*	**YES:** Schizophrenia, learning disorders, autism spectrum disorder, Down syndrome	These clinical conditions have been associated with "ambidexterity" or mixed handedness (e.g. Hauck and Dewey 2001), with swapping hands within an activity being most associated with abnormalities (e.g. Bishop 1990a)

I have compiled these criteria into a checklist using similar questions to be used by kindergarten teachers, schoolteachers, therapists and other professionals working with younger children. It seeks to not only impart important knowledge from the literature but also support a systematic and differentiated procedure when deciding whether a child displays normal variability or atypical handedness. In this regard, the checklist has been reported to be a very useful screening tool.

5.8 Concluding Remarks

This chapter focused on variable hand use, combined under the fabricated term "mixed handedness". Research findings by and large remain inconclusive and diverse, not least because of limited comparability between studies, the one-sided measures used and the focus on hand preference or proficiency rather than handedness with several dimensions. As can be expected, the problems we saw in the *Left-Handedness* research are actually exacerbated in studies on mixed handedness since its members are often even more diverse, undefined and under-researched.

As argued at the beginning of the chapter, mixed handedness is a fabricated rather than a true handedness group, consisting of all those individuals that do not display consistent hand use. Considering that it is left handers (and not right handers) who show a very wide range of manual variability, it seems rather likely that a portion of so-called mixed handers are indeed left handers with a (very) mild degree who, in addition, may have switched handedness due to the right-biassed environment. The need for a clear differentiation between various handedness groups becomes pertinent and a prerequisite for conducting research in this area. Finally, it is important for both research and clinical practice not to focus only on the direction and/or degree of handedness, but to treat handedness as the *polygenetic* and *multidimensional* phenomenon that it has been found to be. This should then be related to the individual's unique constellation of *multivariate* influences.

This chapter concludes the first part of the book, focusing on handedness research and theories in our quest to address some of the questions raised. I will reflect on the first five chapters in a synopsis following this chapter. The second part of the book attempts to incorporate the relevant findings on measuring and capturing handedness in all its dimensions.

References

Armitage M, Larkin D (1993) Laterality, motor asymmetry and clumsiness in children. Hum Mov Sci 12(1–2):155–177

Badzakova-Trajkov G, Häberling IS, Corballis MC (2011) Magical ideation, creativity, handedness, and cerebral asymmetries: a combined behavioural and fMRI study. Neuropsychologia 49(10):2896–2903

Bishop DV (1990a) Handedness, clumsiness and developmental language disorders. Neuropsychologia 28(7):681–690. https://doi.org/10.1016/0028-3932(90)90123-6

Bishop DVM (1990b) Handedness and developmental disorders. Mac Keith Press, Oxford; J.B. Lippincott (Clinics in developmental medicine, 110)

Bookstein FL, Sampson PD, Connor PD, Streissguth AP (2002) Midline corpus callosum is a neuroanatomical focus of fetal alcohol damage. Anat Rec 269(3):162–174. https://doi.org/10.1002/ar.10110

Brouwers EPM, van Baar AL, Pop VJM (2001) Does the Edinburgh postnatal depression scale measure anxiety? J Psychosom Res 51(5):659–663

Bruckert L, Thompson PA, Watkins KE, Bishop DVM, Woodhead ZVJ (2021) Investigating the effects of handedness on the consistency of lateralization for speech production and semantic processing tasks using functional transcranial Doppler sonography. Laterality 26(6):680–705. https://doi.org/10.1080/1357650X.2021.1898416

Bruckner J, Kastner-Koller U, Deimann P, Voracek M (2011) Drawing and handedness of Preschoolers: a repeated-measurement approach to hand preference. Percept Mot Skills 112(1):258–266. https://doi.org/10.2466/04.10.PMS.112.1.258-266

Bryden MP (1977) Measuring handedness with questionnaires. Neuropsychologia 15:617–628

Bryden MP (1987) Handedness and cerebral organization: data from clinical and normal populations. In: Duality and unity of the brain. Springer, pp 55–70

Cantor JM, Klassen PE, Dickey R, Christensen BK, Kuban ME, Blak T et al (2005) Handedness in pedophilia and hebephilia. Arch Sex Behav 34(4):447–459

Capacchione L (2019) The power of your other hand. Unlock creativity and inner wisdom through the right side of your brain. Conari Press, Newburyport

Carlier M, Doyen A-L, Lamard C (2006) Midline crossing: developmental trend from 3 to 10 years of age in a preferential card-reaching task. Brain Cogn 61(3):255–261. https://doi.org/10.1016/j.bandc.2006.01.007

Chase C, Seidler R (2008) Degree of handedness affects intermanual transfer of skill learning. Exp Brain Res 190(3):317–328. https://doi.org/10.1007/s00221-008-1472-z

Christman S (2014) Individual differences in personality as a function of degree of handedness: consistent-handers are less sensation seeking, more authoritarian, and more sensitive to disgust. Laterality 19(3):354–367. https://doi.org/10.1080/1357650X.2013.838962

Christman SD, Butler M (2011) Mixed-handedness advantages in episodic memory obtained under conditions of intentional learning extend to incidental learning. Brain Cogn 77(1):17–22. https://doi.org/10.1016/j.bandc.2011.07.003

Christman SD, Sontam V, Jasper JD (2009) Individual differences in ambiguous-figure perception: degree of handedness and interhemispheric interaction. Perception 38(8):1183–1198. https://doi.org/10.1068/p6131

Collins RL (1985) On the inheritance of direction and degree of asymmetry. In: Cerebral lateralization in nonhuman species, pp 41–71

Corballis MC (1997) The genetics and evolution of handedness. Psychol Rev 104(4):714

Corballis MC, Hattie J, Fletcher R (2008) Handedness and intellectual achievement: an even-handed look. Neuropsychologia 46(1):374–378

Corbetta D, Williams J, Snapp-Childs W (2006) Plasticity in the development of handedness: evidence from normal development and early asymmetric brain injury. Dev Psychobiol 48(6):460–471. https://doi.org/10.1002/dev.20164

Cowell P, Gurd J (2018) Handedness and the corpus callosum: a review and further analyses of discordant twins. Neuroscience 388:57–68

Crow TJ, Crow LR, Done DJ, Leask S (1998) Relative hand skill predicts academic ability: global deficits at the point of hemispheric indecision. Neuropsychologia 36(12):1275–1282. https://doi.org/10.1016/S0028-3932(98)00039-6

Darvik M, Lorås H, Pedersen AV (2018) The prevalence of left-handedness is higher among individuals with developmental coordination disorder than in the general population. Front Psychol 9:1948. https://doi.org/10.3389/fpsyg.2018.01948

Davidson T, Tremblay F (2013) Hemispheric differences in corticospinal excitability and in transcallosal inhibition in relation to degree of handedness. PLoS One 8(7):e70286. https://doi.org/10.1371/journal.pone.0070286

Dellatolas G, Tubert-Bitter P, Curt F (1997) Evolution of degree and direction of hand preference in children: methodological and theoretical issues. Neuropsychol Rehabil 7(4):387–400

Denny K (2008) Cognitive ability and continuous measures of relative hand skill: a note. Neuropsychologia 46(7):2091–2094. https://doi.org/10.1016/j.neuropsychologia.2008.02.004

Denny K, O'Sullivan V (2007) The economic consequences of being left-handed some sinister results. J Hum Resourc 42(2):353–374

Denny K, Zhang W (2017) In praise of ambidexterity: how a continuum of handedness predicts social adjustment. Laterality 22(2):181–194. https://doi.org/10.1080/1357650X.2016.1153107

Domellöf E, Rönnqvist L, Titran M, Esseily R, Fagard J (2009) Atypical functional lateralization in children with fetal alcohol syndrome. Dev Psychobiol 51(8):696–705

Dragovic M, Hammond G (2005) Handedness in schizophrenia: a quantitative review of evidence. Acta Psychiatr Scand 111(6):410–419

Edlin JM, Carris EK, Lyle KB (2013) Memory for hand-use depends on consistency of handedness. Front Hum Neurosci 7:555

Eglinton E, Annett M (1994) Handedness and dyslexia: a meta-analysis. Percept Mot Skills 79(3 Pt 2):1611–1616. https://doi.org/10.2466/pms.1994.79.3f.1611

Elneel FHF, Carter F, Tang B, Cuschieri A (2008) Extent of innate dexterity and ambidexterity across handedness and gender: implications for training in laparoscopic surgery. Surg Endosc 22(1):31–37. https://doi.org/10.1007/s00464-007-9533-0

Fagard J, Corroyer D (2003) Using a continuous index of laterality to determine how laterality is related to interhemispheric transfer and bimanual coordination in children. Dev Psychobiol 43(1):44–56. https://doi.org/10.1002/dev.10117

Fallow KM, Voyer D (2013) Degree of handedness, emotion, and the perceived duration of auditory stimuli. Laterality 18(6):671–692. https://doi.org/10.1080/1357650X.2012.742533

Floris DL, Chura LR, Holt RJ, Suckling J, Bullmore ET, Baron-Cohen S, Spencer MD (2013) Psychological correlates of handedness and corpus callosum asymmetry in autism: the left hemisphere dysfunction theory revisited. J Autism Dev Disord 43(8):1758–1772. https://doi.org/10.1007/s10803-012-1720-8

Forrester GS, Pegler R, Thomas MSC, Mareschal D (2014) Handedness as a marker of cerebral lateralization in children with and without autism. Behav Brain Res 268(6):14–21. https://doi.org/10.1016/j.bbr.2014.03.040

Gabbard C, Hart S, Kanipe D (1993) Hand preference consistency and fine motor performance in young children. Cortex 29(4):749–753. https://doi.org/10.1016/s0010-9452(13)80295-x

Glover V, O'Connor TG, Heron J, Golding J, ALSPAC Study Team (2004) Antenatal maternal anxiety is linked with atypical handedness in the child. Early Hum Dev 79(2):107–118

Goez H, Zelnik N (2008) Handedness in patients with developmental coordination disorder. J Child Neurol 23(2):151–154. https://doi.org/10.1177/0883073807307978

Groen MA, Yasin I, Laws G, Barry JG, Bishop DVM (2008) Weak hand preference in children with down syndrome is associated with language deficits. Dev Psychobiol 50(3):242–250. https://doi.org/10.1002/dev.20291

Hardie SM, Wright L, Clark L (2016) Handedness and social anxiety: using Bryden's research as a catalyst to explore the influence of familial sinistrality and degree of handedness. Laterality 21(4–6):329–347. https://doi.org/10.1080/1357650X.2015.1131712

Hauck JA, Dewey D (2001) Hand preference and motor functioning in children with autism. J Autism Dev Disord 31(3):265–277. https://doi.org/10.1023/a:1010791118978

Hellige, J. B. (2010): Hemispheric specialisation: language, space and sexual differentiation. In: George F. Koob, Michel Le Moal & Richard F. Thompson (Hg.): Encyclopedia of behavioral neuroscience. Burlington: Elsevier Science, 21–26

Hildreth G (1949) The development and training of hand dominance; characteristics of handedness. J Genet Psychol 75(2):197–220. https://doi.org/10.1080/08856559.1949.10533517

Humphrey ME (1951) Consistency of hand usage: a preliminary enquiry. Br J Educ Psychol 21(3):214–225

Isaacs KL, Barr WB, Nelson PK, Devinsky O (2006) Degree of handedness and cerebral dominance. Neurology 66(12):1855–1858. https://doi.org/10.1212/01.wnl.0000219623.28769.74

Jackson J (1905) Ambidexterity. or two-handedness and two-brainedness. Bibliolife

Jasper JD, Christman SD, Clarkson E (2021) Predicting interactions in handedness research: the role of integrated versus independent dual-processes. Laterality

26(6):607–623. https://doi.org/10.1080/1357650X.2021.1879110
Kagerer FA (2015) Control of discrete bimanual movements: how each hand benefits from the other. Neurosci Lett 584(Pt 7):33–38. https://doi.org/10.1016/j.neulet.2014.10.002
Kaploun KA, Abeare CA (2010) Degree versus direction: a comparison of four handedness classification schemes through the investigation of lateralised semantic priming. Laterality 15(5):481–500
Kastner-Koller U, Deimann P, Bruckner J (2007) Assessing handedness in preschoolers: construction and initial validation of a hand preference test for 4-6-year-olds. Psychol Sci 49(3):239–254
Kopiez R, Lee JI (2006) Towards a dynamic model of skills involved in sight reading music. Music Educ Res 8(1):97–120
Kopiez R, Galley N, Lee JI (2006a) The advantage of a decreasing right-hand superiority: the influence of laterality on a selected musical skill (sight reading achievement). Neuropsychologia 44(7):1079–1087
Kopiez R, Weihs C, Ligges U, Lee JI (2006b) Classification of high and low achievers in a music sight-reading task. Psychol Music 34(1):5–26
Kourtis D, de Saedeleer L, Vingerhoets G (2014) Handedness consistency influences bimanual coordination: a behavioural and electrophysiological investigation. Neuropsychologia 58:81–87. https://doi.org/10.1016/j.neuropsychologia.2014.04.002
Kraus E (2003) The handedness profile. The development of a normative profile to determine the extent of handedness in children. Doctoral thesis. La Trobe University, Melbourne
Kraus E (Hg.) (2019) Zwischen Links-& Rechtshändigkeit. Theorie, Diagnostik & Therapie bei Kindern mit wechselndem Handgebrauch. Springer, Berlin
Kuypers HGJM (1982) A new look at the organization of the motor system. Prog Brain Res 57:381–403
LaVoie DJ, Olbinski B, Palmer S (2015) Degree of handedness and priming: further evidence for a distinction between production and identification priming mechanisms. Front Psychol 6:128. https://doi.org/10.3389/fpsyg.2015.00151
Lewin J, Kohen D, Mathew G (1993) Handedness in mental handicap: investigation into populations of Down's syndrome, epilepsy and autism. Br J Psychiatry 163:674–676. https://doi.org/10.1192/bjp.163.5.674
Li D, Li T, Niu Y, Xiang J, Cao R, Liu BO et al (2019) Reduced hemispheric asymmetry of brain anatomical networks in attention deficit hyperactivity disorder. Brain Imaging Behav 13(3):669–684
Lin H-L, Tsuang H-C (2018) Handedness and attention deficit/hyperactivity disorder symptoms in college students. Psychiatry Q 89(1):103–110. https://doi.org/10.1007/s11126-017-9517-8
Luders E, Cherbuin N, Thompson PM, Gutman B, Anstey KJ, Sachdev P, Toga AW (2010) When more is less: associations between corpus callosum size and handedness lateralization. Neuroimage 52(1):43–49. https://doi.org/10.1016/j.neuroimage.2010.04.016
Lust JM, Geuze RH, Wijers AA, Wilson PH (2006) An EEG study of mental rotation-related negativity in children with developmental coordination disorder. Child Care Health Dev 32(6):649
Lyle KB, Orsborn AE (2011) Inconsistent handedness and saccade execution benefit face memory without affecting interhemispheric interaction. Memory 19(6):613–624
Lyle KB, McCabe DP, Roediger III, Henry L (2008) Handedness is related to memory via hemispheric interaction: evidence from paired associate recall and source memory tasks. Neuropsychology 22(4):523
Ma X, Coles CD, Lynch ME, Laconte SM, Zurkiya O, Wang D, Hu X (2005) Evaluation of corpus callosum anisotropy in young adults with fetal alcohol syndrome according to diffusion tensor imaging. Alcohol Clin Exp Res 29(7):1214–1222
Markou P, Ahtam B, Papadatou-Pastou M (2017) Elevated levels of atypical handedness in autism: meta-analyses. Neuropsychol Rev 27(3):258–283
Marlow N, Ni Y, Beckmann J, O'Reilly H, Johnson S, Wolke D, Morris JK (2019) Hand preference develops across childhood and adolescence in extremely preterm children: the EPICure study. Pediatr Neurol 99:40–46. https://doi.org/10.1016/j.pediatrneurol.2019.04.007
McKeever WF, VanDeventer AD (1977) Familial sinistrality and degree of left-handedness. Br J Psychol 68(4):469–471. https://doi.org/10.1111/j.2044-8295.1977.tb01616.x
Michel GF (2021) Handedness development: a model for investigating the development of hemispheric specialization and interhemispheric coordination. Symmetry 13(6):992
Moynihan JB, Breathnach CS (1995) A survey of manual preference, skill and strength in undergraduates. Irish J Psychol Med 12(4):127–131
Mulvey GM, Ringenbach SDR, Jung ML (2011) Reversal of handedness effects on bimanual coordination in adults with Down syndrome. J Intellect Disabil Res 55(10):998–1007
Nastou E, Ocklenburg S, Papadatou-Pastou M (2020) Handedness in ADHD: meta-analyses
Newman S, Malaia E, Seo R (2014) Does degree of handedness in a group of right-handed individuals affect language comprehension? Brain Cogn 86:98–103
Nicholls MER, Chapman HL, Loetscher T, Grimshaw GM (2010) The relationship between hand preference, hand performance, and general cognitive ability. J Int Neuropsychol Soc 16(4):585–592
Niebauer CL, Garvey K (2004) Godel, Escher, and degree of handedness: differences in interhemispheric interaction predict differences in understanding self-reference. Laterality 9(1):19–34. https://doi.org/10.1080/13576500342000130
Obel C, Hedegaard M, Henriksen TB, Secher NJ, Olsen J (2003) Psychological factors in pregnancy and mixed-handedness in the offspring. Dev Med Child Neurol 45(8):557–561. https://doi.org/10.1017/s0012162203001014
Oslejskova H, Dusek L, Makovska Z, Rektor I (2007) Epilepsia, epileptiform abnormalities, non-right-

handedness, hypotonia and severe decreased IQ are associated with language impairment in autism. Epileptic Disord 9 Suppl 1:S9–S18. https://doi.org/10.1684/epd.2007.0154

Papadatou-Pastou M, Tomprou D-M (2015) Intelligence and handedness: meta-analyses of studies on intellectually disabled, typically developing, and gifted individuals. Neurosci Biobehav Rev 56:151–165

Papadatou-Pastou M, Panagiotidou DA, Abbondanza F, Fischer U, Paracchini S, Karagiannakis G (2021) Hand preference and mathematical learning difficulties: new data from Greece, the United Kingdom, and Germany and two meta-analyses of the literature. Laterality 26(5):485–538. https://doi.org/10.31234/osf.io/pc6zh

Peters M (1990) Subclassification of non-pathological left-handers poses problems for theories of handedness. Neuropsychologia 28(3):279–289. https://doi.org/10.1016/0028-3932(90)90021-f

Peters M, Reimers S, Manning JT (2006) Hand preference for writing and associations with selected demographic and behavioral variables in 255,100 subjects: the BBC internet study. Brain Cogn 62(2):177–189. https://doi.org/10.1016/j.bandc.2006.04.005

Porac C (2009) Hand preference and skilled hand performance among individuals with successful rightward conversions of the writing hand. Laterality 14(2):105–121. https://doi.org/10.1080/13576500802299418

Porac C (2016) Laterality. Exploring the enigma of left-handedness. Elsevier Science, Amsterdam. http://www.sciencedirect.com/science/book/9780128012390

Preti A, Lai A, Serra M, Zurrida GG (2008) Mixed handedness prevails among children and adolescents with infantile asthma and diabetes. Pediatr Allergy Immunol 19(8):769–772. https://doi.org/10.1111/j.1399-3038.2007.00703.x

Prichard E, Propper RE, Christman SD (2013) Degree of handedness, but not direction, is a systematic predictor of cognitive performance. Front Psychol 4:9. https://doi.org/10.3389/fpsyg.2013.00009

Propper RE, Lawton N, Przyborski M, Christman SD (2004) An assessment of sleep architecture as a function of degree of handedness in college women using a home sleep monitor. Brain Cogn 54(3):186–197. https://doi.org/10.1016/j.bandc.2004.01.004

Rodriguez A, Waldenström U (2008) Fetal origins of child non-right-handedness and mental health. J Child Psychol Psychiatry 49(9):967–976. https://doi.org/10.1111/j.1469-7610.2008.01923.x

Rodriguez A, Kaakinen M, Moilanen I, Taanila A, McGough JJ, Loo S, Jarvelin M-R (2010) Mixed-handedness is linked to mental health problems in children and adolescents. Pediatrics 125(2):e340–e348. https://doi.org/10.1542/peds.2009-1165

Scharoun SM, Bryden PJ (2014) Hand preference, performance abilities, and hand selection in children. Front Psychol 5:82. https://doi.org/10.3389/fpsyg.2014.00082

Schiffman J, Pestle S, Mednick S, Ekstrom M, Sorensen H, Mednick S (2005) Childhood laterality and adult schizophrenia spectrum disorders: a prospective investigation. Schizophr Res 72(2–3):151–160. https://doi.org/10.1016/j.schres.2004.04.003

Schlaak H (2019) Self-experiment two-handedness. Success with right and left. Tredition, Hamburg

Searleman A, Porac C (2001) Lateral preference patterns as possible correlates of successfully switched left hand writing: data and a theory. Laterality 6(4):303–314

Somers M, Sommer IE, Boks MP, Kahn RS (2009) Hand-preference and population schizotypy: a meta-analysis. Schizophr Res 108(1–3):25–32

Sommer I, Ramsey N, Kahn R, Aleman A, Bouma A (2001) Handedness, language lateralisation and anatomical asymmetry in schizophrenia: meta-analysis. Br J Psychiatry 178:344–351. https://doi.org/10.1192/bjp.178.4.344

Soper HV, Satz P (1984) Pathological left-handedness and ambiguous handedness: a new explanatory model. Neuropsychologia 22(4):511–515. https://doi.org/10.1016/0028-3932(84)90046-0

Steenhuis RE, Bryden MP (1989) Different dimensions of hand preference that relate to skilled and unskilled activities. Cortex 25(2):289–304. https://doi.org/10.1016/S0010-9452(89)80044-9

Surburg PR (1999) Midline-crossing inhibition: an indicator of developmental delay. Laterality 4(4):333–343. https://doi.org/10.1080/713754347

Valera EM, Faraone SV, Murray KE, Seidman LJ (2007) Meta-analysis of structural imaging findings in attention-deficit/hyperactivity disorder. Biol Psychiatry 61(12):1361–1369

van der Knaap LJ, van der Ham IJM (2011) How does the corpus callosum mediate interhemispheric transfer? A review. Behav Brain Res 223(1):211–221

Vingerhoets G, Sarrechia I (2009) Individual differences in degree of handedness and somesthetic asymmetry predict individual differences in left-right confusion. Behav Brain Res 204(1):212–216. https://doi.org/10.1016/j.bbr.2009.06.004

Vuoksimaa E, Koskenvuo M, Rose RJ, Kaprio J (2009) Origins of handedness: a nationwide study of 30,161 adults. Neuropsychologia 47(5):1294–1301. https://doi.org/10.1016/j.neuropsychologia.2009.01.007

Willems RM, van der Haegen L, Fisher SE, Francks C (2014) On the other hand: including left-handers in cognitive neuroscience and neurogenetics. Nat Rev Neurosci 15(3):193–201. https://doi.org/10.1038/nrn3679

Williams SM (1991) Handedness inventories: Edinburgh versus Annett. Neuropsychology 5(1):43

Williams SM (2022) The Edinburgh handedness inventory: a bibliometric return after five years

Yancosek KE (2010) Injury-induced hand dominance transfer. University of Kentucky Libraries, Lexington

Synopsis of Part I

Looking at multidimensional handedness with a particular focus on understanding variable hand use, and considering the multifactorial variables discussed, here is an overall synopsis.

On the one hand, ***Left* and *Right Handedness* are normal human traits** with polygenetic origins for the direction and an inherited degree of handedness. Left handers generally display a much greater variability in their hand use than right handers and also exhibit specific traits not seen in right handers. The right-biassed physical and cultural environmental influences most likely contribute to a reduced incidence of normal or familial *Left Handedness*. Particularly, left handers of milder degree are at risk of becoming converted or switched handers and are likely to be classified in the fabricated mixed handedness group.

On the other hand, and in addition to the complex and individualised interplay between **hereditary** and **environmental** factors forming handedness, in some cases, the so-called **pathological** influencing factors can also impact the handedness direction and degree. This is supported by the body of evidence around risk factors in early development resulting in greater numbers of pathological left and mixed handers. However, risk factors also affect right handers with developmental delay, which have rarely been used as control groups in research. Indeed, these pathological impacts are intricately intertwined with developmental processes and cascades, and the distinction between developmental delay and pathological handedness is often not clear.

Furthermore, the **research** focus often tends to be rudimentary by correlating **unidimensional** indicators for left and mixed handedness with disorders. Correlational studies based on multidimensional handedness and accounting for multivariate influences are rare. In addition, there is a **lack of distinction** between familial left handers and pathological handers, as well as between right handers and converted left handers, which is likely to skew the outcome and conclusions of studies. Indeed, research on left and especially mixed handedness has yielded inconclusive and contradictory results, with both handedness groups being associated with positive as well as negative attributes. Finally, our critical appraisal would not be complete without referring to the **lack of comparability** across studies due to inconsistent and diverse definitions, measures and categorisation of handedness.

Importantly, the multifactorial nature of early risk factors and other influencing impacts on child development are most likely to result in **general developmental delay**, of which handedness may just be one aspect. Therefore, using left or mixed handedness as an indicator for developmental delay and conditions is neither viable nor reliable. Rather, reduced manual lateralisation and *Left Handedness* is one of several *outcomes* or aspects of development that are affected.

For practitioners, these findings mean that children presenting with variable hand use are more likely to be inherently left handed than right handed. Only those right-handed children whose developmental delay has also affected manual lateralisation and specialisation would be mixed handed. In contrast, several groups of left handers, except for those with a strong handedness degree, would display variable hand use, and thus the likelihood for them to be left handed is significantly greater. It is thus critical to **assess handedness multidimensionally,** considering relevant **multivariate factors** specific to an individual. This would allow us to differentiate the assessment outcomes according to specific **types of handedness** since these appear to display very different attributes and distinctive needs affecting intervention.

Part II

Assessment and Analysis: Research and Practice

As an occupational therapist specialised in paediatrics, I repeatedly encountered children with unestablished or mixed handedness. Furthermore, I was confronted with the responsibility to help decide with which hand these children should write at school. I was generally unsure to what extent variable hand use is normal for preschool children, particularly since handedness develops over the first 6 years, and there is evidence of different degrees of handedness irrespective of age. The importance of assessing children to establish whether their variable hand use was normal, an indicator of developmental delay or other conditions prompted me to investigate principles and methods of handedness assessment and analysis.

Assessing Handedness 6

Contents

Handedness could be the result of the researcher's manipulation, if researchers do not take into account the methods by which they explore handedness and the methods that they use to count the results. (Nikolaeva and Vergunov 2018: 656)

6.1 Introduction

Handedness is such a complex phenomenon that the assessment of handedness is not a simple undertaking. As we have seen in Part I, capturing handedness comprehensively requires a multidimensional and multifactorial approach. On the one hand, handedness is a cascade process, evolving from "inconsistent" to "consistent" in early life, so one would expect to see children swapping hands during activities in preschool years (i.e. ⧫**handedness development**). On the other hand, the variability or degree of handedness has been found to be an individualist trait independent of age that continues to be modified over the life span (i.e. ⧫**handedness formation**). Against this background, handedness assessment should capture various handedness dimensions at a particular point in time, informed both by handedness development and formation (i.e. ⧫**handedness status**).

So what are the different dimensions of handedness portrayed in the assessment literature, and how are they measured? What categorisation systems are used in assessments to demarcate different categories based on the degree of handedness? Are multivariate influences considered, and if yes, how? What lessons can be learned from the abundant assessment literature and instruments? These questions guide our exploration of this field.

In this chapter, we review how handedness is generally assessed. I use the term "assessment" to mean testing, measuring, recording or deter-

E. Kraus, *Beyond Left and Right Handedness*, https://doi.org/10.1007/978-3-031-24389-9_6

mining handedness. In particular, we look at assessing handedness, measuring handedness and we consider an overview of common tests and procedures. In addition, I discuss factors influencing handedness assessments, a multidimensional approach to assessing handedness, including relevant recommendations.

6.2 Assessing Handedness: Preference and Proficiency

Handedness is frequently assessed either as hand *preference* or hand *proficiency* or, less typically, as a combination of the two. We will look at these procedures separately.

6.2.1 Assessing Hand Preference

Hand preference refers to one of the two broad dimensions of handedness, where one hand is used in a preferred manner and more frequently than the other in tasks with varying difficulty, demands and experience (see Sect. 1.4 for more details). In general, there are five main approaches to assessing hand preference: *self-assessment questionnaires*, *observation of performing hand preference tasks*, *using the writing hand as an indicator, midline crossing activities* and *third-party assessment.* In this section, I will discuss these approaches and highlight their individual strengths and weaknesses, as well as the lessons that can be learnt from them.

In addition to these five approaches, there have been several propositions on single indicators for hand preference/handedness. For example, the humerus has been considered to be a good anatomical indicator of handedness since the asymmetric measurements between the left and the right correlate to a person's hand preference (Steele 2000). However, this asymmetry could also be a *result* of increased hand use rather than a predictor and has thus been disputed as an indicator (Blackburn 2011). Similarly, the direction of the hair-whorl rotation has been linked to the direction of hand reference/handedness, assuming a biological and genetic basis. Indeed, over 90% of right handers present with a clockwise whorl rotation. Left handers, however, show a mixture of counterclockwise and clockwise directions (Klar 2003). Overall, the results of such proposed predictors of hand preference remain unreliable and will thus not be elaborated here.

Self-Assessment Questionnaires

In self-assessment questionnaires, individuals are asked to rate the frequency of their hand use (and preference) according to a pre-defined Likert scale across a variety of items. The number of rating categories varies between self-assessment questionnaires. For example, some only record hand use as either left or right (direction only), whilst others offer more categories, thereby incorporating the degree of hand preference. A well-known example is the *Edinburgh Handedness Inventory* (Oldfield 1971), using a 5-point Likert scale (Hardie et al. 2016). Each of the ten items can be rated according to these categories: "always right" (+10), "usually right" (+5), "same" (0), "mostly left" (−5) and "always left" (−10). It is argued that multi-point scales can record more subtle differences between the hands (Prichard et al. 2013), so a 5-point scale is more accurate than a 3-point scale. In particular, Peters recommends that self-assessment handedness questionnaires should include skilled *and* unskilled tasks and that they should consist of a range of items to capture a "mass effect of variability" to allow for hand preference grading (Peters 1998).

Since self-assessment questionnaires are very time efficient and do not require many resources compared to performance tests, they are frequently used with large numbers of subjects. However, the disadvantage of self-assessment instruments is their subjectivity. They yield more inconsistent ratings and are influenced by several factors, including the experience (or lack thereof) of a task, the ability to visualise oneself performing the task and the memory of how the task is indeed performed in everyday life (see Bryden et al. 2000). In addition, the number of categories can influence the response of the subject (Brown et al. 2006). For example, Williams adapted the 10-item EHI by removing the items opening a box and using a broom, and added the item using a computer mouse. This version was compared to Annett's Hand Preference quotient, a 12-item questionnaire (AHPQ-12). The EHI-10 showed significantly greater variability in moderate right handers compared to the EHI-8 version, whereas left handers did not. In contrast, AHPQ-12 items revealed an even wider spread. It was concluded that mixed handers are more likely to be identified with a higher number of items, for which AHPQ-12 seemed most suitable (Williams 2022). Based on these considerations, self-assessment questionnaires may be unreliable for certain groups, such as preschool children.

Observation of Performing Hand Preference Tasks

Hand preference can also be recorded whilst observing individuals as they perform a series of activities requiring preferred hand use (e.g. Bruckner 2010). Often the observation-based items are based on self-assessment questionnaires where the child performs the items of the questionnaire whilst being observed by the administrator who records the responses (Scharoun and Bryden 2014). This method can circumvent the self-assessment method's weaknesses by reducing the subjectivity risk. Observation-based assessments are used for preference as well as motor performance over a range of different tasks. They are more time consuming but have been found to be particularly suitable for children. In addition, observations allow a more precise documentation of internal (within-activity) consistency. However, the nature and characteristics of the task to be performed may also influence which hand will be used.

In particular, the following factors have been found to influence the performance of hand preference tasks.

- ***Position of the test item*** (in the centre, to the left or right of the body centre): As we elaborated in Sect. 2.4.2, right-handed people cross the body midline more with their right hand and left handers with their left. All people tend to reach ipsilaterally (on the same side) with their dominant hand (Bryden et al. 2000). Right handers use their right hand almost exclusively when reaching for objects on the right side; left handers also prefer their left hand, but not to the same extent (Surburg 1999).
- ***Visual feedback***: When a task is performed without visual feedback, the use of the non-dominant hand increases (Przybyla et al. 2013). This could be related to the fact that (in right handers) the non-dominant hand usually has better proprioceptive abilities (Adamo and Martin 2009).
- ***Involved musculature***: Particularly left handers are usually strongly lateralised to perform ♦**distal** activities, such as writing, with their left hand and may be less lateralised for ♦**proximal** movements, such as throwing a ball (Nelson et al. 2019), which some left handers do with their right hand (Gilbert and Wysocki 1992; Healey et al. 1986). It thus seems to make a difference whether large and centrally located (proximal) muscle groups are activated, or smaller decentrally located (distal) muscle groups are involved in an activity.
- ***The number of action repetitions***: If the same action or task is repeated several times, one can observe if a person swaps hands *within* the activity. In this book (see Chaps. 7 and 8 on the Handedness Profile), this constancy to perform a task repeatedly with the same hand is referred to as ♦**internal consistency**. It differs from ♦**external consistency**, which measures consistent hand use over several *different* activities (Kraus 2003; Bruckner 2010). The more repetitions there are, the greater the chance that the "other" hand will be used. It has thus been recommended that the number of task repetitions is standardised to ensure good comparability between tasks or items (Cochet and Byrne 2013).
- ***Unimanual and bimanual activities***: Unimanual preference developmentally precedes role-differentiated bimanual (RDBM) preference (see Sect. 1.3). Nelson and colleagues found a strong correlation between uni-

manual and bimanual preference in 70% of children who were then classified as right handed. Only 2% showed a left preference for both types of preference, and 3% showed no preference. The remaining 25% of children showed inconsistent preference across unimanual and bimanual activities (Nelson et al. 2019). This has led to the conclusion that unimanual and bimanual actions are different dimensions of handedness and should be measured separately. In practice, though, this is not typically implemented since unimanual and bimanual items are usually not differentiated when assessing hand preference in children (ibid.).

Using the Writing Hand as an Indicator of Handedness

Assessing handedness by using the writing hand as the only indicator is sometimes used in research, since it is a simple and straightforward variable that can easily be surveyed. However, this has been problematic since handwriting does not differentiate between degrees of handedness and may inflate the number of left or right handers. Also, converted left handers in particular cannot be identified with this method several authors caution that conclusions based on the drawing or writing hand used as a proxy for handedness could be inaccurate (e.g. Nelson et al. 2019).

Crossing the Midline or Contralateral Reaching

As we discussed in Sect. 2.4.1, a form of hand preference assessment involves contralateral reaching across the body midline (Carlier et al. 2006; Scharoun and Bryden 2014; Bishop et al. 1996). The dominant hand crosses the body midline more frequently than the non-dominant hand, and this phenomenon can therefore be used as an indicator of hand preference (Carlier et al. 2006). In addition, research findings suggest that contralateral reaching reflects the *degree* of handedness in particular (Bishop et al. 1996). Some earlier studies indicate that midline crossing is a prerequisite for handedness establishment (see Fisher et al. 2002; Ayres 1972; Provine and Westerman 1979). However, handedness and midline crossing appear to be separate phenomena that are not yet fully understood, and their relationship remains unclear (Scharoun and Bryden 2014; Kraus 2006). Handedness may (also) be a prerequisite for, or at least influence, midline crossing. Indeed, many developmentally delayed children avoid contralateral reaching (e.g. Michell and Wood 1999; Bishop 1990; Surburg 1999).

However, in the clinical setting working with developmentally delayed children, we frequently observe that there is a difference between using the preferred hand in midline and using it for contralateral reaching. For example, children may avoid midline crossing but use a preferred hand in the centre. Conversely, some children cross over with either hand, whereby some also show a preferred hand in the centre whilst others do not. This would confirm the postulate that midline crossing and hand preference are two related but separate phenomena. In this context, it would be critical to supplement a contralateral reaching test with some items or tasks positioned in the centre. So ideally, there should be a preference test without midline crossing and a preference test involving contralateral reaching.

Third-Party Assessment

Numerous studies use a third-party assessment of hand preference. For example, caregivers, parents, relatives or teachers indicate whether their children or pupils are left or right handed and how strong this perceived preference is (e.g. Hill and Khanem 2009). The advantage of this approach is that a significant amount of data can be generated quickly and easily. However, apart from the inherently subjective nature of this method, it does not clearly distinguish between preference and proficiency. Presumably, a general impression of handedness is captured this way. However, Marlow's research team only found a very low agreement between parent reports and handedness scores in children aged 2.5 years, which increased to 67% agreement with children aged 11 years (Marlow et al. 2019). The method of third-party assessment thus appears to be somewhat unreliable in assessing hand preference.

6.2.2 Assessing Hand Proficiency

Hand proficiency refers to the defining dimension of handedness, demonstrating the level of motor performance, skill or aptitude. Different motor tasks are used to measure proficiency performed by each hand. Results of proficiency tests, each performed with the left and right hand, are compared, and the hand with the better performance is considered to be the more proficient one. Even though there are up to ten possible dimensions of measuring motor proficiency, researchers usually resort to measuring either speed or accuracy (Barnsley and Rabinovitch 1970). Other motor dimensions, such as strength, for example, are rarely implemented since it is considered to be a weak predictor of handedness (Brown et al. 2006).

As with hand preference, several factors influence the outcome of proficiency as well as the extent of the asymmetry, including the following:

1. *The level of task complexity*: Similar to the influencing factors of preference, the difference in motor performance increases with task complexity (Alphonso et al. 2008).
2. *Visual feedback*: Without the possibility of visual feedback, the performance of both hands decreases on a continuum as one percentage. As mentioned earlier, this seems to affect the dominant hand in particular, thereby increasing the relative performance of the non-dominant hand (Przybyla et al. 2013).
3. *Practice effect*: Practice and training influence the execution of highly specialised and complex motor activity (Peters 1998; Koeneke et al. 2009). The hand with more practice and experience yields better performance results, increasing the difference between the hands. Such highly specialised and trained actions include writing and drawing (which correlate highly with Tracing and Dotting tasks) since they are repeatedly practised from preschool onwards. Unpractised and untrained motor tasks that do not show such practice effects include tapping (Carlier et al. 1993).
4. *Unimanual or bimanual*: The role division between the hands adds extra complexity to proficiency, making it more challenging to measure (e.g. Gonzalez and Nelson 2021); this may be the reason why unimanual proficiency is assessed more often than bimanual motor skills.

Some researchers have indeed combined hand preference and proficiency, using questionnaires and behavioural measures. For example, Das and colleagues looked at 113 self-reported right, left and mixed handers and compared to the self-reports with a modified seven-item EHI as well as proficiency items using the grooved pegboard, finger tapping and grip strength. The combined results show a more differentiated continuous grading of handedness, where the hand preference degree from the questionnaire correlates more strongly with proficiency measures. The authors conclude that this mixture is suitable for estimating the degree of handedness in left and right handers (Das et al. 2021).

Overall, some of these proficiency items show a higher correlation with handwriting, such as tracing tasks (e.g. Provins and Cunliffe 1972; Provins and Magliaro 1993), and other items seem to be more independent of training effects such as tapping or peg-moving tasks. Tracing tasks could be classified as being more trained because of a high correlation with writing. It also transpires that proficiency measured is usually unimanual rather than bimanual and that either speed or accuracy is usually documented.

So, what can we learn about hand proficiency as a measure? Several researchers have recommended that proficiency assessments should contain *a range of different requirements*, to obtain a multidimensional view of motor performance (Brown et al. 2004; Corey et al. 2001). This is important since different motor performances do not necessarily correlate highly, probably because various dimensions are involved (Brown et al. 2006). In addition, age and gender should be considered, as these factors may also significantly influence proficiency levels (ibid.). Finally, it has been recommended that hand proficiency rather than hand preference should be used as a measure for mixed handedness (Williams 1991, 2022—see Sect. 5.5.1).

6.3 Measuring Handedness

Broadly speaking, handedness can be measured in two ways: on a continuum or according to categories. In particular, Merni and colleagues distinguish between three types of models: (1) a *continuum* ranging from left to right, (2) a limited number of *unordered categories* and (3) a limited number of *ordered* (prioritised) *categories* (Merni et al. 2014). When comparing the three models, they found that ordered categories were the most reliable measure (ibid.). In research practice, a combination of continuums and categories is frequently used, whereby the cut-off point of the categories is often defined arbitrarily. We will look at measuring handedness on a continuum and according to categories separately.

6.3.1 Measuring Handedness on a Continuum

A widely used formula that measures differences between the hands on a continuum is the ⧫**laterality quotient** (LQ).[1] This measures the size of the difference between the hands on a continuum as one percentage. We will refer to this as ⧫**inter-hand differences** (IHDs), thereby portraying the degree of right-left asymmetry as a percentage.

The laterality quotient is typically calculated for hand ***preference*** by subtracting the number of left-handed responses from the number of right-handed responses to calculate the difference between the hands. The result is then divided by the sum of responses and multiplied by 100 to obtain a percentage. A negative score indicates more left-handed responses (Oldfield 1971). Thus, it is very useful to have one number representing inter-hand differences, and if laterality quotients of various dimensions of handedness are calculated, they can be more easily compared. Here are fictional examples of using the formula of the laterality quotient for right- and left-handed individuals, with Example 1 based on 10 preference items, and Example 2 on 20 items:

1. $\text{LQ}(\text{Preference}): \frac{R-L}{R+L} = \frac{8-2}{8+2} = \frac{6}{10} \times 100 = \mathbf{60\%\,more\ right}$

2. $\text{LQ}(\text{Preference}): \frac{R-L}{R+L} = \frac{6-14}{6+14} = \frac{-8}{20} \times 100 = \mathbf{-40\%\,more\ left}$

A preference laterality quotient (LQ-Pref) of 100% is considered to be the highest possible degree of left- or right-hand preference. Between 80 and 100% can be considered as strongly established hand preference, between 60 and 79% moderately established hand preference and below 60% mildly established or variable hand preference. A value of 0% would indicate no difference between hands. These cut-off points were based on a study with more than 1500 people, where the average of strongly established (consistent) left and right handers obtained laterality quotients of 80%. Consequently, individuals with a score below 80% would be classified as mildly established (inconsistent) handers (Prichard et al. 2013).

For ***proficiency***, the difference between the hands can also be calculated according to the principle of the laterality quotient. It has been referred to as the ⧫**dominance index** (DI) (Schilling 2009; Schönthaler 2020). The DI expresses the ratio of the right hand's performance concerning the overall performance. A DI of 100 represents very strongly established *Right Handedness*, a DI of 0 represents very strongly established *Left Handedness* and a DI of 50 means that both hands achieved the same test results. The following formula is used to calculate the DI:

$$\mathbf{DI} = \frac{\textbf{results of the right hand} \times \mathbf{100}}{\textbf{results of the R + L hand}}$$

[1] There are different variations of the laterality quotient (also referred to as laterality index). Whilst the principle is the same, i.e. obtaining one score to indicate the difference between left and right rather than two separate scores for each hand, there are several variations. Vingerhoets has conducted a Delphi study with over 100 handedness experts and found no consensus (Vingerhoets 2022).

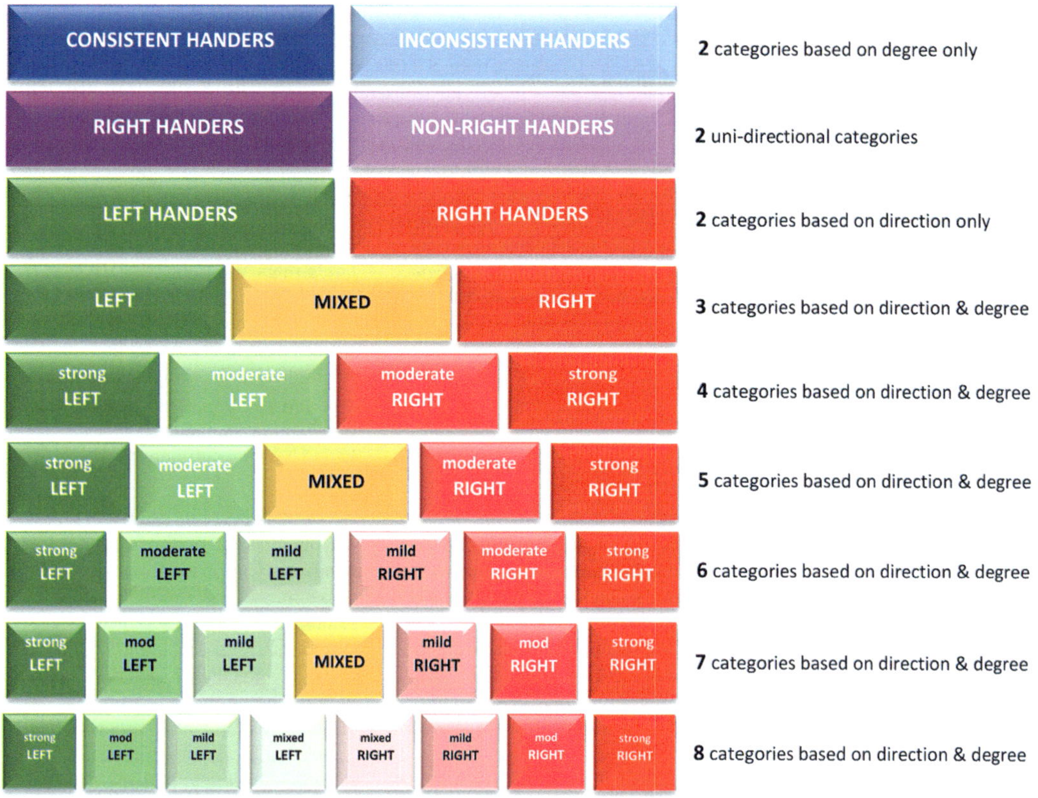

Fig. 6.1 Overview of different categorisation possibilities of handedness

6.3.2 Measuring Handedness According to Categories

As discussed in Chap. 1 (Sect. 1.4.2), the number for classifying handedness tends to range from two to eight categories, as summarised in Fig. 6.1.

These categories are usually based on a continuous measure, such as the laterality quotient. Clearly, the more categories used, the more specific the handedness group, provided that there are significant differences between them.[2] However, as we have seen there is no consensus on a standardised cut-off point to demarcate the categories, and the subsequent handedness groups thus differ considerably between studies.

[2]This was investigated in the context of developing the Handedness Profile, where I found significant differences between eight categories based on the inter-hand differences using laterality quotients for both preference and proficiency (see Chap. 8). Annett found similar support for her eight handedness categories (Annett 1994).

6.4 Overview of Commonly Used Tests and Procedures

We now turn to some commonly used handedness assessments. Table 6.1 displays a range of standardised tests and procedures for assessing hand preference and hand proficiency, focusing mainly on those frequently used in clinical and educational settings as well as research. In the case of preference tests, I differentiate between self-assessment questionnaires, observation-based preference tests and midline crossing preference tests.

Table 6.1 Summary of commonly used handedness tests in research and practice

Test/assessment Authors, year	Description of method and content	Comments
Preference: Third-party assessment		
Home Handedness Questionnaire (HHQ) for Preschoolers (Nelson et al. 2019)	There are two sub-scales: 15 items assessing unimanual manipulation and 15 items that assess role-differentiated bimanual manipulation (RDBM) (one hand stabilises an object whilst the other hand manipulates it). Parents observe and record each action twice non-consecutively, scoring up to 30 data points for the unimanual and bimanual tasks (60 data points overall)	The items/actions are based on being (1) familiar to parents and easy to administer; (2) accessible and common to be performed in households; and (3) clear in identifying and eliciting the target manual action. The HHQ identified most children as right-handed whilst also showing variability across the different items: About one-quarter of children in the sample showed mixed preferences between unimanual and bimanual tasks, indicating that handedness was still developing
Preference: Self-assessment questionnaires		
Edinburgh Handedness Inventory (EHI) (Oldfield 1971) Hand preference by self-assessment (questionnaire)	Includes ten items related to everyday life: writing, drawing, throwing, brushing teeth, cutting with scissors, eating with a spoon, lighting a match, sweeping with a broom, cutting with a knife and opening a box. In its original form, the test had only two response categories (right or left); adapted versions usually score on a 5-point Likert scale (e.g. Niebauer et al. 2004)	**Scoring**: A laterality quotient (LQ) is calculated based on the responses to hand use. The EHI is frequently used in research, and it generally has high reliability and factor stability (McFarland and Anderson 1980). The EHI has often been adapted for use with children by omitting certain items (e.g. Hill and Bishop 1998; Hill and Khanem 2009); letting parents complete questionnaires (e.g. Hill and Khanem 2009); or by performing and observing the items (e.g. Karapetsas and Vlachos 1997)
Waterloo Handedness Questionnaire (WHQ) (Bryden 1977) Hand preference by self-assessment (questionnaire)	In the first version, 60 tasks had to be rated according to a 5-point scale (always left hand—usually left hand—no preference—usually right hand—always right hand). Based on this first test version, variants with different numbers of items were developed. The items refer to distal and proximal activities and those with high and low skill requirements	An adapted form of the WHQ with 36 or 20 items has been used with children 3 years of age and older (e.g. Bryden and Roy 2005; Bryden et al. 2007a, b). The items are read to younger children under 12 years and explained. Children are also asked to imagine or imitate the activity in question **Scoring**: If the child indicates a preference for one hand for a specific task, he/she is asked whether he/she *always* or *usually* uses that hand. Thus, the 5-scale response format is maintained. Parents are asked to rate their hand preference if children are under 4 years of age. The 32-item version has high test-retest reliability and factor stability (Steenhuis et al. 1990)[a]

Table 6.1 (continued)

Test/assessment Authors, year	Description of method and content	Comments
Preference: Observed performance of preference tasks		
Handpräferenztest (HAPT) for 4–6-year-old children (Bruckner et al. 2011) Testing hand preference by observing task performance	It is a standardised and normed test with good validity. It incorporates consistency within a task through 3 trials for each item. The test consists of 16 items, 8 of which are "precise" (e.g. throwing a ball, drawing, stamping, sweeping, fishing, opening a can, picking up chain and bead) and 8 "automated" (e.g. waving, rolling dice, picking up sticker and reward, using a light switch, opening zipper). The assessment is embedded in a child-orientated adventure journey and takes place in a standing position with the child	**Scoring**: The number of right- and left-hand reactions are counted, and a laterality quotient is calculated. Separate norm tables are available for girls and boys, where the percentile rank can be obtained. Other tables, also divided by gender, age and binary handedness, provide information on the degree of hand preference. The values are categorised into average, above-average and below-average categories. No laterality quotients are used The items are differentiated into precise and automated categories (rather than bimanual/unimanual or trained/untrained tasks)—the logic of this categorisation is not always clear. Since the child's standing position during the assessment changes the stability compared to sitting at a table, task performance could be influenced and may not be entirely comparable to hand use when the child is sitting
Sattler Method for Handedness Clarification (S-MH)® (Sattler 2008) Observation and background information for clarification of handedness	The S-MH includes very detailed, qualitative background information (questionnaire-based interview, often in the presence of the child). These results are incorporated into the interpretation. In addition, 25 items assessing hand preference are child-appropriate, playful and repeatedly performed without a stipulated number of repetitions. Items are divided according to bimanual, unimanual, trained and untrained characteristics. The assessment is recorded by video	**Scoring**: Video analysis is used as a basis for interpretation. The frequency of hand use is counted and categorised into bimanual, unimanual, and trained and untrained groups. Items are standardised, but the number of executions is not. Administration of this assessment requires official training, experience and practice, and a relatively broad scope exists for interpretation. Since the S-MH only assesses hand preference, results are often supplemented with quantitative data from the hand dominance test (HDT)
WatHand Cabinet Test (WHCT) (Bryden et al. 2000, 2007a; Scharoun and Bryden 2015) Hand preference (observed performance) with consistency value	A box with a flap and a handle contains eight different objects or actions that the child performs: (1) open the flap of the box (four times in total), (2) use a toy hammer, (3) hang a ring on a hook, (4) throw a ball on a target made of Velcro, (5) open a lock with a key, (6) use a screwdriver, (7) press a button and (8) operate a candy dispenser	**Scoring:** Laterality quotients are calculated for the following aspects: *skill score* for items that require manual dexterity; *consistency score* based on opening the flap four times; *bimanual score* for candy dispenser and flap task; and a *total score*. Since the test does not require a high level of language comprehension, it can also be used with younger children. The WHCT has been tested for validity and reliability (Scharoun and Bryden 2012).[b] Each item was performed four times in later administration to obtain a more comprehensive score (Scharoun and Bryden 2015)

(continued)

Table 6.1 (continued)

Test/assessment Authors, year	Description of method and content	Comments
Hand Preference Demonstration Test (HPDT) (Soper and Satz 1984) Hand preference (observed performance) with consistency measurement	Eight items are each offered three times in random order: eat with a spoon, drink from a cup, brush teeth, draw with a pencil, throw a ball, use a hammer, pick up raisins or similar and pick up a 10-cent piece	**Scoring:** The administrator presents each item with alternating hands to avoid a left or right bias. However, it is possible that the child imitates this behaviour and also picks up the items with either hand. A consistency measurement within an action or a task is possible because the items are performed three times
Preschool Handedness Inventory (PHI) (Tan 1985) Hand preference (observed performance)	The following activities are performed: open and close a box, take a pencil out of a box and put it back in, draw, cut with scissors, hammer with a hammer, pour with a pitcher, put beans in a bottle, build a tower with cubes, catch bean bag with one hand and throw bean bag with one hand. The objects are presented in the centre of the visual field	**Scoring:** The use of the right hand is counted with 0 points, left hand with 2 points and both hands with 1 point. This results in a value between 0 (extremely right handed) and 26 (extremely left handed). Each item is performed only once
Preference: Tasks crossing the centre of the body		
Space Visualization Contralateral Use (SVCU) Score (part of the Sensory Integration and Praxis Tests (SIPT)) (Ayres 1989) Overview of different categorisation possibilities of handedness	As part of the SIPT, the SVCU is a test of spatial perception. It involves crossing the body midline based on the frequency of contralateral reaching. The two blocks are each placed in line with the child's shoulders. Only one block fits into the shaped hole, positioned centrally behind the two blocks. The child picks up the matching block with the right hand (ipsilateral response) or the left hand (contralateral response). The contralateral and ipsilateral reaching frequency is recorded over 30 tasks with increased difficulty	**Scoring:** The child's writing hand was identified in a previous SIPT subtest, and this hand is referred to as the "dominant hand". How often this hand crosses the body midline (number of contralateral responses) is counted. This value can then be calculated as a percentage. There are age norms for children between 4 and 11 years It is important to know that this test was not designed to determine handedness but midline crossing. Assessing hand dominance based only on the writing hand is questionable. It is based on the assumption that contralateral reaching provides insight into the state of hemispheric lateralisation and specialisation
Quantification of Hand Preference (QHP) Task (Bishop et al. 1996) Midline crossing test of the body midline	Subjects pick up cards with pictures of objects (e.g. car, bird, aeroplane) arranged in seven positions, with three cards each in a semicircle to the right, left and centre. The cards are then placed in a box in the centre and the hand used is noted. The order of the cards is random, but the starting point is the card in the middle (position 4)	**Scoring**: Left-hand use is calculated as −0.50 and right-hand use as +0.50. Categorization is according to LATB (laterality/bishop): LATB <0 is considered left handed and LATB >0 is considered right handed. The number of times the hand is used in the body's centre is also calculated as the degree of handedness; its value ranges from 0 (no crossing) to 18 (all possible contralateral responses are made)
Preferential Reaching Task (Brown et al. 2006; Bryden et al. 2000) Midline crossing test of the body midline	Seven round logs (10 cm × 5 cm) are used to perform various activities: pointing at objects, picking them up, knocking them over, throwing them and sticking them into an opening. The logs are placed in a semicircle in front of the subject, and the activities are performed one handed. In an alternative version of the test for younger subjects (3–20 years), a suitable container for the objects was used and integrated into the task	**Scoring**: The principle of the laterality quotient is used so that positive values represent a preference for the right hand and negative values represent a preference for the left hand. Furthermore, a so-called switch point score is calculated at which the test person switches hands. In this test, crossing the hemispace (midline crossing) is used—the further a person crosses the centre of the body, the more pronounced the degree of handedness

Table 6.1 (continued)

Test/assessment Authors, year	Description of method and content	Comments
Proficiency: Unimanual untrained tasks		
Grooved pegboard test (Wang et al. 2011; Petrigna et al. 2020) Peg-moving task	This standardised motor skill test consists of a board with 25 holes. Metal rods or pegs are placed in the holes in a specific order. To insert the pegs, they must first be rotated. It has a good test-retest reliability (0.91 and 0.85 for right and left hands, respectively), but the administration time is relatively long, and the test is challenging for younger children (Wang et al. 2011). There are sets of normative data: adult: 15 years 0 months and above; adolescent: 9 years 0 months to 14 years 12 months; and children: 5 years 0 months to 8 years 12 months (Trites 1977)	**Scoring**: 3 values are produced: Time in seconds, number of errors (dropped sticks) and number of correctly inserted sticks. The test is normed for different age groups distinguishing between genders and between the dominant and non-dominant hands. It is a dexterity test, not a specific handedness test, and there are no separate values for left and right handers
Speed dot-filling test (Tapley and Bryden 1985) Dotting	A paper and pencil test in which dots are to be placed in given circles as fast as possible. The test proceeds in four rounds; in the first and fourth rounds, the preferred hand is used, and in the second and third, the non-preferred hand. Twenty seconds is given for each of the rounds	**Scoring**: All correctly placed points are counted, and values for the left and right hands are formed. The difference between the hands is then expressed with another value: the right-handed and left-handed value is divided by the total value
Annett's pegboard (Annett 1970) Inserting pegs	The test consists of two boards with ten holes each. Whilst standing, the children insert pegs successively and as quickly as possible, first with the right hand and then with the left. The time is recorded. If a peg falls, the trial is repeated. Older children do five trials; younger children perform three trials	**Scoring**: 3 values are determined: right hand, left hand and a difference-between-the-hands value. This difference value is an index that reflects the direction and degree of hand asymmetry
Finger tapping (Peters and Durding 1978) Tapping	Subjects tap a switch as fast as possible with the index finger for 10 s whilst the rest of the hand is held still. A small box (815 cm × 25 cm × 3 cm) with a mounted microswitch with a lever is used	**Scoring**: The time interval is activated at the first press and records the number of pressed responses for 10 s. The test is performed with children aged 5–13 years
Peg-moving task (Annett 1970, 1985, 2002) Moving pegs	The peg-moving task is used with adults and children. Ten wooden pegs are moved from the back row of holes to the front row of holes as quickly as possible on a wooden board. Three trials are performed alternately with each hand whilst standing. If a peg falls, the pass is repeated. The time is noted for each trial	**Scoring**: The average for the right and left hand is calculated. The difference between the hands is established using the principle of the laterality quotient. Negative values indicate *Left Handedness*, and positive values *Right Handedness*
Zurich Neuromotor Test (Largo et al. 2007) Inserting and moving pegs	A standardised and normed motor skill test for children 5–16 years old. The pegboard has two versions: younger children (5–10 years) insert pegs; older children (11–16 years) turn the pegs before insertion. Sequential and repetitive finger and hand movements are thought to represent untrained motor performance	**Scoring**: The time for 20 repetitions is measured. In addition, the extent of contralateral co-movements is evaluated as a so-called difference component. There is a speed measurement but no accuracy measurement. The norm values only refer to the dominant and non-dominant hand, and there is no separate data for left and right handers

(continued)

Table 6.1 (continued)

Test/assessment Authors, year	Description of method and content	Comments
Proficiency: Unimanual trained tasks		
Hand Dominanz Test (HDT) (Steingrüber 2011) Tracing and Dotting	The HDT consists of three subtests: *tracing between two lines, dotting circles* and *dotting squares*. Younger children (ages 6–10) have 30 s for the tasks, performed once with the right hand and once with the left; older children and adults (ages 11–70) have 15 s The HDT is a norm-referenced test with good test-retest and inter-rater reliability. However, the correlation of the test results with the children's self-assessment is low	**Scoring**: A *difference* score is calculated for each of the subtests. These difference scores together result in the total score with a standard and a percentile rank, which can be assigned to a five-level categorisation. Only motor accuracy is measured—the quality of the lines and dots is not considered. Also, it assesses trained proficiency (dotting and tracing correlate highly with writing)
Lateralitäts/Präferenz Dominanz Test (LDT/PDT) (Schilling 2009) Dotting test	The PTK-LDT is a paper-pencil test for children aged 5–12 years. A clown figure is presented on a test sheet (mirror-inverted for the left and right hands) with a total of 150 small circles arranged along its outline. Using a fine liner, the child places dots in these circles as quickly and accurately as possible	**Scoring**: Speed and accuracy are taken into account, and a motor function quotient is calculated for right- and left-hand performance, respectively. A dominance index (DI) is determined on a scale of 0–100. Norms are available for the LDT/PDT separately for age and gender. The test-retest reliability is very high, and the correlation with the parents' assessment of handedness is high. It assesses trained proficiency (dotting and tracing correlate highly with writing)
Motor Accuracy Test (MAcc) of the Sensory Integration and Praxis Test (SIPT) (Ayres 1989) Tracing task	The MAcc consists of a butterfly-shaped tracing task presented on an A3 paper to be performed with each hand. The hand that picks up the pen first and starts tracing is referred to as the "dominant" hand. Tracing must be performed without lifting the fine liner and should be completed with each hand within about 1 min	**Scoring**: The time is recorded, and errors are calculated based on deviations from the centre line. Errors are offset against time—the longer the time, the more error points. This produces comparable values for each hand. Like all SIPT tests, this test is normed for children between the ages of 4 and 11
Proficiency: Bimanual untrained tasks		
Bimanual circle drawing (Carson et al. 1997; Semjen et al. 1995) Drawing bimanual circles simultaneously	Two circles (10 cm in diameter) are drawn with both hands simultaneously, in three different directional modes: symmetrical "inward" (the left hand moves clockwise and the right hand counterclockwise), symmetrical "outward" (the left hand moves counterclockwise and the right hand clockwise) and asymmetrical/parallel (both hands move clockwise or counterclockwise). There are two versions: one at the preferred speed and one as fast as possible. About 10 s is given for each direction	The test was used in a research study, concluding that the dominant hand draws better circles and maintains direction, especially in the parallel movements (both hands clockwise or against). In the parallel movements, particularly in the fast version, a "transient departure from the required mode of coordination" (Carson et al. 1997) is seen. It refers to a turning point where the non-dominant hand mirrors the direction of the dominant hand. The dominant hand also seems to lead more

Table 6.1 (continued)

Test/assessment Authors, year	Description of method and content	Comments
Proficiency: Uni- and bimanual untrained tasks		
Purdue Pegboard (Tiffin 1948) Inserting pegs with one and both hands, assembly task	In the first trial, pegs are inserted separately with the right and left hands for 30 s each. In the second trial, this task is performed with both hands simultaneously (30 s). The third trial consists of a bimanual assembly task (60 s)	**Scoring**: Time is taken for each trial to be completed. There are standard values for 5- to 16-year-old children, whereby boys and girls have separate norms. This test assesses untrained proficiency. Speed is measured, but not accuracy. It is assumed that more skilled children also score faster. The primary goal of the test is to assess manipulation and dexterity rather than handedness

[a] In a study, the items of the Edinburgh Handedness Inventory and the Waterloo Handedness Questionnaire were combined to form the E-WHQ with 22 items, and a 5-point scale was used. Results showed 5% lower accuracy compared to the single inventories, the test-retest reliability was weak and it did not predict the dominant hand strongly. The authors concluded that the E-WHQ was not suitable for predicting hand preference (Flindall and Gonzalez 2019)

[b] Nelson et al. critically appraise the WHCT, stating that it distinguishes different types of actions but the bimanual tasks are not easily comparable since some require sequential unimanual steps and others simultaneous cooperation, and it is not commercially available (Nelson et al. 2019)

6.5 Factors Influencing Handedness Assessment

As we have seen from the previous chapters, multivariate influences affect the direction and degree of handedness, particularly during handedness development over the first 6 years, but also during the continuous handedness formation across the life span. In this section, I attempt to make relevant influences more tangible so that they can be incorporated as practical guidelines for a comprehensive handedness assessment.

We will first explore the intricate relationship between *handedness and motor abilities* more carefully, since these affect handedness in a specific way in the context of clinical practice and is thus of particular importance to practitioners working with children. We will then look at specific *task characteristics* that affect the extent of asymmetries and *specific influencing factors* affecting the assessment of handedness.

6.5.1 Motor Abilities Influencing Handedness and Its Assessment

In addition to obtaining inter-hand differences in preference and proficiency, it is important to capture how *well* the task is performed on both sides, i.e. obtaining a *level* of proficiency. For example, if a child shows small ♦**inter-hand differences**, it could mean that both hands perform equally well or equally poorly, subsequently requiring a very different approach to intervention.

So exactly how are degrees of handedness and motor function related in everyday life? It seems logical to assume that an average or above-average motor ability on both sides is advantageous for functioning in everyday life. Explicit left and right handers are likely to display a clear and constant distribution of the roles between the hands, with the dominant hand leading and being more active and the non-dominant hand taking the supporting and stabilising role. Conversely, mild or variable left and right handers with good motor proficiency will probably use the non-dominant hand more often and very effectively. This results in a highly ergonomic performance where it often seems arbitrary which hand is used. So, one could conclude that good proficiency facilitates bimanual coordination and cooperation, and a high degree of handedness assists in clear and consistent division of manual roles.

But what happens if there are motor dysfunctions, particularly if these affect the dominant hand? How does this affect the relationship between motor abilities and handedness? Hypothetically, there are four possibilities:

(a) Motor dysfunctions and disorders could *coexist* independently and coincidentally to a handedness status. This means that there is no direct relationship between handedness and motor skills: regardless of whether a person is left or right handed or how strongly established her/his handedness, motor dysfunctions may or may not be present (Kraus 2019).

(b) Motor dysfunction or disorders caused by early brain insult (i.e. damage before, at or after birth—see Sect. 3.5) could *causally* change the direction of handedness. If the dominant hand is impaired and affected, it is likely that the non-dominant hand will be used for more complex and demanding motor activities. This process is referred to as ♦**handedness reshaping**[3] (rather than handedness conversion), characterised by large inter-hand differences particularly in proficiency. In severe cases, it would resemble cerebral palsy hemiplegia, but frequently the affected side is only mildly affected. Individuals with an inherently high degree of handedness would probably still perform undemanding, simple and spontaneous tasks with their dominant hand, whilst the more demanding, complex and trained activities would be performed with the non-dominant but better hand. With a lesser degree of handedness, it is likely that the performance of most activities will be performed with the non-dominant and less affected hand.

(c) If there is motor dysfunction on both sides, this could also trigger variable hand use. This is typically the case in developmentally delayed children. The child attempts to perform an activity using one hand but does not succeed, tries to do it with the other hand but that is also unsuccessful and swaps back, etc. (see also Bishop 1990). The degree of handedness would presumably also influence this manual pattern: the lesser the degree, the more frequent the change of hand use.

(d) Motor abnormalities could be the *result* of sociocultural environmental switching or ♦**converted handedness**, e.g. when the non-dominant hand is trained for writing (Searleman and Porac 2001; Porac 1996; Sattler and Marquardt 2006) (see also Sects. 3.4.2 and 4.5). Although there is evidence that the non-dominant hand can achieve a very high motor level through training (e.g. Walker and Henneberg 2007), this is based on studies in which certain motor aspects or steps were practised, which do not withstand the complexity of writing. The MRI studies on converted left handers (e.g. Searleman and Porac 2001; Klöppel et al. 2007, 2010) clearly show bilateral activation of both hemispheres of the brain, which presumably leads to reduced efficiency. Even if motor abilities are inherently good on both sides, the non-dominant hand is unlikely to perform at the same potential proficiency level as the dominant hand, even with extensive practice. Consequently, this could also result in motor abnormalities of the non-dominant writing hand and in subsequent hand swapping.

In addition, certain conditions are associated with reduced laterality and thus variable hand use, such as autism, Down syndrome or schizophrenia (see Sects. 3.6, 4.4.1 and 5.5.2). It would therefore be important to either exclude or confirm these conditions as a possible cause for mixed handedness.

6.5.2 Task Characteristics Influencing Handedness Assessments

For an overview, task characteristics affecting manual asymmetry have been formulated as counterparts, as was suggested by Cochet and

[3] Handedness reshaping refers to a change of handedness direction and degree based on early pathological motor impact, whereas handedness conversion is based on a change in handedness direction due to environmental factors.

Byrne (2013). I have summarised these and supplemented them with findings from other authors and my clinical practice in Table 6.2.

Using a visual summary, the characteristics increasing or decreasing manual asymmetry can be presented differently (see Fig. 6.2).

6.5.3 Specific Factors Influencing Handedness Assessment Outcomes

In addition to task demands, specific factors influence the outcome when assessing handed-

Table 6.2 Task characteristics that may influence asymmetrical hand use

Increased asymmetry	Decreased asymmetry
Manipulative activities involving an object or tool show higher asymmetry in hand use than non-manipulative activities (Cochet and Byrne 2013)	*Non-manipulative* activities performed with empty hands show lower asymmetry in hand use (Cochet and Byrne 2013)
Demanding activities that require high dexterity show a stronger preference pattern (Fagard and Lockman 2005; Mamolo et al. 2004; Steenhuis and Bryden 1989)	*Non-demanding* activities that require a low level of skill exhibit less severe asymmetries (Fagard and Lockman 2005; Mamolo et al. 2004; Steenhuis and Bryden 1989)
Unimanual (one-handed) activities are less complex; therefore, it is presumably easier to automate unimanual actions through practice and repetition (Kraus 2003)	*Bimanual* (two-handed) activities assume a division of labour between the hands (e.g. a working hand and a holding hand in role-differentiated bimanual movement RDBM) and thus map asymmetries in hand use most clearly (Fagard and Lockman 2005)
Practised activities correspond reasonably well with demanding and complex activities, such as drawing or writing, because they are subject to a strong practice effect (Steenhuis and Bryden 1989)	*Unskilled* activities are mostly unfamiliar and can be challenging or easy. However, the extent of practice here may be influenced by factors such as gender-specific activities (Steenhuis and Bryden 1989)
Trained activities are not only practised as such, but they are practised with a specific hand. They are usually activities that have a high cultural value, such as greeting with the right hand (Sattler and Klußmann 2014; Sattler 2002)	*Untrained* activities are considered spontaneous and not influenced by the environment. The requirements may vary in complexity. The subdivision between trained and untrained serves primarily to identify environmental influences on the formation of handedness (Sattler 2002, 2008)

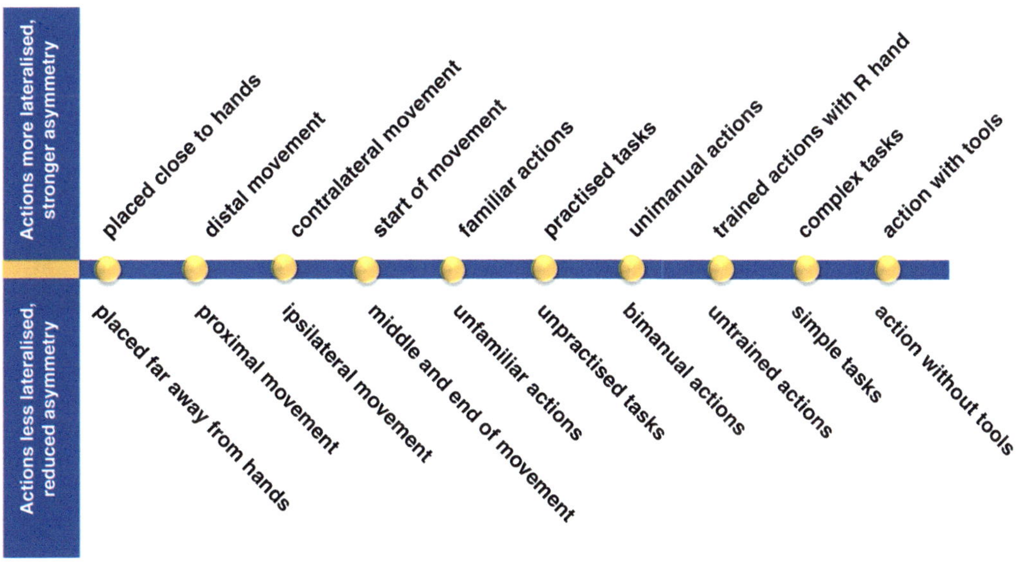

Fig. 6.2 Visualisation of specific features that increase or decrease manual asymmetry

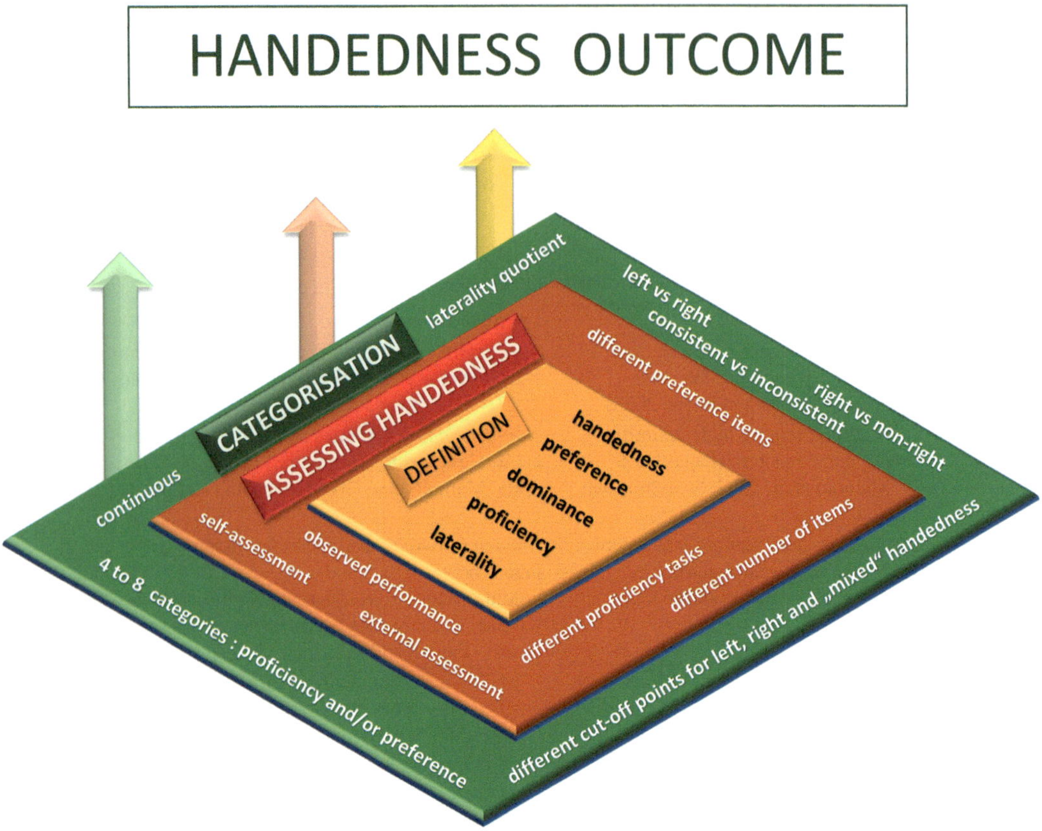

Fig. 6.3 Summarising multiple factors influencing the assessment of handedness

ness. These differ from the general influencing factors on handedness, which we have dealt with in detail over the last chapters, such as hereditary and pathological factors. Instead, these factors are concerned with the definition of handedness, its assessment method and categorisation, as illustrated in Fig. 6.3.

In terms of *definition*, a handedness assessment might measure only preference or proficiency; it might focus more on laterality or include laterality items that measure sidedness rather than handedness. Sometimes, the term "dominance" is used, and this term, too, may involve a variety of interpretations. Looking at the *assessment items* of preference and proficiency, the number and type of items strongly influence the outcome, as does the methodology (e.g. self-assessment or observation). Finally, the type of *categorisation* into handedness groups according to the particular cut-off points will also determine the handedness outcome, whereby the degree of handedness may not be considered. The influence of research factors on the outcome is not included in the diagram, including the number of subjects, sample selection, research design and experimental conditions.

6.6 A Multidimensional Approach to Assessing Handedness

What can we learn from the multiple studies investigating handedness assessment measures and procedures? Moreover, how do we deal with incorporating different handedness dimensions, measures, categorisation and influencing factors into assessing handedness in practice, particularly with children? We will first look at some general lessons learned and relevant recommendations from the literature for a practice-based approach to handedness.

6.6.1 Learning Lessons from the Literature

Firstly, we need to ensure that the ***choice of test procedures is congruent with the aims***. For example, a self-assessment preference questionnaire seems appropriate if the objective is to capture the incidence of handedness in a country. Conversely, an observational approach to hand preference and proficiency seems most suitable if we aim to assess handedness in children.

Secondly, since most handedness assessments have been developed in a research context, it is understandable that the focus needs to be restricted to address specific research questions. It is the nature of many research studies to focus on a particularly narrow and limited aspect of the construct investigated. Indeed, some studies on handedness assessments have tried to overcome this tendency. For example, based on open data initiatives, Ruck and colleagues were able to access data of 1179 typically developed subjects by looking at three different handedness measures. They compared the Edinburgh Handedness Inventory (EHI), nine-hole pegboard and grip strength. These three measures correlated poorly, with about 10% of subjects having one of the measures opposite to the others and over 65% of left handers having at least one mismatch. The authors conclude that it is crucial to establish ***direction, degree and consistency of handedness*** in future studies (Ruck and Schoenemann 2021), in addition to ***several handedness measures.***

Thirdly, there is a tendency for research studies on handedness to assess typically developed and functioning adults (apart from the developmental and correlational studies between handedness and disorders). Consequently, many results may not be directly transferrable to the paediatric clinical context. In particular, children are confined to cascades of developmental processes that can be influenced considerably by their context and their occupations. This places a great responsibility on practitioners making decisions that influence developmental processes such as handedness development and formation. A practice-based approach incorporating critical clinical decision-making affecting children's future development and handedness establishment thus requires a holistic understanding of their problems within their unique and complex milieu. So, a ***multidimensional approach*** is needed if the goal is to understand the complexity of mixed handedness in children with developmental problems. This is also confirmed by various authors who argue that a person's handedness is indeed reflected in multiple dimensions (Gonzalez and Nelson 2021; Peters 1998; Marcori et al. 2019). In addition to capturing multidimensional handedness, our approach should be ***multifactorial***, including recording background factors such as familial *Left Handedness*, possible injury to the dominant side or hemisphere, sociocultural influences and developmental milestones.

Finally, we should seek to ***synthesise relevant information*** and bring the diverse factors around handedness together, considering the various strengths and weaknesses. For example, a general weakness of current handedness tests is that they often confine handedness to being either preference or proficiency; predominantly use unimanual items; neglect internal consistency within the same tasks; do not differentiate between trained and untrained tasks; and do not include contralateral reaching as a preference measure. Incorporating all of these aspects would be the aim of a multidimensional assessment for clinical practice, for which a set of *guidelines* are needed. In particular, handedness should include observation-based preference and proficiency measures. Additionally, there should be a *variety* of preference and proficiency items that include simple and complex tasks and bimanual and unimanual activities that are practised/trained as well as unpractised/untrained.

6.6.2 Summarising Recommendations from the Literature

Several authors made recommendations for the ***observation-based (observed performance) assessment of hand preference and proficiency*** (e.g. Bear et al. 1986). The specific advice of different authors is summarised here:

- Assessments of hand preference should involve a relatively **high number of different everyday activities** (Ida et al. 2000; Peters 1998; Steenhuis and Bryden 1989), and they should include different levels of performance (Steenhuis and Bryden 1989; Ida et al. 2000).
- Hand preference test items should not only consist of **practised** items with high test-retest reliability since these are often subject to a practice effect. Instead, it should also comprise **unpractised** items, which usually have lower reliability (Annett 1998; Olsson and Rett 1989; Steenhuis and Bryden 1989).
- An activity, action or task should be assessed concerning its nature and context, including training and practice effects and complexity, thereby considering its **proximal-distal** and **unimanual-bimanual** characteristics (see also Steenhuis and Bryden 1989).
- Categorisation should not only be binary (left and right) but rather **multi-categorial** and provide means to capture the degree of handedness (Jäncke et al. 1998; Peters 1998).
- **Inter-hand differences** (i.e. differences between the hands) should be measured separately (Barnsley and Rabinovitch 1970) for each handedness dimension and compared in the analysis (Kraus 2003, 2019).
- Some researchers consider a laterality quotient below 60% as the threshold for unestablished (mixed) handedness or ambidexterity (Bear et al. 1986; Schachter et al. 1987; Annett 1998). Other authors refer to a threshold value of 80% (Christman 2014; Prichard et al. 2013). A **standardised cut-off point** would indeed be very useful.
- Preference should initially be displayed on a **continuum**, such as **laterality quotients**, rather than binary categories (Bishop et al. 1996).
- The **spatial factor** (contralateral or ipsilateral) should be controlled (Colman et al. 2017). Although there is evidence of a correlation between **crossing the body midline** and hand preference, they are two different phenomena (Kraus 2006). Therefore, preference items should be placed in the centre (Kraus 2003, 2019) in addition to assessing contralateral reaching.
- **Proficiency** should always be measured based on **accuracy *and* speed**, not just one of these measures (Fitts 1954; Steingrüber 2011).

These recommendations based on empirical research are very useful for a practice-based approach to handedness, since they can be used as guiding principles for handedness assessment in clinical practice.

6.6.3 Formulating Guidelines for a Practice-Based Handedness Assessment

Based on the above, a number of assumptions and recommendations are particularly relevant and important to clinical practice. Accordingly, I have formulated 12 guidelines for practitioners and their professional reasoning when assessing handedness and analysing the results. These guidelines also underpin the Handedness Profile 2018:

1. Handedness is a highly complex phenomenon, interacting with the genetic predisposition of direction and degree of handedness, the motor disposition and the general adaptability of a person, as well as the physical and sociocultural environment and task demands.
2. Each person has a unique constellation of laterality and, in particular, an individual *Handedness Profile* that is particularly expressed in the degree of handedness across its different dimensions and aspects.
3. There are three major determining handedness factors: genetic predisposition, environmental factors and confounding motor-related (pathological) factors.
4. Knowledge of these determining factors can help understand an individual's handedness within her/his context.
5. Handedness consists of two main dimensions: preference (centred and midline crossing, unimanual and bimanual) and proficiency (unimanual and bimanual). Crossing the midline

and bimanual cooperation are further aspects of hand preference and hand proficiency, respectively.

6. The combination of a high number of activities with different task characteristics best represents both preference and proficiency. Subsequently, task demands and features should include a combination of the following: easy–difficult; simple–complex; automated–spontaneous; practised–unpractised; trained–untrained; proximal–distal; and unimanual–bimanual.
7. The *preference* measurement of handedness is revealed not only in preferred hand use, but also in the consistency this is done within an activity.
8. Motor *proficiency* is measured most reliably when speed and accuracy are calculated together.
9. Writing is the most significant activity when assessing handedness, as it is a most complex task intricately intertwined with cognitive, fine motor, language and affective processes. Writing, therefore, has a unique standing and is not to be equated with other activities. Writing is also the defining activity for switched/converted handedness.
10. Converted handedness has neurophysiological consequences, which in turn can lead to problems or switching repercussions. Each switched person copes differently, some adapting better and some worse to the change of handedness direction.
11. In the case of children with diagnosed conditions, disorders or delays, a comprehensive handedness assessment can help reveal underlying problems and determining factors. This knowledge can help to make informed decisions about the writing hand and other activities.
12. A better understanding through a systematic differentiation of handedness dimensions can support clinical decision-making and inform the intervention process. Similarly, it may provide greater clarity regarding different groups and their characteristics when used in research.

6.7 Concluding Remarks

There are clear recommendations from the literature that handedness assessments should comprise multiple measures of various dimensions of handedness, incorporating the direction, degree, consistency and bimanual tasks. In addition to using standardised measures, a practice-based approach should also include hereditary, background and sociocultural factors. In particular, we need to be able to differentiate the variability between strongly established left and right handers whilst also assigning them to multiple categories based on degrees of handedness. In addition, we should consider the various factors influencing assessment procedures and outcomes. Combining these aspects would thus result in a comprehensive multidimensional and multivariate approach to assessing handedness.

Building the bridge between research and practice, three types of synthesis would be helpful for a practice-based approach to handedness. Firstly, explicitly summarising the different dimensions of handedness to be measured and linking them to the co-determinants of handedness discussed in Chap. 3. Secondly, to facilitate an overview and a deeper understanding of handedness in the context of clinical practice, it would be useful for practitioners to perceive handedness on a continuum ranging from a typical human trait to a trait linked to medical conditions. Finally, formulating clear guidelines for assessing handedness comprehensively and reliably can escort and direct practitioners during the diagnostic stage. The following chapter will attempt to meet these goals.

References

Adamo DE, Martin BJ (2009) Position sense asymmetry. Exp Brain Res 192(1):87–95. https://doi.org/10.1007/s00221-008-1560-0

Alphonso K, Roy EA, Bryden PJ, Balkowski B, Mayer M, Kuehner Z (2008) Preference and performance measures of handedness: the effect of task complexity. Brain Cogn 67:11. https://doi.org/10.1016/j.bandc.2008.02.014

Annett M (1970) A classification of hand preference by association analysis. Br J Psychol 61(3):303–321. https://doi.org/10.1111/j.2044-8295.1970.tb01248.x

Annett M (1985) Left, right, hand, and brain. The right shift theory. L. Erlbaum Associates, London

Annett M (1994) Handedness as a continuous variable with dextral shift: sex, generation, and family handedness in subgroups of left- and right-handers. Behav Genet 24(1):51–63. https://doi.org/10.1007/BF01067928

Annett, M. (1998): The stability of handedness. In: Kevin J. Connolly (Hg.): The psychobiology of the hand: Cambridge University Press, 63–76

Annett M (2002) Handedness and brain asymmetry. The right shift theory. Psychology Press, Hove

Ayres AJ (1972) Sensory integration and learning disorders. Western Psychological Services, Los Angeles

Ayres J (1989) Sensory integration and praxis test. Western Psychological Services, Los Angeles

Barnsley RH, Rabinovitch MS (1970) Handedness: proficiency versus stated preference. Percept Mot Skills 30(2):343–362. https://doi.org/10.2466/pms.1970.30.2.343

Bear D, Schiff D, Saver J, Greenberg M, Freeman R (1986) Quantitative analysis of cerebral asymmetries: fronto-occipital correlation, sexual dimorphism and association with handedness. Arch Neurol 43(6):598–603

Bishop DVM (1990) Handedness and developmental disorders. Mac Keith Press, Oxford; J.B. Lippincott (Clinics in developmental medicine, 110)

Bishop DV, Ross VA, Daniels MS, Bright P (1996) The measurement of hand preference: a validation study comparing three groups of right-handers. Br J Psychol 87(Pt 2):269–285. https://doi.org/10.1111/j.2044-8295.1996.tb02590.x

Blackburn A (2011) Bilateral asymmetry of the humerus during growth and development. American journal of physical anthropology 145(4):639–646.

Brown SG, Roy EA, Rohr LE, Snider BR, Bryden PJ (2004) Preference and performance measures of handedness. Brain Cogn 55(2):283–285. https://doi.org/10.1016/j.bandc.2004.02.010

Brown S, Roy E, Rohr L, Bryden P (2006) Using hand performance measures to predict handedness. Laterality 11(1):1–14. https://doi.org/10.1080/1357650054200000440

Bruckner J (2010) Erfassung der Handpräferenz bei Kindern von 4 bis 6 Jahren & entwicklungspsychologische Relevanz der differenzierten Erfassung der Handpräferenz im Kindergartenalter. http://othes.univie.ac.at/13855/

Bruckner J, Deimann P, Kastner-Koller U (2011) HAPT 4-6. Handpräferenztest für 4-6-jährige Kinder. Hogrefe, Göttingen

Bryden MP (1977) Measuring handedness with quetionnaires. Neuropsychologia 15:617–628

Bryden PJ, Roy EA (2005) A new method of administering the grooved pegboard test: performance as a function of handedness and sex. Brain Cogn 58(3):258–268. https://doi.org/10.1016/j.bandc.2004.12.004

Bryden PJ, Pryde KM, Roy EA (2000) A performance measure of the degree of hand preference. Brain Cogn 44(3):402–414. https://doi.org/10.1006/brcg.1999.1201

Bryden PJ, Roy EA, Rohr LE, Egilo S (2007a) Task demands affect manual asymmetries in pegboard performance. Laterality 12(4):364–377. https://doi.org/10.1080/13576500701356244

Bryden PJ, Roy EA, Spence J (2007b) An observational method of assessing handedness in children and adults. Dev Neuropsychol 32(3):825–846. https://doi.org/10.1080/87565640701539667

Carlier M, Duyme M, Capron C, Dumont AM, Perez-Diaz F (1993) Is a dot-filling group test a good tool for assessing manual performing in children? Neuropsychologia 31(3):233–240

Carlier M, Doyen A-L, Lamard C (2006) Midline crossing: developmental trend from 3 to 10 years of age in a preferential card-reaching task. Brain Cogn 61(3):255–261. https://doi.org/10.1016/j.bandc.2006.01.007

Carson RG, Thomas J, Summer JJ, Walters MR, Semjen A (1997) The dynamics of bimanual circle drawing. Q J Exp Psychol A 50A(3):664–683

Christman S (2014) Individual differences in personality as a function of degree of handedness: consistent-handers are less sensation seeking, more authoritarian, and more sensitive to disgust. Laterality 19(3):354–367. https://doi.org/10.1080/1357650X.2013.838962

Cochet H, Byrne RW (2013) Evolutionary origins of human handedness: evaluating contrasting hypotheses. Anim Cogn 16(4):531–542. https://doi.org/10.1007/s10071-013-0626-y

Colman HA, Remington RW, Kritikos A (2017) Handedness and graspability modify shifts of visuospatial attention to near-hand objects. PLoS One 12(1):e0170542. https://doi.org/10.1371/journal.pone.0170542

Corey DM, Hurley MM, Foundas AL (2001) Right and left handedness defined: a multivariate approach using hand preference and hand performance measures. Neuropsychiatry Neuropsychol Behav Neurol 14(3):144–152

Das B, Meltzer J, Armstrong B (2021) Quantitative assessment of handedness and cerebral lateralization. JNS 2(1):6–22. https://doi.org/10.33137/jns.v2i1.34660

Fagard J, Lockman JJ (2005) The effect of task constraints on infants' (bi)manual strategy for grasping and exploring objects. Infant Behav Dev 28(3):305–315. https://doi.org/10.1016/j.infbeh.2005.05.005

Fisher AG, Murray EA, Bundy AC (2002): Sensorische Integrationstherapie. Theorie & Praxis. 2., durchgesehene Auflage. Berlin, Heidelberg, s.l.: Springer Berlin Heidelberg (Rehabilitation & prävention). https://doi.org/10.1007/978-3-662-09864-6

Fitts PM (1954) The information capacity of the human motor system in controlling the amplitude of movement. J Exp Psychol 47(6):381–391. https://doi.org/10.1037/h0055392

Flindall JW, Gonzalez CLR (2019) Wait wait, don't tell me: handedness questionnaires do not predict hand preference for grasping. Laterality 24(2):176–196. https://doi.org/10.1080/1357650X.2018.1494184

Gilbert AN, Wysocki CJ (1992) Hand preference and age in the United States. Neuropsychologia 30(7):601–608. https://doi.org/10.1016/0028-3932(92)90065-T

Gonzalez SL, Nelson EL (2021) Factor analysis of the home handedness questionnaire: unimanual and role differentiated bimanual manipulation as separate dimensions of handedness. Appl Neuropsychol Adult 28(2):173–184

Hardie SM, Wright L, Clark L (2016) Handedness and social anxiety: using Bryden's research as a catalyst to explore the influence of familial sinistrality and degree of handedness. Laterality 21(4–6):329–347. https://doi.org/10.1080/1357650X.2015.1131712

Healey JM, Liederman J, Geschwind N (1986) Handedness is not a unidimensional trait. Cortex 22(1):33–53. https://doi.org/10.1016/S0010-9452(86)80031-4

Hill LE, Bishop DVM (1998) A reaching test reveals weak hand preference in specific language impairment and developmental co-ordination disorder. Laterality 3(4):295–310. https://doi.org/10.1080/713754314

Hill EL, Khanem F (2009) The development of hand preference in children: the effect of task demands and links with manual dexterity. Brain Cogn 71(2):99–107. https://doi.org/10.1016/j.bandc.2009.04.006

Ida Y, Mandal MK, Bryden MP (2000) Factor structures of hand preference questionnaires: are "skilled" and "unskilled" factors artifacts? In: Side bias: a neuropsychological perspective. Springer, pp 175–190

Jäncke L, Peters M, Schlaug G, Posse S, Steinmetz H, Müller-Gärtner H (1998) Differential magnetic resonance signal change in human sensorimotor cortex to finger movements of different rate of the dominant and subdominant hand. Brain Res 6(4):279–284. https://doi.org/10.1016/s0926-6410(98)00003-2

Karapetsas AB, Vlachos FM (1997) Sex and handedness in development of visuomotor skills. Percept Mot Skills 85(1):131–140

Klar AJS (2003) Human handedness and scalp hair-whorl direction develop from a common genetic mechanism. Genetics 165(1):269–276

Klöppel S, Vongerichten A, van Eimeren T, Frackowiak RSJ, Siebner HR (2007) Can left-handedness be switched? Insights from an early switch of handwriting. J Neurosci 27(29):7847–7853. https://doi.org/10.1523/JNEUROSCI.1299-07.2007

Klöppel S, Mangin J-F, Vongerichten A, Frackowiak RSJ, Siebner HR (2010) Nurture versus nature: long-term impact of forced right-handedness on structure of pericentral cortex and basal ganglia. J Neurosci 30(9):3271–3275

Koeneke S, Battista C, Jancke L, Peters M (2009) Transfer effects of practice for simple alternating movements. J Motor Behav 41(4):347–356

Kraus E (2003) The handedness profile. The development of a normative profile to determine the extent of handedness in children. Doctoral Thesis. La Trobe University, Melbourne

Kraus E (2006) Ist das Überkreuzen der Körpermittellinie ein Indikator für die Handpräferenz bei Kindern? Ergoscience 1(3):100–109. https://doi.org/10.1055/s-2006-927098

Kraus E (Hg.) (2019) Zwischen Links-& Rechtshändigkeit. Theorie, Diagnostik & Therapie bei Kindern mit wechselndem Handgebrauch. Springer, Berlin

Largo RH, Fischer JE, Caflisch JA, Jenni OG (2007) Züricher Neuromotorik Test

Niebauer CL, Christman S, Reid S, Garvey K (2004). Interhemispheric interaction and beliefs on our origin: Degree of handedness predicts beliefs in creationism versus evolution. *Laterality: Asymmetries of Body, Brain and Cognition* 9(4):433–447

Mamolo CM, Roy EA, Bryden PJ, Rohr LE (2004) The effects of skill demands and object position on the distribution of preferred hand reaches. Brain Cogn 55(2):349–351. https://doi.org/10.1016/j.bandc.2004.02.041

Marcori AJ, Monteiro PHM, Okazaki VHA (2019) Changing handedness: what can we learn from preference shift studies? Neurosci Biobehav Rev 107:313–319

Marlow N, Ni Y, Beckmann J, O'Reilly H, Johnson S, Wolke D, Morris JK (2019) Hand preference develops across childhood and adolescence in extremely preterm children: the EPICure study. Pediatr Neurol 99:40–46. https://doi.org/10.1016/j.pediatrneurol.2019.04.007

McFarland K, Anderson J (1980) Factor stability of the Edinburgh handedness inventory as a function of test-retest performance, age and sex. Br J Psychol 71(1):135–142. https://doi.org/10.1111/j.2044-8295.1980.tb02739.x

Merni F, Michele D, Rocco, Soffritti G (2014) Assessment of handedness using latent class factor analysis. Laterality 19(4):405–423. https://doi.org/10.1080/1357650X.2013.845572

Michell D, Wood N (1999) An investigation of midline crossing in three-year-old children. Physiotherapy 85(11):607–615. https://doi.org/10.1016/S0031-9406(05)66041-5

Nelson EL, Gonzalez SL, El-Asmar JM, Ziade MF, Abu-Rustum RS (2019) The home handedness questionnaire: pilot data from preschoolers. Laterality 24(4):482–503. https://doi.org/10.1080/1357650X.2018.1543313

Nikolaeva E, Vergunov E (2018) Handedness: manual lateral parameter–or the result of the Researcher's manipulation. In: KnE Life Sciences, pp 648–659

Oldfield RC (1971) The assessment and analysis of handedness: the Edinburgh inventory. Neuropsychologia 9(1):97–113. https://doi.org/10.1016/0028-3932(71)90067-4

Olsson B, Rett A (1989) Linkshändigkeit. Hans Huber, Bern

Peters M (1998) Description and validation of a flexible and broadly usable handedness questionnaire. Laterality 3(1):77–96. https://doi.org/10.1080/713754291

Peters M, Durding BM (1978) Handedness measured by finger tapping: a continuous variable. Can J Psychol 32(4):257

Petrigna L, Pajaujiene S, Gaetano MI, Thomas E, Paoli A, Bianco A, Palma A (2020) The execution of the grooved pegboard in a dual-task situation. A pilot study. Heliyon 6:1–4

Porac C (1996) Attempts to switch the writing hand: relationships to age and side of hand preference. Laterality 1(1):35–44. https://doi.org/10.1080/713754205

Prichard E, Propper RE, Christman SD (2013) Degree of handedness, but not direction, is a systematic predictor of cognitive performance. Front Psychol 4:9. https://doi.org/10.3389/fpsyg.2013.00009

Provine RR, Westerman JA (1979) Crossing the midline: limits of early eye-hand behavior. Child Dev 50(2):437–441

Provins KA, Cunliffe P (1972) The reliability of some motor performance tests of handedness. Neuropsychologia 10(2):199–206. https://doi.org/10.1016/0028-3932(72)90060-7

Provins KA, Magliaro J (1993) The measurement of handedness by preference and performance tests. Brain Cogn 22(2):171–181

Przybyla A, Coelho CJ, Akpinar S, Kirazci S, Sainburg RL (2013) Sensorimotor performance asymmetries predict hand selection. Neuroscience 228(Pt. 2):349–360. https://doi.org/10.1016/j.neuroscience.2012.10.046

Ruck L, Schoenemann PT (2021) Handedness measures for the human connectome project: implications for data analysis. Laterality 26(5):584–606. https://doi.org/10.1080/1357650X.2020.1866001

Sattler JB (2002) Linkshändige & umgeschulte linkshändige Kinder sowie Kinder mit wechselndem Handgebrauch in der Ergotherapie. Ergother Rehab (41):21–29

Sattler JB (2008) Händigkeitsabklärung SMH nach der Sattler-Methodik. Testverfahren mit Item-Karten, Kopiervorlagen & um-fassendem Dokumentationsbogen. Auer Verlag, Donauwörth

Sattler JB, Klußmann A (2014) Leitlinie Händigkeit. - Bedeutung & Untersuchung / 002/017 - S1. Unter Mitarbeit von DGAUM, AWMF, zuletzt aktualisiert am 06.2020

Sattler JB, Marquardt C (2006) Rückschulung bei erwachsenen umgeschulten Linkshändern. In: Motorik, Zeitschrift für Motopädagogik & Mototherapie, pp 121–127

Schachter SC, Ransil BJ, Geschwind N (1987) Associations of handedness with hair color and learning disabilities. Neuropsychologia 25(1B):269–276. https://doi.org/10.1016/0028-3932(87)90137-0

Scharoun SM, Bryden PJ (2012) Test-retest reliability of the Wathand cabinet test in children and adults. J Exercise

Scharoun SM, Bryden PJ (2014) Hand preference, performance abilities, and hand selection in children. Front Psychol 5:82. https://doi.org/10.3389/fpsyg.2014.00082

Scharoun SM, Bryden PJ (2015) Is strength of handedness reliable over repeated testing? An examination of typical development and autism spectrum disorder. Front Psychol 6:17

Schilling F (2009) Punktiertest & Leistungs-Dominanztest für Kinder (5–12 Jahre). Der Linkshändertest. 1. Aufl. Modernes Lernen, Dortmund

Schönthaler E (2020) Die Händigkeit des Kindes. In: Schönthaler E (Hg.): Grafomotorik & Händigkeit. Ergotherapie bei Kindern. 2. Auflage. Thieme, Stuttgart, pp 188–220

Searleman A, Porac C (2001) Lateral preference patterns as possible correlates of successfully switched left hand writing: data and a theory. Laterality 6(4):303–314

Semjen A, Summers J, Cattaert D (1995) Hand coordination in bimanual circle drawing. J Exp Psychol 21(5):1139–1157

Soper HV, Satz P (1984) Pathological left-handedness and ambiguous handedness: a new explanatory model. Neuropsychologia 22(4):511–515. https://doi.org/10.1016/0028-3932(84)90046-0

Steele J (2000) Skeletal indicators of handedness. Human Osteology 307–23

Steenhuis RE, Bryden MP (1989) Different dimensions of hand preference that relate to skilled and unskilled activities. Cortex 25(2):289–304. https://doi.org/10.1016/S0010-9452(89)80044-9

Steenhuis RE, Bryden MP, Schwartz M, Lawson S (1990) Reliability of hand preference items and factors. J Clin Exp Neuropsychol 12(6):921–930. https://doi.org/10.1080/01688639008401031

Steingrüber HJ (2011) H-D-T. Hand-Dominanz-Test ; Manual. 3., überarb. & neu normierte Aufl. Göttingen [u.a.]: Hogrefe

Surburg PR (1999) Midline-crossing inhibition: an indicator of developmental delay. Laterality 4(4):333–343. https://doi.org/10.1080/713754347

Tan LE (1985) Laterality and motor skills in four-year-olds. Child Dev 56(1):119–124

Tapley SM, Bryden MP (1985) A group test for the assessment of performance between the hands. Neuropsychologia 23(2):215–221. https://doi.org/10.1016/0028-3932(85)90105-8

Tiffin J (1948) The Purdue pegboard. Lafayette Instrument Company, Lafayette

Trites RL (1977) Neuropsychological test manual. Royal Ottawa Hospital, Ottawa

Vingerhoets, Guy (2022): Laterality indices consensus initiative (LICI). Some results of the Delphi expert survey. 8th north sea laterality conference on brain asymmetry. University of Bergen. Bergen, Norway, 2022

Walker L, Henneberg M (2007) Writing with the non-dominant hand: cross-handedness trainability in adult individuals. Laterality 12(2):121–130. https://doi.org/10.1080/13576500600989665

Wang Y-C, Magasi SR, Bohannon RW, Reuben DB, McCreath HE, Bubela DJ et al (2011) Assessing dexterity function: a comparison of two alternatives for the NIH toolbox. J Hand Ther 24(4):313–321. https://doi.org/10.1016/j.jht.2011.05.001

Williams SM (1991) Handedness inventories: Edinburgh versus Annett. Neuropsychology 5(1):43

Williams SM (2022) The Edinburgh handedness inventory: a bibliometric return after five years

Constructing a Multidimensional Assessment: The Handedness Profile 2003

7

Contents

Handedness establishment is decisive in the development of manual skill and occupational performance, and unestablished handedness has been associated with developmental delay. Furthermore, evidence exists that motor and learning problems could occur if a child's handedness is misclassified. The accurate assessment of handedness of preschool children by paediatric occupational therapists is therefore important. However, unestablished handedness has received little attention within the occupational therapy literature, and there is a lack of comprehensive handedness assessments designed to investigate unestablished handedness and related neuromotor behaviours. (Kraus 2003: xv)

7.1 Introduction

The above quote was the opening paragraph of my doctoral thesis, reflecting years of practice with children that demonstrated atypical variable hand use. In my quest to capture the handedness status as accurately as possible, I encountered many unforeseen challenges during my initial five research studies. I created a battery of handedness tests by attempting to solve these challenges and meet the need in clinical practice.

In the next two chapters, we will look at the development of the assessment I subsequently developed, the *Handedness Profile.* I will reflect on its various aspects and summarise the respective studies. There are two phases in which the Handedness Profile was developed. This chapter focuses on the first phase (where I wrote my doctoral thesis), in which I explored specific research questions. In particular, I conceptualised, developed and evaluated five handedness subtests; collected normative data; and constructed a tool for analysis, the *Category Profile* (Kraus 2003). The second phase involves a number of studies that validate the Handedness Profile to the current version of 2018, which will be presented in the next chapter.

7.2 Research Studies Developing a Multidimensional Assessment

Guided by these initial contemplations, I first explored how variable hand use was evident in 5-year-old Australian preschool children. I assumed

E. Kraus, *Beyond Left and Right Handedness*, https://doi.org/10.1007/978-3-031-24389-9_7

that handedness is subject to a developmental process and only becomes established between the ages of 6 and 9 years, based on the literature (e.g. McManus et al. 1988; Ross et al. 1992).

7.2.1 Study I: Assessment of the Extent of Handedness in 5-Year-Old Preschool Children

Background

In Study I, I addressed the question of how well existing test procedures can reveal the extent of handedness, and how this would relate to other related developmental aspects. The study assumed that data of typically developed left- and right-handed girls and boys would provide a point of reference when evaluating children with unestablished handedness. Another assumption was that whilst all individuals display some handedness variability, children under the age of 6 would show notably greater variability since they were still developing their handedness. I assessed handedness in 120 Australian 5-year-old preschool children based on these assumptions. In addition, Ayres, a psychologist and occupational therapist, had linked handedness establishment to crossing the body midline as well as bimanual coordination as a type of sensory integration disorder (Ayres 1972). I thus investigated these variables as well to see if they correlated with the degree of handedness.

Test Material

The handedness variability was assessed using a combination of four test procedures. (1) The "Edinburgh Handedness Inventory" (EHI) (Oldfield 1971) was used to assess *hand preference*, consisting of a mixture of items with different test-retest reliabilities (McFarland and Anderson 1980). However, I modified the EHI as a performance-based preference measurement, as this has been found to be the most reliable method for children (Longoni and de Gennaro 1992; Rigal 1992). Another adaptation was performing multiple trials of each preference item (four times) to measure ♦**internal consistency**. Finally, the bimanual item "sweeping with a (long) broom" was. The original item the only item not performed sitting at the table but standing, and it required gross proximal movement from the shoulder, which is less lateralised (Healey et al. 1986; Mäki-Marttunen et al. 2014). Instead, I replaced it with the bimanual item using a hand brush and dustpan, which involves more distal (and more lateralised) movement.

In addition to the everyday functional tasks of the EHI, a **Midline Crossing Test** seemed viable to assess hand preference in combination with contralateral reaching. I could only find one standardised procedure, the "Space Visualization Contralateral Use Score" (SVCU), generated during the visual-spatial subtest "Space Visualisation" of the standardised battery of tests called the "Sensory Integration and Praxis Tests—SIPT"[1] (Ayres 1989). It is documented in the test how often the preferred hand[2] is used to pick up shapes placed to the left and right of the child's centre.

To cover the other dimensions of handedness, performance or ♦**proficiency** (as is referred to it consistently in this book), a unimanual and a bimanual motor task were chosen. For **unimanual motor proficiency**,[3] I used another subtest of the SIPT, the "Motor Accuracy (MAcc) Test", consisting of a tracing task performed by each hand, taking into account both speed and accuracy of the child's response. Tracing is a common task to assess motor proficiency (Stirling et al. 2013; Bishop 1990) and thus seemed appropriate. For **bimanual performance**, I tested bilateral motor integration of the two upper extremities using the "Bilateral Motor Coordination Test" (BMC) of the SIPT, where bilateral movement is rated according to a 3-point scale (average, bor-

[1]The SIPT is commonly used in occupational therapy praxis to evaluate possible sensory integration dysfunction. It is based on normative data for children aged 4–11 years.

[2]The "preferred hand" is based on the first hand chosen by the child when performing the proficiency test (MAcc) described below.

[3]The term "performance" is used in the doctoral thesis—it is synonymous with the term "proficiency" used in this book and the current Handedness Profile.

derline, below average). The normative data of 5-year-olds were used to assess the level of performance.

Method

One hundred and twenty-two 5-year-old typically developed Australian preschool children were recruited and tested with the instruments described. The gender ratio was evenly distributed ($N = 61$ each), and there were 18 left-handed children based on parents' and teachers' report and confirmed by the study. For the EHI, a laterality quotient (LQ) was used to measure inter-hand differences by subtracting left-hand responses from right-hand responses. The three SIPT subtests were scored as standardised.

Results and Discussion

The direction of hand preference seemed viable with an incidence of 14.7% left handers. However, the modified EHI preference test results revealed different variability between left- and right-handed subjects, with a ceiling effect on right-handed children. In fact, the vast majority of right-handed children revealed a very high degree of hand preference with an average LQ of 85%, so the extent/degree of handedness could not be described as variable, a rather unexpected finding in 5-year-olds. In contrast, the preference distribution of left-handed children was much broader, with an average LQ of −62%. This difference between left and right handers is in concordance with many research studies where left handers show significantly greater variability than their right-handed counterparts. However, the group of 18 left handers was too small for generalisation. In the MAcc *proficiency* test, no differences were found between left and right handers nor between boys and girls. In addition, the inter-hand differences were unexpectedly small, especially in right handers. In the *SVCU midline crossing*, 20% avoided contralateral reaching entirely, and the remaining subjects had inter-hand differences of 35% in right handers (i.e. crossed over 35% more with the right hand) and −33% in left handers (i.e. crossed over 33% more with the left hand). The average bimanual motor coordination (BMC) test score was 23%, with girls performing slightly better than boys (27–20%), this difference approaching significance.

Since the same SVCU and BMC subtests were standardised for a wide age range (4–11-year-olds) (Ayres 1989), it was probably not surprising that 5-year-old children performed relatively low in these tests. They belonged to the younger group where bilateral coordination is still in an early developmental stage. Although low scores may be typical for that age group, the lack of variability in the results limited the ability to discriminate comprehensively between typically developed children and those with problems crossing the body midline and bilateral coordination.

Conclusion

All tests were statistically skewed and failed to show the expected variability and diversity of the multidimensional handedness phenomenon as described in the literature. Whilst it could be argued that the EHI and the MAcc test were too "simple" and therefore resulted in ceiling effects, the SVCU Midline Crossing Test and the bilateral motor coordination test (BMC) appeared to be too difficult for 5-year-olds. I concluded that these tests were not sensitive enough for this age group to display the expected variability cited in research studies on hand use in and various degrees of handedness.

7.2.2 Study II: Comparing Handedness Variability in Different Age Groups

Background

Based on the results of the first study, it seemed reasonable to conduct a second study with similar questions, but younger children and some different testing procedures. Firstly, I hypothesised that 3- and 4-year-olds would display an even greater variability since their handedness development would be less advanced. Expectedly, one would see the development of handedness extent or degree across age groups. Secondly, the modified EHI and MAcc tests for preference and proficiency could be used again since they were "too easy" for 5-year-olds and would likely show a more normal spread in younger children. Thirdly, the SVCU midline crossing and BMC tests that already seemed "too difficult" for 5-year-olds would be even more difficult for younger children. Also, I concluded that the BMC of the SIPT was not suitable for asymmetric role differentiation between the hands, since a "good" response of the test items requires simultaneous *coordination* between both arms and hands instead of a leading hand. So I developed new tests for crossing the body midline, as well as for bimanual *cooperation* involving a leading hand.[4]

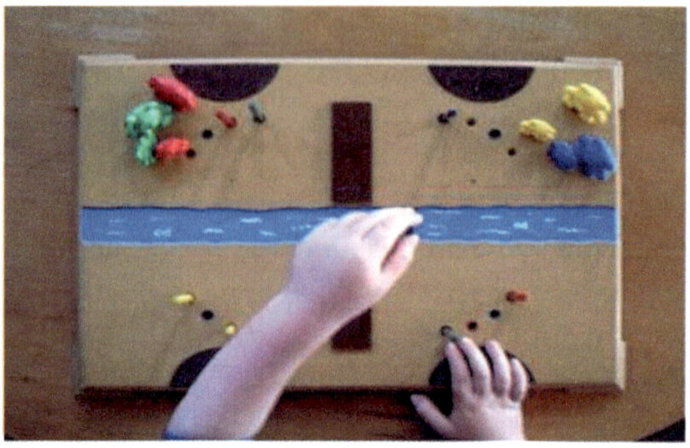

Photo: Kraus, 2003

Fig. 7.1 The Midline Crossing Test (MCT) of the Handedness Profile (Photo by Kraus 2003)

Test Development

Midline Crossing Test: Based on the concept of the "Test of Manual Midline Crossing" used in a study to assesses midline crossing in 2- to 6-year-old children (Stilwell 1987), I developed a peg game. It consisted of a total of 32 possible responses in ♦**ipsilateral** (same side—12x), ♦**contralateral** (opposite side—12x) and centre responses (8x). To make the repetitive peg-moving activity attractive to young children and ensure that their attention was not directed to the hand used, I invented a story with colourful bears that needed the child's help to build a fence with matching-coloured pegs (see Fig. 7.1). The centre responses were used as a control to differentiate between midline crossing and hand preference. For example, a child could pick up pegs ipsilaterally on the left and the right, thus avoiding crossing the body midline and showing no hand preference. In the centre, however, he/she might consistently use one hand when contralateral reaching is eliminated, possibly displaying some degree of preference. This, in turn, could indicate that midline crossing avoidance might or might not be (co)responsible for the observed variable hand use.

Bimanual Cooperation Test: In everyday bimanual activities, the dominant hand usually takes a leading and more active role, and the non-dominant shows a more assistive and stabilising function.[5] It is also seen in bimanual movement patterns not related to functional activities. For example, studies on bimanual coordination have used bimanual simultaneous circle drawing in different directions, using mirror and parallel movement patterns (Carson et al. 1997; Fagard and Pezé 1992; Semjen et al. 1995). Findings show that circles drawn with the dominant hand in typically developed adult left and right handers are rounder and more accurate. The dominant hand also tends to lead and displays more consistent pressure than the non-dominant hand. During parallel bimanual movement, particularly when demands are accentuated by increased speed and excluded vision, the dominant hand is more likely to maintain the original drawing direction. In contrast, the non-dominant hand tends to revert to mirroring the movement of the dominant hand.

Based on these findings, I developed a test of simultaneous circle drawing for my study. To make it more interesting for young children, I used a mechanical drawing toy, Etch-A-Sketch,[6] similar to other researchers who worked with children (Steese-Seda et al. 1995; Fagard 1990; Fagard and Pezé 1992). The two knobs of the

[4]In my Ph.D. studies, I used the term "bimanual coordination". In the course of developing the current Handedness Profile, this has changed into the term "bimanual cooperation" to better represent the specific aspect of bimanual coordination that involves the role differentiation of the hands.

[5]This has been termed as role-differentiated bimanual manipulation (RDBM) (Babik 2014).

[6]The Etch-A-Sketch is a rectangular toy with two knobs in the lower corners. When these are turned, a stylus draws a solid line by displacing aluminium powder on the back of the screen.

Etch-A-Sketch were adapted by attaching discs of 8 cm, each with a small bear and a swivel mechanism. This allowed the child to draw bimanual circles in all direction combinations (outward, inward, to the right and the left) by holding the bears (see Fig. 7.2). If both hands moved at an equal pace and synchronised perfectly, a slope of 45° would result. If the right hand moved faster, the slope would be steeper, and if the left hand was leading, the slope would be flatter. If the hands did not move at the same time, the line would display "steps" rather than a gradient. The degrees of the slopes were measured and recorded for each of the four directions.

Method

In Study II, I recruited 91 typically developed preschool children: 30 3-year-olds, 31 4-year-olds, and 30 5-year-olds. Of these, eight children were left handed (9%). Parents and educators/teachers confirmed that all children had a clear direction for handedness and absence of developmental delay or problems according to inclusion criteria. Children with unestablished handedness were excluded. The distribution of girls to boys was approximately equal in all age groups. The following tests were conducted: the *modified EHI preference test*, the MAcc test for hand performance/proficiency, the new *Midline Crossing Test (MCT)* and the new *Bimanual Coordination Test (BCT)*. The laterality quotient (LQ) was calculated for all tests to ensure the comparability of the results.

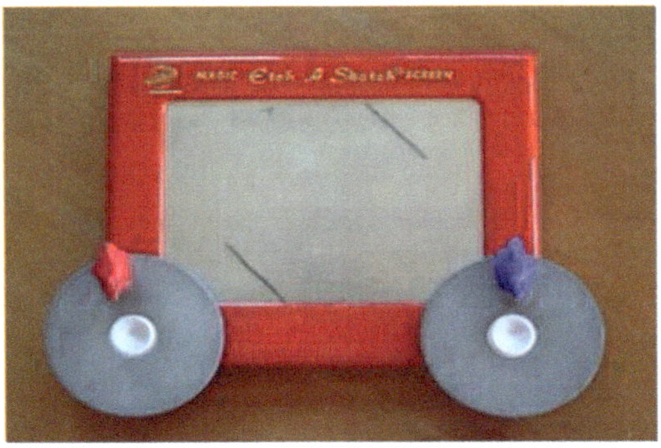

Photo: (Kraus, 2003)

Fig. 7.2 The Bimanual Coordination (BMC) Test with the Etch-A-Sketch of the Handedness Profile (Kraus 2003)

Results and Discussion

Girls showed greater lateralisation than boys in the modified EHI preference test, with a tendency towards significance. However, an analysis of variance (ANOVA) showed no significant differences between the three age groups. On the contrary, the average LQ of the 83 right-handed children was 84% (compared to 85% in Study I), and for the eight left-handed children 50% (compared to 62% in Study I). On the MAcc proficiency test, 3-year-olds showed larger inter-hand differences than the older children, and the differences between the age groups were significant. The distribution of the results was similar to Study I: it was skewed and showed a ceiling effect on left and right handers, and small inter-hand differences in 4- and 5-year olds. The MCT showed significantly more contralateral responses than the SVCU in Study I. Crossing the midline also increased with age: the LQ average for 3-year-olds was 52%, in 4-year-olds 60%, and in 5-year-olds 63% (compared with the SVCU average of 34% in Study I). Similarly, the results of the new BCT showed a normal distribution instead of the floor effect of the BMC in Study I: the LQ average BCT was 67% overall with significant differences between the age groups, compared to an LQ of 23% in Study I.

Conclusion

The findings of Study II led me to conclude that the two newly developed tests (MCT and BCT) were suitable and sufficiently sensitive to investigate the research questions exploring normal variability of handedness in typically developed preschool children. In contrast to data distributions of the SVCU and BMC in Study I, the MCT and BCT showed statistically unskewed normal distributions. The modified EHI preference and MAcc proficiency test were expected to capture a developmental increase in proficiency over the three age groups. However, the EHI produced similar results to the first study with little variability. In the MAcc test, age differences were found but the inter-hand differences (IHD) between the hands were relatively small for the older children, in contrast to the very large preference IHDs and the expected developmental progression. The larger IHDs in younger children were even more puzzling, contrary to the well-known premise that lateralisation (as represented by inter-hand differences) increases with age (De Agostini et al. 1992; Mandell et al. 1984). Thus, whilst the new subtests MCT and BCT seemed sufficiently sensitive and suitable for capturing a developmental profile of preferred contralateral reaching and bimanual in young children. The modified EHI preference and the MAcc proficiency test were not.

Table 7.1 Differences between left and right handers in new/modified tests

Modified test	Significance
FHPT total (preference)	0.001[a]
Untrained items (preference)	0.039[b]
Trained items (preference)	0.000[a]
Internal consistency (preference)	0.037[b]
Ability: hammering and tapping (performance)	0.020[b]
Skill: tracking and puncturing (performance)	0.004[a]
MCT (midline crossing)	0.038[b]
BCT (bimanual coordination)	0.009[a]

[a] Significant at 0.01
[b] Significant at 0.05

7.2.3 Study III: Comparing Existing and Modified Tests for Typically Developed 6-Year-Olds

Background

Based on the previous results, I developed new tests for preference and proficiency to replace the EHI and the MAcc. There was a clear need to compare the conventional tests with the new ones whilst other variables remained stable.

Test Development

Preference test: Since the items of the EHI have been validated and are arguably the most frequently preference items in handedness research, ensuring better comparability of results, it seemed reasonable to keep these items. However, there was a need to cover a larger range of everyday actions, so I supplemented the EHI items with additional items, ensuring a balance between trained and untrained and unimanual and bimanual tasks. Several authors have stressed incorporating different task characteristics when assessing handedness (Bryden et al. 1996; Provins and Cunliffe 1972). I hypothesised that a mixture of such items would be more likely to demonstrate the individual and developmental based degree or variability of handedness. Thus, in addition to the 10 EHI items, 14 items were added to make up the new "Functional Hand Preference Test" (FHPT). Twelve of the total 24 items were considered to be ♦**trained**, and 12 ♦**untrained**,[7] half of which consisted of bimanual and unimanual tasks, respectively (see Table 7.1). In addition, each of these items was performed four times in order to evaluate the level of ♦**internal consistency** (within an item or task). LQs were calculated for the total FHPT as well as for trained vs. untrained and unimanual vs. bimanual tasks.

As described in Sect. 1.4, the preferred hand is not necessarily the better one. Motor proficiency is typically assessed in handedness research using tracing or dotting tasks (Carlier et al. 1993, 1996). Both Tracing and Dotting correlate highly with writing and are thus subject to a strong practice effect (see Annett 1992; Tapley and Bryden 1985). For this reason, such tasks are unlikely to detect converted handedness. For example, if a switched left hander has automated right-handed writing through extensive practice, the right hand probably performs better in Tracing and Dotting than the dominant left hand (see also Coren 1992; Peters 1992, 1998; Peters and Murphy 1992).

The question of how to capture motor proficiency not affected by practice or training effects prompted me to develop additional tests. First, an additional motor task were needed.

[7]Trained items refer to activities or movement sequences that have been subjected to a particular (right) sided bias or training, resulting in practising a specific (left or right) hand (e.g. shake hands or write with the right hand). With repeated practice, movements are often automated. Such trained activities have a high cultural value, and they do not necessarily demand a high level of skill.

Two proficiency tests were likely to be unaffected by training. *Tapping* and *hammering* have been shown to be motor actions not influenced by practice (e.g. Peters 1990; Watter and Burns 1995). Tapping is controlled distally (i.e. movement comes from the wrist as in finger tapping (Watter and Burns 1995)), whilst hammering is controlled from the shoulder (i.e. proximally—see Peters 1990). The distinction between proximal and distal is relevant to handedness since there is evidence that distal movements are generally more lateralised than proximal ones (ibid.). Also, as seen in clinical practice, motor problems in children often consist of a combination of different motor aspects. For example, some fine motor skills might be related to a lack of shoulder stability, whilst in other cases, more distal interferences like tremors interfered with proficient movement. It thus seemed a good idea to include both Hammering and Tapping in the untrained proficiency test (hammering test and tapping test), which I collectively termed "**Ability**".

The trained proficiency tasks I referred to "**Skill**". They also consisted of two tasks, Tracing and Dotting, using a bear figure to make the tasks more child-orientated (i.e. bear tracing test (BTT) and bear dotting test (BDT)). The BTT was similar to the MAcc, combining speed and accuracy measures for the laterality quotient, as is the case for all proficiency subtests.

Method

For Study III, I recruited 60 typically developed 6-year-old children: 30 left handers and 30 right handers (half boys and half girls). Inclusion criteria were the absence of any developmental delay or condition and unmistakably established handedness as confirmed by parents and teachers. The test battery included all the conventional tests of the first two studies: MAcc, SVCU, BMC test and modified EHI. In addition, all of the newly developed subtests were administered: *Functional Hand Preference Test (FHPT)*, Tracing and Dotting (*Skill tests*), Hammering and Tapping (*Ability tests*), *Midline Crossing Test (MCT)* and *Bimanual Cooperation Test (BCT)*.

Results and Discussion

The results of the newly developed tests did not indicate significant gender differences in the performance level between left and right handers. However, the degree of handedness as a basis for differentiation between various groups of *Left* and *Right Handedness* was significant (see Table 7.1), whereby the trained items were highly significant and the untrained items moderately significant.

In contrast to the modified EHI, the distribution of left and right handers in the FHPT preference test showed normal distributions. Also, the LQ values in the FHPT had comparatively lower averages and a more even dispersion (left handers: EHI −67% and FHPT −46%; right handers: EHI 89% and FHPT 70%). Nevertheless, the FHPT also showed a clear tendency that right handers were generally more lateralised and had higher internal constancy and lower variability than left handers. The literature supports these findings (see Sect. 4.3).

The MAcc test again displayed a ceiling effect with a comparatively narrow dispersion for proficiency. In comparison, the new *Skill tests* (Tracing and Dotting) showed a normal and broader distribution for both tests as calculated by performance LQs (*left handers*: MAcc −1% and average skills −8%; right handers: MAcc 4% and average skill 11%). Contrasting the Tracing and Dotting subtests, there were minimal differences between the tests in right handers, whilst in left handers, there was a higher error rate in the dotting test compared to the tracing test.

In the new *Ability test* (Hammering and Tapping), the average difference between the hands was also greater for right handers (right handers LQ 16%; left handers LQ −10%). This is also in concordance with other research findings (e.g. Peters 1990). Two of the 30 left handers performed better with the right hand, and three left handers showed no difference between the hands, compared to one right-handed child. The average for hammering was higher than for tapping, indicating that 6-year-old children find hammering easier than tapping.

The new crossing midline test *MCT* also produced a normal distribution with a higher average compared to the SVCU. For left handers, the

SVCU LQ average was −25% and −34% on the MCT. Right handers achieved an SVCU LQ of 27% and 55% for the MCT. These results are also consistent with the literature (e.g. Atwood and Cermak 1986; Cermak and Ayres 1984; Cermak et al. 1980). Left handers crossed less with their dominant left hand than right handers with their right, and only left handers used their non-dominant right hand to cross over.

The new BCT showed did not show a floor effect for bimanual proficiency, displaying a significantly higher performance level than the original BMC test (left handers: BMC −27%, BCT −61%; right handers BMC 27%, BCT 57%). The inter-hand differences were much smaller in this test for left handers (LQ −2%) than for right handers (LQ 22%), which is again in agreement with the literature (Fagard 1991; Fagard and Corroyer 2003).

Conclusion

This study demonstrated that the new subtests showed a significantly greater variability of the handedness dimensions in more normal distributions than the conventional tests. Furthermore, the results were consistent with the literature. Thus, I could conclude that the newly developed tests formed a suitable basis for a developmentally sensitive instrument assessing handedness in children, taking the direction and the degree of handedness across various dimensions into account.

7.2.4 Study IV: Constructing a Normative Basis for the Handedness Profile

Background

For further analysis, I grouped the seven developed subtests for the different handedness dimensions into five test procedures: (1) functional (everyday) hand **preference** with trained and untrained tasks (FHPT); (2) trained proficiency (consisting of an average of Tracing and Dotting); (3) **midline crossing** (MCT); (4) untrained proficiency (**Ability** consisting of an average of Hammering and Tapping); and (5) **bimanual cooperation** (BCT). These subtests formed the assessment battery called the Handedness Profile.

Based on the literature, I assumed that calculating the laterality quotients (LQ) of the different tests would provide a basis for comparing the degree of handedness and the level of performance across the different handedness dimensions. So, I categorised them according to percentiles to use them as benchmarking references for children with unestablished handedness. The normative data of the 60 typically developed left- and right-handed 6-year-olds of Study III were used, implementing a classification system. Whilst it is most common to define the cut-off point of a normal bell-shaped distribution at 68%, some authors have proposed a narrower range of 50%, where the cut-off values for the norm have been proposed to lie between the 25th and the 75th percentiles (Munro 1997; Lezak 1995). This ranking would allow better differentiation between and within subgroups of handedness, particularly since the available data set is small. In addition, percentile ranks provide information about how a given test result or score relates to the norm, which is important information when interpreting test results. For example, a child's score falling into the 85th percentile indicates that 85% of the children of the same age are at or below the same value. Conversely, a score falling in the fifth percentile designates that 95% of children at this age achieve higher values. For the Handedness Profile, scores falling between the 24th and 10th percentiles were described to be "borderline" and scores between the first and the ninth percentiles as below average, orientating the percentiles according to classic psychometric conversion tables, where scores below the 25th percentile are considered borderline and those below 9% sub-average (e.g. Novick 1980). Based on these percentiles, I constructed eight categories based on the laterality quotients quantifying inter-hand differences of left and right handers, so that groups could be clearly compared and categorised.

There is no consensus in the literature specifying the number of categories that should be used to classify handedness (see Annett 1992; Bishop 1990) or the cut-off points of such categories.

Fig. 7.3 Categories 1–8 based on degrees of handedness according to percentiles (Kraus 2003)

Explicit LEFT	Moderate LEFT	Mild LEFT	Variable LEFT	Variable RIGHT	Mild RIGHT	Moderate RIGHT	Explicit RIGHT
L+	L	L-	VL	VR	R-	R	R+
75th - 100 percentile	25th - 74th percentile	10th - 24th percentile	0 - 9th percentile	0th - 9th percentile	10th - 24th percentile	25th - 74th percentile	75th - 100 percentile

Category percentiles	L+ 75th - 100th	L 25th - 74th	L- 10th - 24th	VL 1 - 9th	0	VR 1 - 9th	R- 10th - 24th	R 25th - 74th	R+ 75th - 100th
Interhand Differences (IHD)	Large IHD			Small IHD					Large IHD
Untrained PREFERENCE (FHPT)	-76 to -100	-40 to -17	-3 to -39	-1 to -2	0	1 to 26	27 to 47	48 to 75	76 to 100
Trained PREFERENCE (FHPT)	-80 to -100	-42 to -79	-18 to -41	-1 to -17	0	1 to 69	70 to 77	78 to 93	94 to 100

Fig. 7.4 Excerpt of LQ scores of the FHPT, categorised according to percentiles

Initially, a five-group classification seemed adequate: explicit left and right handers, moderately left and right handers and mixed handers. However, one would not be able to distinguish between those mixed handers with left- or right-sided tendencies that might be very slight. Also, the sensitivity of scales is increased by a higher number of categories (e.g. Finstad 2010), so more handedness groups would likely represent the degree of handedness more accurately. Therefore, I decided, similar to Annett (1970, 1976)), to use an eight-group classification system for the degree of handedness (Fig. 7.3).

As far as the *level of performance/proficiency* was concerned, I thought it to be sufficient to use a three-group category system indicating whether the performance was average (25th–100th percentile), borderline (10th–24th percentile) or sub-average (0–9th percentile). The goal of the Handedness Profile was to establish degrees of handedness with reference to whether proficiency was adequate.

Method

The laterality quotient averages and ranges for each subtest in Study III were calculated based on the data set of the 60 typically developed left and right handers. The ranges were then categorised according to the percentile ranks defined above. The categories were numbered from 1 (very left) to 8 (very right) so that an average category value could be obtained, the overall "Profile Score" of the Handedness Profile. An example of the range of LQs for *hand preference* from the subtest of untrained FHPT part is shown in Fig. 7.4.

If we look at the top 25% of scores (i.e. 75th–100th percentiles) in untrained FHPT tasks, we see that explicit left handers (L+) show average LQs between −76 and −100%. Incidentally, this is identical to explicit right handers (R+) with LQs between 76 and 100%. The moderate left hander category (L) in untrained FHPT tasks ranges from −40 to −17% between the 25th and 74th percentiles, compared to the moderate right hander category (R) with values between 48 and 75%. Here, it becomes clear that the ranges differ between subtests and categories of left and right handers, with differences with differences being generally significantly larger in the latter.

To calculate the inter-hand differences for *hand proficiency*, the DI for proficiency was adapted (see Sect. 6.3.1). Whilst the principle of R – L remains the same and thus ensures high comparability with the preference (*LQ-Pref*), it is also important to compare the performance level in terms of how "good" a hand performs, not only in relation to the other hand, but also the "perfect" performance level. The proficiency of each hand is thus a ratio of the maximum or best possible score, calculated as a percentage thereof, comprising the proficiency laterality quotient (*LQ-Prof*). In this way, the LQ-Prof allows us to measure the difference between the hands and how well the hands perform, using the same continuum as for hand preference. 100% is the maximum proficiency possible for the right hand, and –100% is the maximum proficiency for the left hand.

Results and Discussion

Two databases of preliminary norms were created according to the 8-point classification system. The first data set shows the degree of handedness based on inter-hand differences measured with the LQ for left and right handers. Statistical analyses showed that the differences between the eight groups were significant. This means that the degree of handedness can be dependably grouped into these eight categories, even based on the relatively small sample of this study. The second data set broadly indicates the proficiency level of the respective subtests based on average performance values. An LQ average ranging between the 25th and 100th percentile is considered in the average performance range for 6-year-old children; an LQ falling between the 10th and 24th percentiles is considered borderline, and values below the 10th percentile are sub-average. Again, the three groups significantly differed from each other. Figures 7.5 and 7.6 illustrate the categorised scores for each of the five subtests according to the eight categories for all 60 subjects. One can see clearly that the left handers use their right hand much more frequently than the right handers use their left hand.

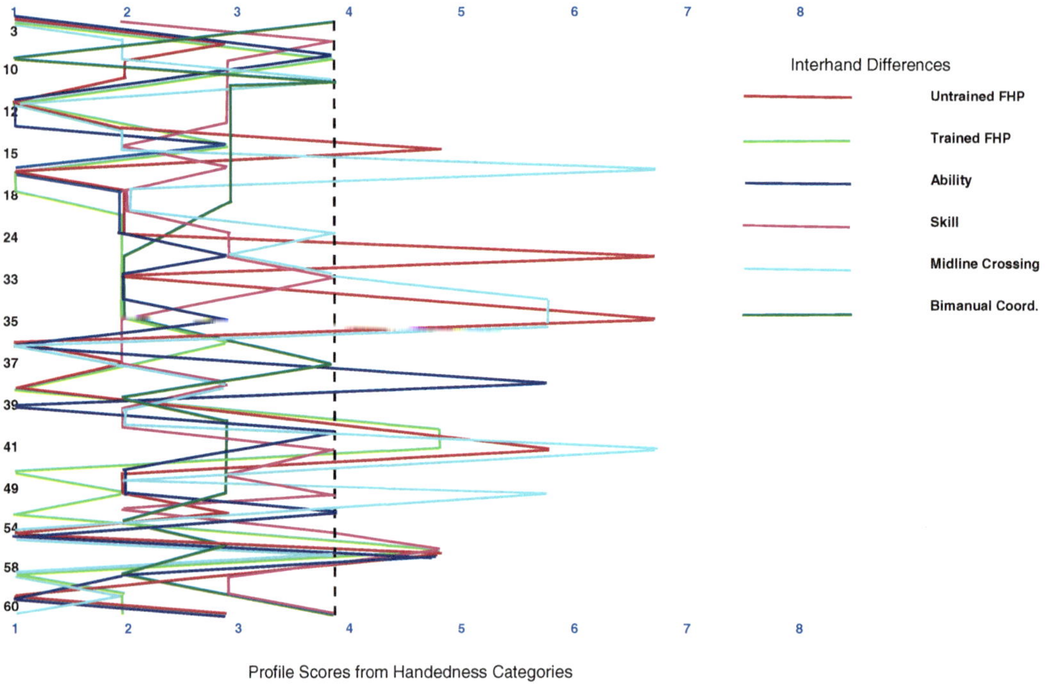

Fig. 7.5 Individual profile scores for typically developed left-handed children (n=30)

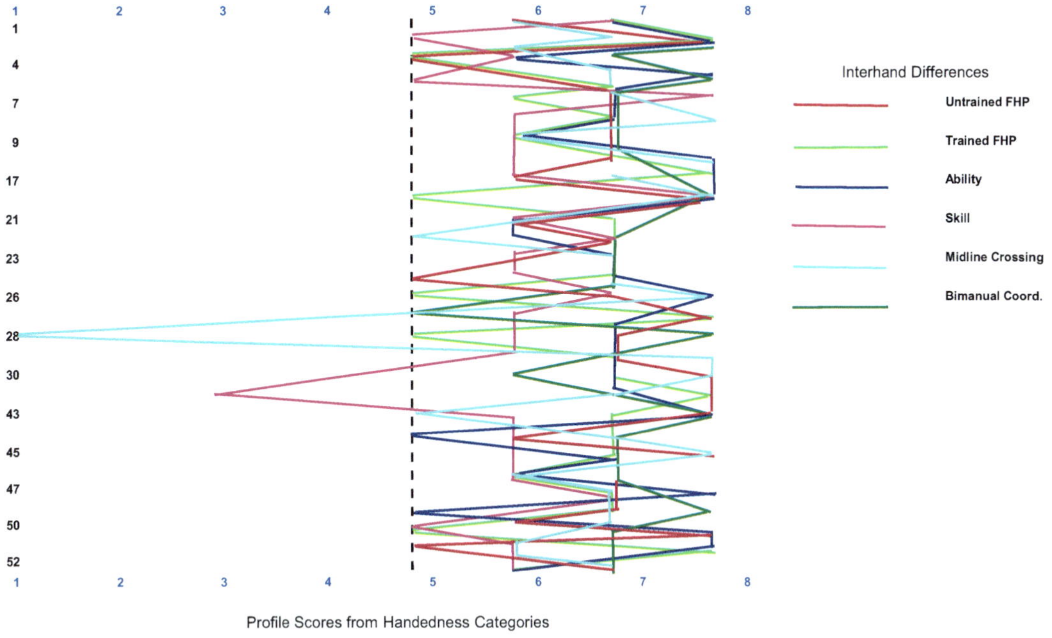

Fig. 7.6 Individual profile scores for typically developed right-handed children (n=30)

The following figures (Figs. 7.7, 7.8, 7.9, 7.10, 7.11, 7.12, 7.13, and 7.14) show an average categorisation profile for each of the eight categories. On the right side, the degree and direction of handedness are profiled in eight colour-coded categories for all subtests, whilst the left side depicts the three categories for the proficiency level. Shades of green are used for the left, and shades of red for the right hand. Between the two, the LQ scores are usually summarised and recorded (not included in these average profiles).

Conclusion

The categories of the eight-group classification system for the direction and degree of handedness as well as those of the three-group classification system for the proficiency level showed significant differences between the groups. They were thus deemed suitable as a basis for the assessment and interpretation of the Handedness Profile. This normative pilot study was based only on data from 6-year-old children. Larger normative studies are required to cover more age groups (particularly the developmental phases between 4 and 7 years), as well as adults.

7.2.5 Study V: Assessing Children with Unestablished[8] Handedness

Background

Now that a suitably sensitive assessment was available to assess and categorise handedness multidimensionally, I wanted to find out how the Handedness Profile could be applied to children with unclear handedness. How would such profiles differ from the normative ones? Were there certain patterns or indicators that could reveal atypical handedness profiles, and if yes, were there different types?

[8] In my thesis, I used the terms "unestablished" and "unclear" rather than mixed handedness.

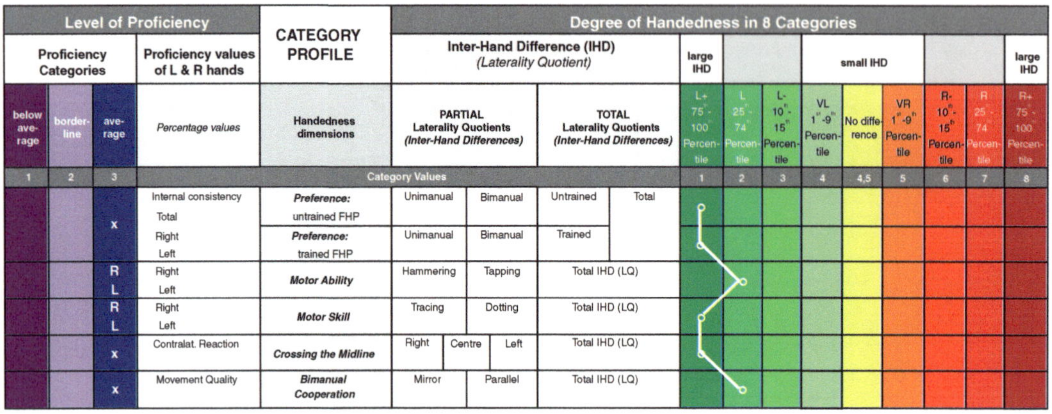

Fig. 7.7 Categorisation profile for explicit left degree (L+)

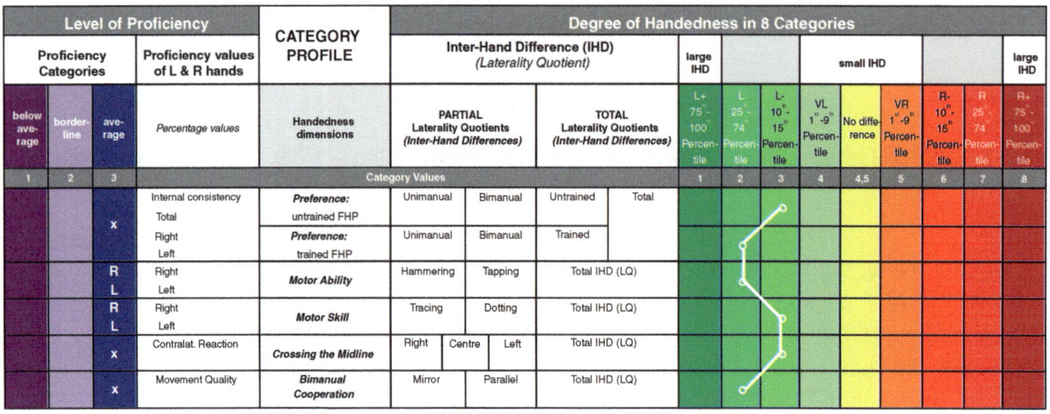

Fig. 7.8 Categorisation profile for moderate left degree (L)

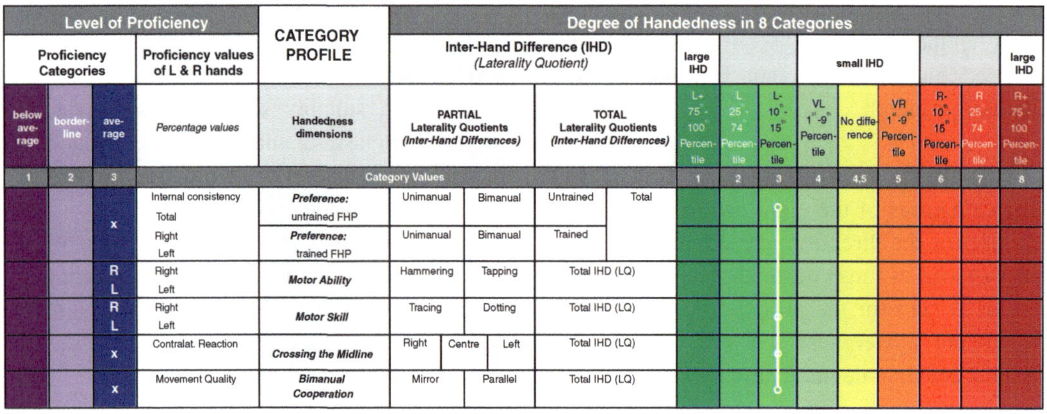

Fig. 7.9 Categorisation profile for mild left degree (L−)

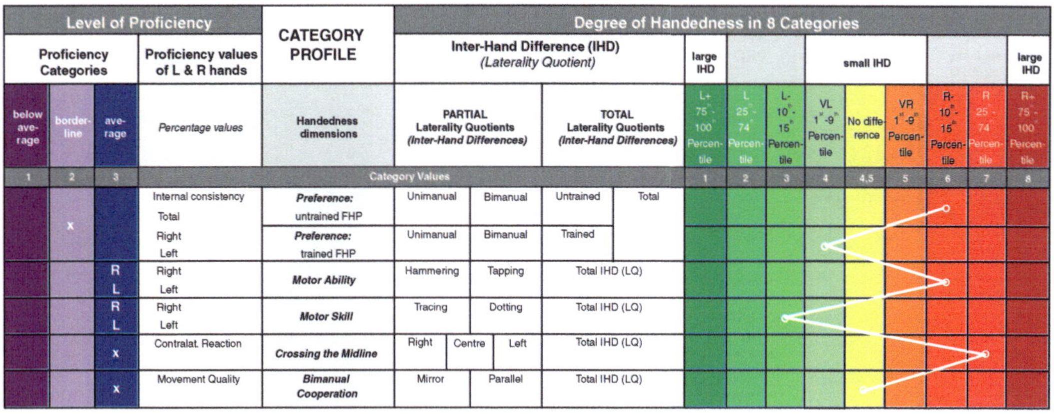

Fig. 7.10 Categorisation profile for variable left degree (VL)

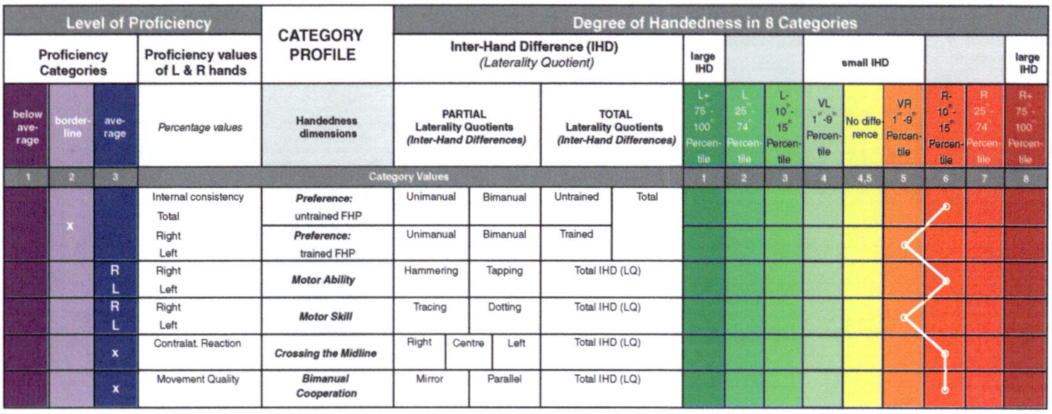

Fig. 7.11 Categorisation profile for variable right degree (VR)

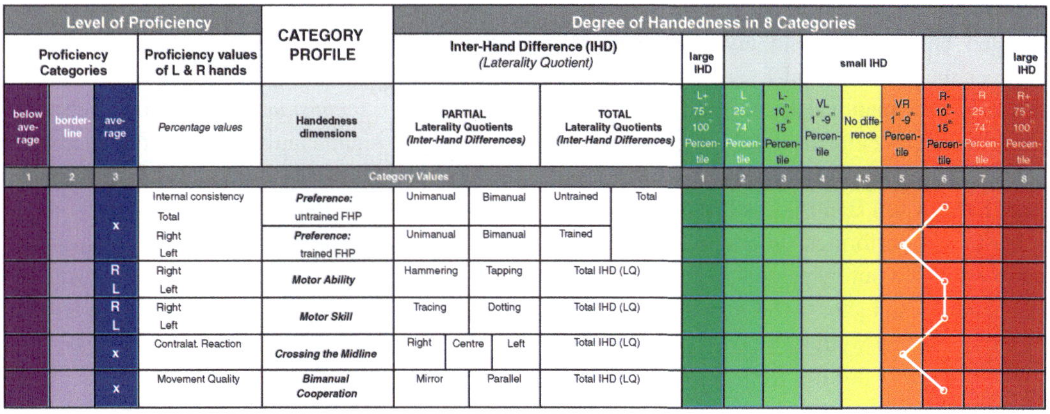

Fig. 7.12 Categorisation profile for mild right degree (R−)

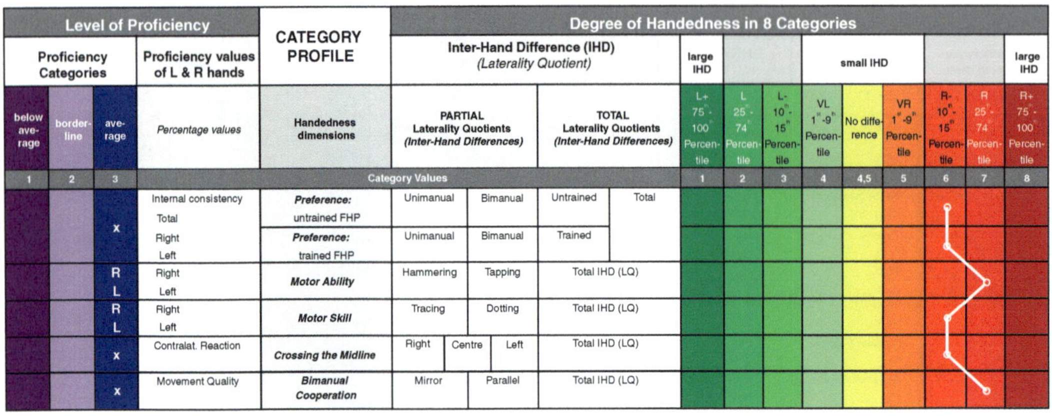

Fig. 7.13 Categorisation profile for moderate right degree (R)

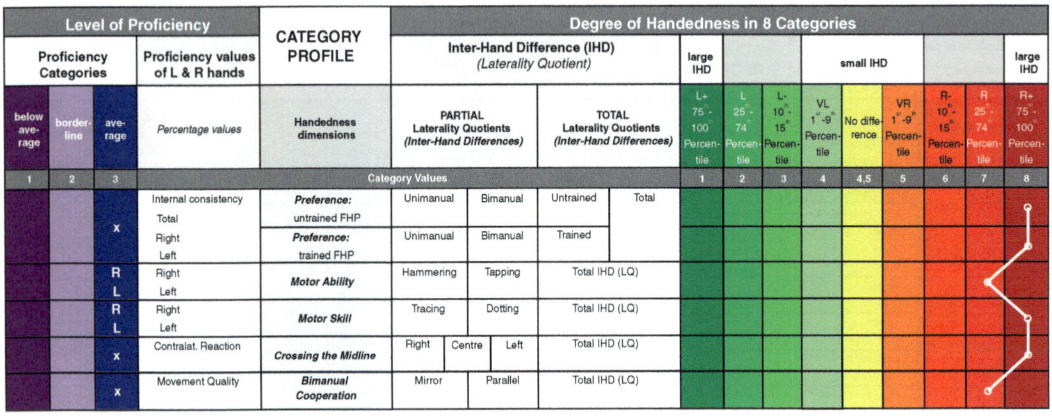

Fig. 7.14 Categorisation profile for explicit right degree (R+)

Method

I tested 68 children with atypical handedness between the ages of 5 and 7 years within the context of my occupational therapy practice. Atypical handedness was defined as children showing variable hand use with no clear indication of the dominant hand. A full Handedness Profile with all five subtests was performed. In addition, a questionnaire was filled out by parents to gather influencing handedness factors. The handedness profiles of these children were then compared with those of the normative profiles from Study IV, and differences were documented.

Results and Discussion

Children with atypical handedness exhibited profiles that differed significantly from the normative profiles (Study IV). Certain characteristics could indeed be identified as features of this group (see also Fig. 7.15):

- *Internal inconstancy*: Atypical children changed significantly more within activities and thus scored lower on internal consistency.
- *Incongruence*: Refers to a profile where some of the test results are performed more or better with the left hand, and others more or better with the right hand, so that there is a mixture of left and right laterality quotient across the subtests.
- *Very large inter-hand differences*: Many atypical children presented with large inter-hand differences (i.e. large LQ values), indicating that one hand was used excessively more or performed significantly better than the other.
- *Very small inter-hand differences*: Other atypical children showed very small inter-hand

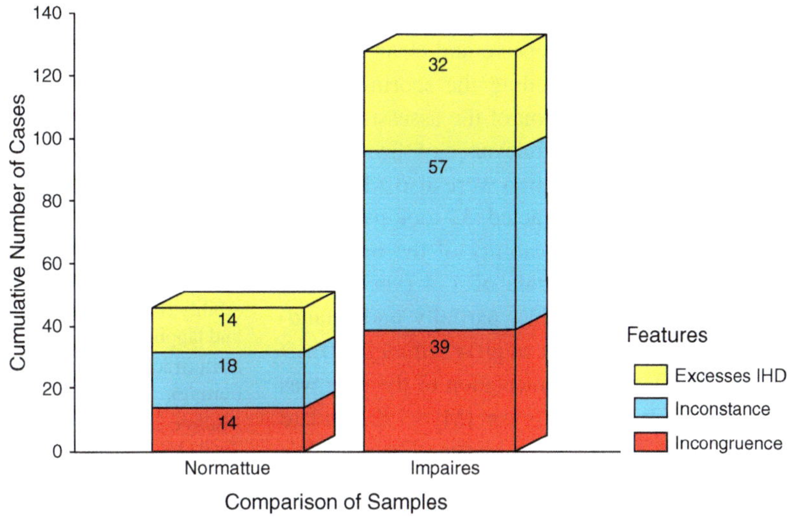

Fig. 7.15 Comparing handedness characteristics of atypical and normative profiles (Kraus 2003)

differences (i.e. small LQ values), indicating that both hands were used to the same extent and/or performed similarly.

- *Avoiding midline crossing:* Many atypical children did not engage in contralateral reaching, neither with the dominant hand nor with the non-dominant one.
- *Motor deficit*: Most children display motor problems in the unimanual proficiency tests and in the Bimanual Coordination/Cooperation Test.
- *A medical diagnosis* of a condition such as developmental delay was usually present.

Conclusion

Study V demonstrated that the Handedness Profile could display the variability of hand preference and proficiency. It could differentiate clearly between various aspects of handedness, particularly concerning the specific characteristics listed above. These atypical profiles support the importance of capturing different dimensions of handedness as a basis for further analysis and interpretation. Furthermore, the descriptive data from the parent questionnaire was helpful when contemplating possible reasons and causes for variable hand use of a child. For example, family history of *Left Handedness*, difficulties around birth resulting in minimal brain injury or evidence of switching handedness can substantiate or complement the quantitative data of the Handedness Profile. Together, the data often indicated that the reason for unestablished handedness appeared to be either normal variability, pathological or switched handedness. I concluded from these five PhD studies, against the background of the rich and diverse knowledge from the literature, that the Handedness Profile would be a suitable tool in clinical practice to identify and understand unclear handedness in children.

7.3 Validating the Handedness Profile

After completing my Ph.D. in 2003, I continued to develop the Handedness Profile by conducting some funded research as well as supervising academic research on a later versions leading up to the current Handedness Profile (2018) that will be described in Chap. 8, further validating and refining it. Even though the sample size of the studies tended to be small, the findings and recommendations were helpful to fine-tune my thinking and optimise the Handedness Profile further. These research projects are summarised here chronologically to provide a short overview.

7.3.1 Practicability Study (2010)

In this study, Schübl surveyed experts in paediatric occupational therapy that had been trained to use the Handedness Profile. Participants were asked about the instrument's applicability, with a focus on how comprehensive and clear the individual tests were, including the scoring procedure. The implementation of the assessment, the time it required and the relevance of the results to the subsequent intervention were also addressed. Of the 150 experts contacted, 33 took part in the survey. The comprehensibility of the individual tests was rated on a scale of 1–4 (very understandable, understandable, partially understandable, not understandable at all) (Schübl 2010).

In general, the implementation of the tests was rated as comprehensible (mean [M] = 1.8; standard deviation [SD] = 0.5). The Midline Crossing Test was considered to be the most comprehensible (M = 1.7; SD = 0.5) and the bimanual cooperation test as the least comprehensible (M = 2.1, SD = 0.5). It was interesting to note that the experts with less professional experience (<12 years) rated the practicability somewhat better than experts with more professional experience (>12 years). This result indicates that professional experience is not necessarily a prerequisite for the effective application of the Handedness Profile. The scoring of the Handedness Profile was also rated as comprehensible on average, particularly when supported by a digitised scoring software (M = 1.8; SD = 0.6) (see Chap. 8). Regarding the estimated time to conduct and score the assessment, there was a wide variety of views, probably due to different clinical contexts and time constraints. For example, 52% of the experts rated the time required for implementing and evaluating the profile as insufficient; 48%, however, thought that the effort was appropriate in terms of the information obtained.

The results show that the Handedness Profile was seen to be a helpful instrument for clarifying children with variable hand use. Most participants agreed with the statement that "the results of the Handedness Profile help me to understand the child's handedness". Overall, 88% of the experts surveyed rated the usability of the Handedness Profile as high (Schübl 2010).

Table 7.2 Inter-rater and test-retest reliability of the inter-hand differences of the Handedness Profile subtests (Grath et al. 2013: 40)

Test domain	Test-retest reliability (*N* = 24)	Inter-rater reliability (*N* = 24)[a]
FHPT		
Total	0.99	1.0
Untrained	0.97	0.89
Trained	0.99	1.0
Ability (hammering and tapping)	0.81	0.79
Skill (tracing and dotting)	0.89	0.89
Midline Crossing Test[a] (MCT)	0.84	0.71

Source: Grath et al. (2013). Pearson-Korrelationskoeffizienten. Compiled by the authors. No values were available for the Bimanual Cooperation Test (BCT)

[a] Crossing midline test: *N* = 23

7.3.2 Reliability Study (2013)

Grath and colleagues conducted a study to evaluate the test reliability and inter-rater reliability of the Handedness Profile. They used 12 left-handed and 12 right-handed children aged 5–6 years (11 boys and 13 girls). The children were tested twice by HP-trained[9] therapists with a 6-week break in between, and the assessment was video recorded. To determine inter-rater reliability, the tests were evaluated separately by two trained therapists. Classifying the results of each child into the 8 handedness categories, test-retest values were found to correlate highly (rs = 0.91). The therapist's inter-rater reliability values were also high (rs = 0.95), as were the laterality quotients and the proficiency levels for the individual tests (see Tables 7.2 and 7.3) (Grath et al. 2013).

The tables reveal that the internal consistency of the FHPT across repeated testing does not agree so well with the first test (test-retest reliability). It is speculated that the repeated performance of the test changed the spontaneous and unbiased attitude of the child. Since high test-retest values were found for the laterality quotients, the authors suggest that the variability of handedness in 5- to 6-year-old children is mainly

[9] Therapists or HP users can do a 5-day training course for the Handedness Profile (HP): day 1—theory and research background; day 2—implementation of the HP tests; day 3—practising implementation; day 4—scoring the HP using software; and day 5—interpretation of HP in terms of handedness types.

Table 7.3 Inter-rater and test-retest reliability of proficiency levels of Handedness Profile subtests (Grath et al. 2013: 44)

Test domain and performance values	Test-retest reliability ($N = 24$)	Inter-rater reliability ($N = 24$)
FHPT		
Internal consistency	0.57	0.83
Ability		
Right	0.78	0.52
Left	0.85	0.77
Skills		
Right	0.75	0.95
Left	0.82	0.96
Midline crossing test[a] (MCT)		
Contralateral reactions	0.57	0.97

Source: Grath et al. (2013). Pearson-correlation coefficient. Compiled by the authors. No values were available for the Bimanual Cooperation Test (BCT)
[a] Midline Crossing Test: $N = 23$

expressed by an internal inconsistency (i.e. changing hand use within the same task). The Ability tests (Hammering and Tapping) showed slightly lower values for test-retest and inter-rater reliability than the other tests. This may be because users need to count and sometimes estimate the number of strokes made, which is more error-prone when hammering or tapping is very fast or irregular.[10] The inter-rater reliability values for bimanual cooperation were also somewhat reduced, which could also be explained by the more subjective nature of the rating procedure. The values of the Midline Crossing Test displayed a rather wide scattering of the data, suggesting that the children tested were not consistent in their contralateral reaching behaviour. This is in accordance with the literature (see Sects. 1.3 and 3.6.3). The authors also speculated that children at this age might have different concentration spans, which fluctuate in relatively undemanding tasks like the MCT test, particularly when repeated a second time. The MCT also showed the lowest correlation for the inter-rater reliability of the laterality quotients. The literature, too, reports a significant variability in crossing the midline, even in adults. Even though the sample size does not allow for generalisation, the authors concluded that the Handedness Profile appears to be an objective and reliable instrument for the assessment of handedness in children (Grath et al. 2013).

7.3.3 Comparing Left- and Right-Handed 4- to 7-Year-Old Children During Simultaneous Bimanual Circle Drawing (2013)

Söller investigated 20 typically developed children (10 left and 10 right handed), between the ages of 4 and 7 years. The children performed the revised Bimanual Cooperation Test (see Sect. 8.4.5) with bimanual circle drawing in four different directions: two mirror movement variations (outward and inwards) and two parallel movement variations (to the right and to the left). The study aimed to determine whether certain patterns could be identified in left and right handers and the level of movement quality preschool children demonstrate when drawing circles, as seen in Fig. 7.16 (Söller 2013).

Söller observed that all children changed direction more often with their non-dominant hand. Furthermore, the inter-hand differences during the different directions seemed higher in right handers than in left-handed children. These observations correspond to the findings of Semjen and colleagues (Semjen et al. 1995) and Carson and team (Carson et al. 1997), who evaluated adults in bimanual circle drawing. In addition, irrespective of the children's handedness, so-called outer types and inner types could be identified (outer types succeed better in making circles using the outward variation, whilst inward types performed better in the inward variation) (Söller 2013).

All children found parallel movements particularly difficult and changed direction with the non-dominant hand much more often in this variation compared with the mirror movement variations. These results are also in accordance with other research findings on bimanual circle drawing (Carson et al. 1997; Semjen et al. 1995).

[10] Since the digitisation of the test, this problem of subjectivity has been reduced.

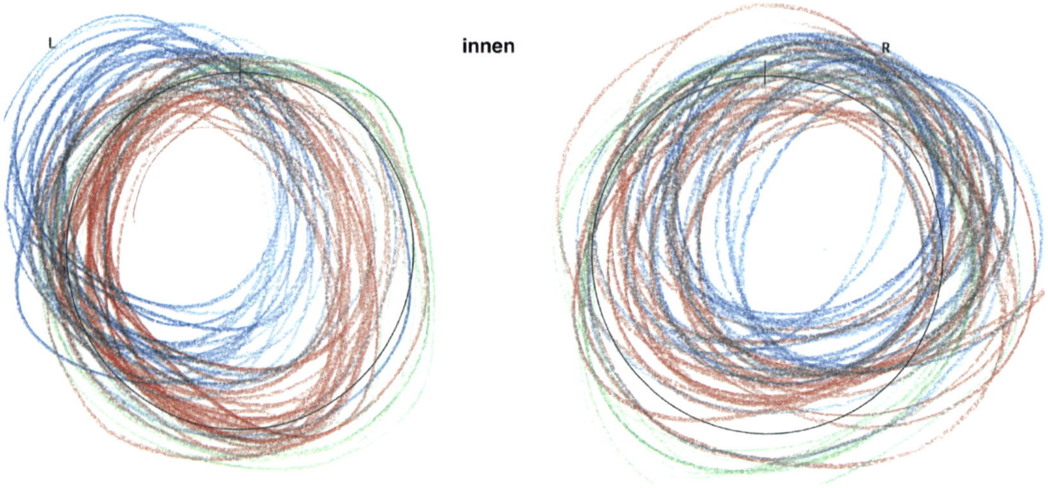

Fig. 7.16 Example of a bimanual circles "inside type", performed by a six-year old typically-developed left handed girl (Söller 2013). *Source*: (Kraus, 2014)

7.3.4 Features of Laterality in Preschool Children (2015)

Heimrod investigated the relationship between degrees of handedness and other laterality traits. The relationship between laterality (sidedness) and handedness has attracted the attention of many researchers (Heimrod 2015). As we have seen in the previous chapters, laterality of the modalities (in particular feet, eyes, and ears) shows varying and limited correlations with handedness. Some authors, however, have found that footedness, in particular, corresponds with handedness (Grouios et al. 2009; Martin and Machado 2005). Other laterality features are frequently used in occupational therapy practice to assess laterality, with inconclusive correlations to handedness.

Twenty typically developed children with clear handedness at the age of 5–6 years (ten left handers and ten right-handed children) were tested with a 30-item laterality checklist developed to provide optional and additional information for the Handedness Profile (Kraus 2018). Results were compared with the child's parents' and teachers' external reports of the child's handedness using a 5-point scale (very left, moderate left, mixed, moderate right, very right). Unfortunately, this study could only distinguish between left and right handers because of the small number of subjects.

More than half of the 30 items did not show a correlation with handedness. The following laterality features showed a very high significance ($p \leq 0.001$) when correlated with the reported handedness:

- Kicking a ball (starting position feet together and ball stationary in the centre)
- Tearing paper (leading hand)
- Folding paper (leading hand)
- Placing small beads in a row with both hands and recording the leading hand
- Looking through a telescope

These laterality features showed a high significance ($p \leq 0.05$):

- Hitting a softball with one hand (starting position with both hands behind back)
- Catching a rod with one hand (starting with both hands facing each other 8 cm apart)
- Stepping on a step (starting position feet together in front of the step)

Left-handed children tended to be less strongly lateralised overall than right-handed children.

However, the numbers are too small to generalise these findings (Heimrod 2015).

7.3.5 Digitising the Handedness Profile: dig-TEMA Project (2015)

In an IFAF[11]-funded project, "digital Test and Evaluation System for Manual Actions" (dig-TEMA), software and hardware were developed to digitise aspects of the Handedness Profile (Kraus and Hufnagl 2013, 2017). A software was developed for the parent questionnaire, the preference test and the Midline Crossing Test. For the motor tests, various hardware options were explored to capture the speed and accuracy for Hammering and Tapping. In addition, Tracing and Dotting were performed on a tablet. In one of the studies, we tested children aged 4–7 years on both the manual and the digital versions of the Handedness Profile using a tablet. We found that the performance of younger children and children with motor deficits was not consistent with the paper-pen version, particularly with the non-dominant hand. We postulated that the discrepancy might be due to a lack of proprioceptive feedback when using a digital pen and a tablet. Typically, children with emerging or deficient motor skills compensate with increased pressure, which is not possible in the same way on a tablet on paper (Kraus et al. 2019).

7.3.6 Comparing Manual and Digital Scoring of the Handedness Profile (2015)

Allweiss compared the reliability and measurement error of the digital and conventional analysing methods (Allweiss 2015). The digitised image analysis calculates errors of the scanned-in worksheets of the motor tests (tracing, dotting, hammering, tapping and bimanual cooperation). These measurements should be much more accurate, specific and time-efficient than the conventional manual method that requires manual scoring according to specified criteria. This study aimed to determine whether the digital evaluation method provides reliable results comparable with the conventional analysis. The results could be used to replace the conventional scoring with the digitised one. The study's design corresponds to a so-called judge agreement study (judge 1 = human; judge 2 = computer) (Allweiss 2015).

A total of 37 typically developed children aged 4–7 years participated in the study. Of the 37 children, 26 were female, and 11 were male, 9 were left handed, and 28 were right handed. Since the test administration as such was not digitised and remained unchanged, the participating children could be tested using the conventional paper worksheets, which were then used for comparison with the digital version for analysis.

The results indicate that the digital evaluation method for the tracing, dotting, Hammering and Tapping tests is reliable and provides highly consistent results with the conventional method. Allweiss concluded that digital image analysis could indeed replace the laborious conventional analysis method. However, the imaging analysis of the Bimanual Cooperation Test showed insufficient agreement with the conventional method, so analysis using imaging is not recommended for this test. Also, the two methods of analysis should not be used in parallel because of the wide range of differences between the individual pairs of mean values. Overall, the dig-TEMA software could contribute to a more reliable version of the paper-based motor skill tests. For the use in clinical practice, Allweiss recommended that new normative data be collected using digital imaging analysis (Allweiss 2015).

7.3.7 Laterality Features and Handedness in Adults (2019)

Whilst it is clear that many laterality features do not correlate highly with the direction of hand-

[11] IFAF: Institut für Angewandte Forschung Berlin, Germany.

edness, little research has been conducted to investigate how degrees of handedness relate to sidedness. So, in a similar but larger study, the same 30 laterality features were given in the form of a questionnaire to 90 adult participants aged between 18 and 73 years (Scherbel 2019). In addition, a self-assessment questionnaire based on the 24 items of the FHPT (Kraus 2003) was filled out by all participants. Scherbel investigated whether and to what extent a correlation exists between the laterality traits and the degree of hand preference. Findings supported such a correlation: the higher the degree of hand preference, the stronger the laterality of a person, regardless of the handedness direction. Furthermore, it was found that the degree of handedness was significantly higher than the degree of laterality of the other body parts, such as foot or eye (Scherbel 2019). Based on this study, the author concluded that a laterality trait checklist is a useful additional indicator when assessing degrees of handedness (Scherbel 2019).

7.3.8 Follow-Up Digitisation Study: manDAAD Project (2019)

Since evidence-based practice is of great importance in the field of health professions, valid and reliable test instruments are indispensable. However, the implementation, evaluation and interpretation of tests and assessments in healthcare professions are still carried out without much IT support. Tests are often based on subjective rating procedures and observations that may or may not be according to specified criteria. Subsequently, subjective interpretations and inconsistent results are often obtained. This, in turn, reduces the reproducibility, comparability and thus reliability of those instruments. The project "dig-TEMA" summarised above exemplified the digitisation of an assessment using the Handedness Profile as a standardised multidimensional instrument (Kraus and Hufnagl 2013; Kraus et al. 2019). In a follow-up IFAF-funded research project, manDAAD (manuelle Fertigkeiten: Digitalisierung von Assessments). The overall goal was to illustrate how the various aspects of an assessment could be digitised: performing the assessment, scoring and calculating the results, documentation of work and protocol sheets, and supporting interpretation with automated summaries and graphs. It aimed to be a good-practice example for the digital documentation and evaluation of a standardised and validated assessment in clinical practice.

In a first step, we examined whether and how the subtests of the Handedness Profile, especially the motor tests, could be digitised. We examined hardware solutions such as touchscreen and multi-touch displays, Wii Technology and motion sensors. A program was developed for the skill tests (Tracing and Dotting) to perform the tests on a tablet PC. The digital version of this test was intended to improve the previously subjectively assessed motor quality in the form of movement flow, regularity, stability, acceleration and pressure. This would generate more differentiated and reliable data significantly. In addition, software was developed to record the documentation of the Handedness Profile on a computer or laptop, with automated calculations of the laterality quotients (see Fig. 7.17).

Two studies investigated to what extent the digitised version of the Tracing and Dotting correlated with the conventional paper version. Study 1 included 25 children with established handedness between 4 and 10 years, with and without motor abnormalities. Study 2 included 20 children with clear handedness of the same age group and with and without motor abnormalities. In addition, in two focus groups, trained users ($N = 14$) were interviewed about the documentation and evaluation software for comments or suggestions for optimisation (Kraus and Hufnagl 2013, 2017).

In the focus groups, the practicability of the digital documentation and evaluation software was discussed, with good overall rating by participants (ibid.). The digital imaging analysis in the scoring process was thought to improve the reliability of the instrument by minimising human error.

In summary, it can be confirmed that digitisation of motor tests shows good potential to assess

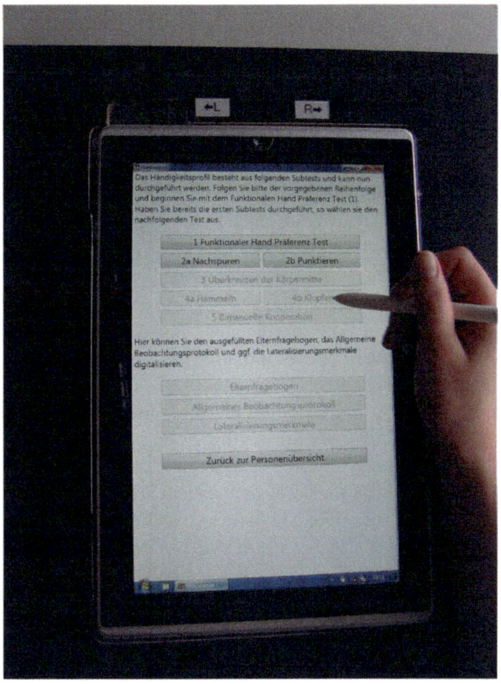

Fig. 7.17 Digitised documentation of the Handedness Profile (Kraus and Hufnagl 2013) (Photo Kraus)

the aspects of motor function in more detail, more objectively and with greater time efficiency. Kraus et al. 2019; Kraus and Schübl 2020).[12]

7.4 Concluding Remarks

This chapter summarises a number of research studies developing, evaluating and validating the current Handedness Profiles. The findings support the construct of the Handedness Profile, indicating that it is a sufficiently sensitive assessment that can significantly differentiate between various categories as well as dimensions of handedness. Since 2003, the Handedness Profile has been implemented in occupational therapy practice in Germany, Austria, Switzerland and South Africa by hundreds of trained therapists. Based on regular feedback from practitioners and evaluation, I continue to date to refine, standardise and validate the instrument. In addition, I conducted and coordinated research projects to evaluate the practicability, investigate the inter-rater reliability or correlate digitised and manual scoring versions of the Handedness Profile. These studies and numerous revisions of the administration and scoring procedures have helped further develop the multidimensional assessment. The current Handedness Profile 2018 is presented in the following chapter.

[12]In another IFAF-funded project "manDAAD" (Kraus and Schübl 2020), alternatives are now being developed with which motor quality can be measured digitally in a different way (e.g. by a digital pen; Kraus and Hufnagl 2017; Kraus and Schübl 2020).

References

Allweiss TC (2015) The digitalised handedness profile: reliability and measurement error of the digital and the conventional methods of analysis. Masterthesis. Hochschule für Angewandte Wissenschaften Hamburg, Hamburg

Annett M (1970) A classification of hand preference by association analysis. Br J Psychol 61(3):303–321. https://doi.org/10.1111/j.2044-8295.1970.tb01248.x

Annett M (1976) A coordination of hand preference and skill replicated. Br J Psychol 67(4):587–592

Annett M (1992) Five tests of hand skill. Cortex 28(4):583–600. https://doi.org/10.1016/s0010-9452(13)80229-8

Ayres AJ (1972) Sensory integration and learning disorders. Western Psychological Services, Los Angeles

Ayres J (1989) Sensory integration and praxis test. Western Psychological Services, Los Angeles

Babik I (2014) Development of handedness for role-differentiated bimanual manipulation of objects in relation to the development of hand-use preferences for acquisition. Dissertation. The University of North Carolina at Greensboro, Greensboro

Bishop DVM (1990) Handedness and developmental disorders. Mac Keith Press, Oxford, Philadelphia; J.B. Lippincott (Clinics in developmental medicine, 110)

Bryden MP, Bulman-Fleming MB, MacDonald V (1996) The measurement of handedness and its relation to neuropsychological issues. In: Manual asymmetries in motor performance, pp 57–81

Carlier M, Duyme M, Capron C, Dumont AM, Perez-Diaz F (1993) Is a dot-filling group test a good tool for assessing manual performing in children? Neuropsychologia 31(3):233–240

Carlier M, Spitz E, Vacher-Lavenu MC, Villéger P, Martin B, Michel F (1996) Manual performance and laterality in twins of known chorion type. Behav

Genet 26(4):409–407. https://doi.org/10.1007/BF02359485
Carson RG, Thomas J, Summer JJ, Walters MR, Semjen A, Summers J, Cattaert D (1997) The dynamics of bimanual circle drawing. Q J Exp Psychol Sect A 50A(3):664–683
Cermak SA, Ayres AJ (1984) Crossing the body midline in learning-disabled and normal children. The American Journal of Occupational Therapy 38(1):35–39
Cermak SA, Quintero EJ, Cohen PM (1980) Developmental age trends in crossing the body midline in normal children. The American Journal of Occupational Therapy 34(5):313–319
Coren S (1992) The left-hander syndrome. The causes and consequences of left-handedness. Free Press, New York
De Agostini M, Paré C, Goudot D, Dellatolas G (1992) Manual preference and skill development in preschool children. Dev Neuropsychol 8(1):41–57
Fagard J (1990) The development of eye-hand co-ordination. In: Bard MFC, Hay L (ed) Development of eye-hand co-ordination across life span, pp 262–282
Fagard J (1991) Synchronisation and desynchronisation in bimanual co-ordination: a developmental. Perspective 81:305–322
Fagard J, Corroyer D (2003) Using a continuous index of laterality to determine how laterality is related to interhemispheric transfer and bimanual coordination in children. Dev Psychobiol 43(1):44–56. https://doi.org/10.1002/dev.10117
Fagard J, Pezé A (1992) Coupling and lateralization in bimanual coordination at 7, 8, and 9 years of age. Dev Neuropsychol 8(1):69–85
Finstad K (2010) Response interpolation and scale sensitivity: evidence against 5-point scales. J Usability Stud 5(3):104–110
Grath S, Lumper C, Schiffman J (2013) Darstellung der Test-Retest-Reliabilität & Inter-Rater-Reliabilität des Händigkeitsprofils nach Kraus. Bachelorarbeit. FH Campus Wien University of Applied Sciences, Wien
Grouios G, Hatzitaki V, Kollias N, Koidou I (2009) Investigating the stabilising and mobilising features of footedness. Laterality 14(4):362–380
Healey JM, Liederman J, Geschwind N (1986) Handedness is not a unidimensional trait. Cortex 22(1):33–53. https://doi.org/10.1016/S0010-9452(86)80031-4
Heimrod S (2015) Muss ein linkshändiges Kind auch linksfüßig sein? Eine Pilotsstudie zu Lateraliserungsmerkmalen bei Kindern 5–6 Jahre. BSc. Alice Salomon Hochschule Berlin, Berlin
Kraus E (2003) The handedness profile. The development of a normative profile to determine the extent of handedness in children. Doctoral thesis. La Trobe University, Melbourne
Kraus E (2018) Manual zum Händigkeitsprofil. Berlin
Kraus E, Hufnagl P (2013) Entwicklung eines digitalen Test- & Evaluierungssystems für Manuelle Aktionen (dig-TEMA). Quartalsberichte. Unter Mitarbeit von Alice Salomon University of Applied Sciences & Hochscule für Technik & Wirtschaft Berlin. Hg. v. IFAF. Institut für Angewandte Forschung IFAF. Berlin
Kraus E, Hufnagl P (2017) Manuelle Fertigkeit: Digitalisierung des Assessments, Auswertung & Dokumentation. Abschlussbericht. Hg. v. Alice Salomon Hochschule Berlin. IFAF. Berlin
Kraus E, Schübl C (2020) Digitalisierung in den Gesundheitsberufen: Therapeutische Diagnostik durch den Einsatz digitaler Technologien. Alice SoSe 2020:98–99
Kraus E, Hufnagl P, Allweiss T (2019) Ist das Nachspuren auf einem Tablet vergleichbar mit dem Nachspuren auf Papier? Eine explorative Pilotstudie. Ergoscience 14(4):134–146
Lezak MD (1995) Neuropsychological assessment. Oxford University Press, New York
Longoni AM, de Gennaro L (1992) Reliability of a handedness performance test in right and left handed children: a research note. J Child Psychol Psychiatry 33(4):771–778. https://doi.org/10.1111/j.1469-7610.1992.tb00912.x
Mäki-Marttunen V, Villarreal M, Leiguarda RC (2014) Lateralization of brain activity during motor planning of proximal and distal gestures. Behav Brain Res 272:226–237
Mandell RJ, Nelson DL, Cermak SA (1984) Differential laterality of hand function in right-handed and left-handed boys. Am J Occup Ther 38(2):114–120. https://doi.org/10.5014/ajot.38.2.114
Martin WLB, Machado AH (2005) Deriving estimates of contralateral footedness from prevalence rates in samples of Brazilian and non-Brazilian right-and left-handers. Laterality: Asymmetries of Body, Brain and Cognition 10(4):353–368
McFarland K, Anderson J (1980) Factor stability of the Edinburgh handedness inventory as a function of test-retest performance, age and sex. Br J Psychol 71(1):135–142. https://doi.org/10.1111/j.2044-8295.1980.tb02739.x
McManus IC, Sik G, Cole DR, Mellon AF, Wong J, Kloss J (1988) The development of handedness in children. Br J Dev Psychol 6(3):257–273. https://doi.org/10.1111/j.2044-835X.1988.tb01099.x
Munro BH (1997) Correlation. In: Statistical methods for health care research, pp 224–245
Novick MR (1980) Statistics as psychometrics. Psychometrika 45(4):411–424
Oldfield RC (1971) The assessment and analysis of handedness: the Edinburgh inventory. Neuropsychologia 9(1):97–113. https://doi.org/10.1016/0028-3932(71)90067-4
Peters M (1990) Subclassification of non-pathological left-handers poses problems for theories of handedness. Neuropsychologia 28(3):279–289. https://doi.org/10.1016/0028-3932(90)90021-f
Peters M (1992) How sensitive are handedness prevalence figures to differences in questionnaire classification procedures? Brain Cogn 18(2):208–215. https://doi.org/10.1016/0278-2626(92)90079-2

Peters M (1998) Description and validation of a flexible and broadly usable handedness questionnaire. Laterality 3(1):77–96. https://doi.org/10.1080/713754291

Peters M, Murphy K (1992) Cluster analysis reveals at least three, and possibly five distinct handedness groups. Neuropsychologia 30(4):373–380. https://doi.org/10.1016/0028-3932(92)90110-8

Provins KA, Cunliffe P (1972) The reliability of some motor performance tests of handedness. Neuropsychologia 10(2):199–206. https://doi.org/10.1016/0028-3932(72)90060-7

Rigal RA (1992) Which handedness: preference or performance? Percept Mot Skills 75(3):851–866. https://doi.org/10.2466/pms.1992.75.3.851

Ross G, Lipper E, Auld PAM (1992) Hand preference, prematurity and developmental outcome a school age. Neuropsychologia 30(5):483–494

Scherbel M (2019) Der Zusammenhang von Lateralitätsmerkmalen & dem Ausprägungsgrad der Händigkeit bei Erwachsenen. BSc. Fresenius University of Applied Sciences, Munich

Schübl C (2010) Das Händigkeitsprofil: Eine Untersuchung zur Anwendbarkeit eines neuen Befundinstruments in der Ergotherapie. Alice Salomon Hochschule Berlin, Berlin

Semjen A, Summers J, Cattaert D (1995) Hand coordination in bimanual circle drawing. J Exp Psychol 21(5):1139–1157

Söller L (2013) Gibt es Unterschiede zwischen Links- & Rechtshändern im Alter von 4–7 Jahren bei der Durchführung der bimanuellen Kreise? Bachelorarbeit. Alice Salomon Hochschule Berlin, Berlin

Steese-Seda D, Brown WS, Caetano C (1995) Development of visuomotor coordination in school-age children: the bimanual coordination test. Dev Neuropsychol 11(2):181–199

Stilwell JM (1987) The development of manual midline crossing in 2-to 6-year-old children. The American Journal of Occupational Therapy 41(12):783–789

Stirling LA, Lipsitz LA, Qureshi M, Kelty-Stephen DG, Goldberger AL, Costa MD (2013) Use of a tracing task to assess visuomotor performance: effects of age, sex, and handedness. J Gerontol Ser A Biol Med Sci 68(8):938–945. https://doi.org/10.1093/gerona/glt003

Tapley SM, Bryden MP (1985) A group test for the assessment of performance between the hands. Neuropsychologia 23(2):215–221. https://doi.org/10.1016/0028-3932(85)90105-8

Watter P, Burns Y (1995) Repeatability of three fine motor tests. Aust J Physiother 41(1):21–26

Developing the Handedness Profile 2018

8

Contents

The Handedness Profile (HP) is well structured, the data makes sense, and children and young people have fun doing it. The HP provides an excellent overview of untrained as well as trained tasks in the FHPT. (Participant A)[1]

The Handedness Profile has several useful tools, including a clearly structured template with laterality quotients that facilitate analysis and consultation. I find the diversity of the aspects examined very convincing. (Participant B)

The HP has a clear structure and is a compact system in itself. It covers many aspects of handedness, but does not claim that there is "the" answer. In addition, aspects of the environment are taken into account in the interpretation. The Digital Scoring Template facilitates the evaluation. (Participant C)

8.1 Introduction

Since constructing the basic Handedness Profile 2003 in my doctoral thesis, hundreds of therapists have been trained to administer, score, anal-

[1]These are quotes from participants in a practicability study where 103 Handedness Profile-trained occupational therapists evaluated the instrument and its tools between 2018 and 2021. *Participant A = HPA060420/11.20.01; Participant B = HPA022022/17.06.42; Participant C = HPA122018/16.03.26.*

E. Kraus, *Beyond Left and Right Handedness*, https://doi.org/10.1007/978-3-031-24389-9_8

yse and interpret the Handedness Profile. I conduct training courses which include a comprehensive section on theory and research to contextualise and substantiate the structure and procedure of the assessment for the administrators. I also offer long-term coaching to therapists with difficult handedness cases. This has enabled me to remain in touch with clinical practice and continue to collect data using the Handedness Profile. The feedback from practitioners has been largely positive, as can be seen in the above quotes. In most cases, the multidimensional and differentiated results allow practitioners to understand variable hand use and make appropriate clinical decisions regarding intervention.

This chapter presents the *current* Handedness Profile (2018). As part of my academic work in Germany since 2005, handedness remained one of my main research areas, I translated the Handedness Profile (HP) from English to German. After some adaptation, all items and protocol sheets were standardised, and a 120-page manual was developed. Three of the original five subtests have essentially remained the same from the earlier HP version, whilst the administration of two subtests was modified. In addition, a Digital Scoring Template was developed to support administrators. The regular feedback from practitioners have led to continuous adjustments and optimisations to make the instrument more user-friendly and accurate (Kraus 2003, 2018). I also compiled the *Laterality Profile* as a separate instrument with 30 sidedness items based on actions that are typically performed differently by left and right handers. In addition, several tools for analysis and interpretation were generated. All of these aspects of the Handedness Profile 2018 are disclosed in this. In the last part, we revisit the literature by comparing the Handedness Profile to other handedness assessments before we focus on clinical practice where trained HP administrators evaluated the Handedness Profile.

8.2 Overview of the Handedness Profile 2018

The current Handedness Profile exceeds the parameters of regular assessments since it also offers additional information and tools that aim to support therapists with clinical decision-making. The different parts of the Handedness Profile are illustrated in Fig. 8.1, and each will be discussed in greater detail.

The Handedness Profile 2018 consists of three parts:

- The first part consists of qualitative **multivariate information** related to the co-determinants of handedness proposed in Chap. 7. This information is gathered by the *Parent Questionnaire* filled out prior to the assessment. In addition, the qualitative observations made by the administrator on the motor performance and abilities throughout the test are documented in the *Observation Protocol, Checklists* and (if required) *Laterality Profile*.
- The second part consists of **multidimensional subtests** assessing preference and proficiency. Preference subtests are divided into the *Functional Hand Preference Test (FHPT)*, consisting of two parts, trained and untrained items, and the *Midline Crossing Test*. The proficiency subtests consist of trained proficiency or *Skill* (assessed by Tracing and Dotting tasks), and untrained proficiency or *Ability* (assessed by Hammering and Tapping). The *Bimanual Cooperation Test* is also untrained, comprising simultaneously drawn bimanual circles in different directions.
- The third part p the **HP Tools** developed for the quantitative analysis (i.e. the Category Profile), for advanced analysis (the Cluster Table with HP Stairs) and for intervention (i.e. Differential Check and the HP Axes).

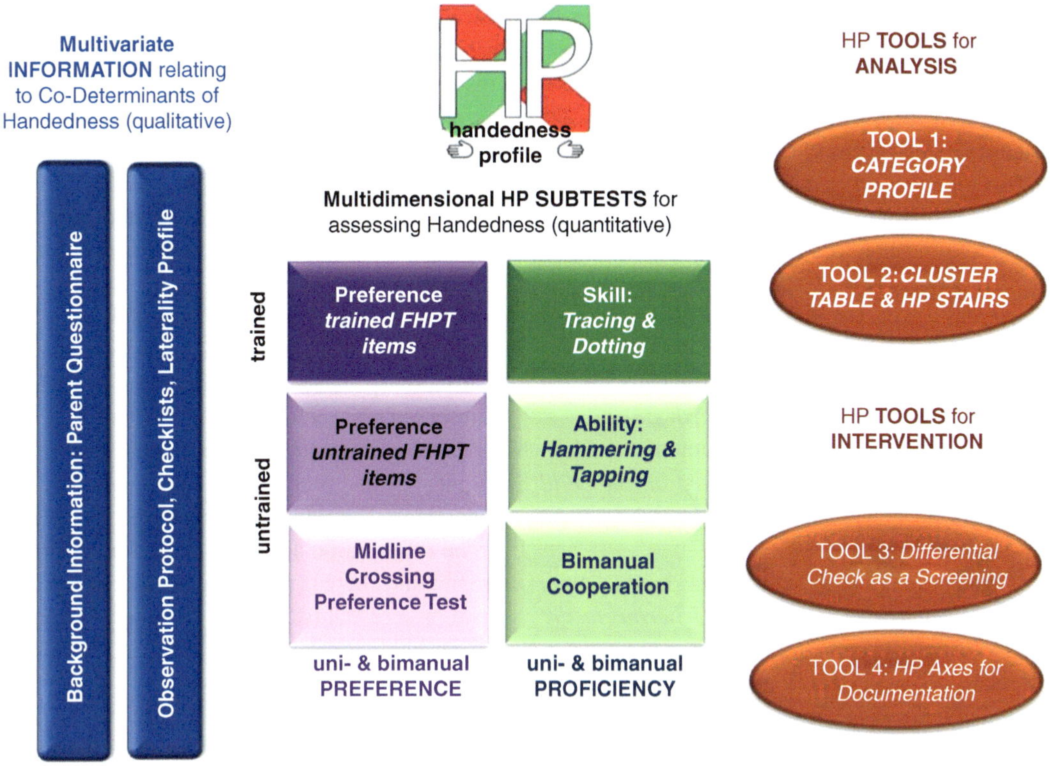

Fig. 8.1 Three aspects of the Handedness Profile: Multivariate Information, Multidimensional Subtests and Tools for Analysis (Kraus 2018, 2019)

In addition to the HP tools, the scoring procedure of the Handedness Profile has been digitised using a digital template and a handedness code, which will be introduced briefly. We will now look at these three parts in more detail.

8.3 Multivariate Information Relating to Co-determinants of Handedness (*Qualitative Data*)

A background questionnaire for parents is the main instrument used to collect information on inheritance, environmental factors and pathological motor impact, the three co-determinants proposed in Chap. 7. Information on developmental milestones and related material is also included. In addition, the movement quality can be assessed throughout the assessment and may be very useful. This is done by structured clinical observations using checklists. Therefore, additional tools are needed, and those developed for the Handedness Profile will be briefly presented here.

8.3.1 Parent Questionnaire

Incorporating relevant social and physical environmental influences, genetic predisposition to *Left Handedness*, possible pathological factors and developmental parameters are critical to obtaining a holistic and comprehensive understanding of children and their context. In addition to the information on the child's background and medical history collected by the Parent Questionnaire, a supporting parent interview is recommended to follow up on some of the information provided.

It is important to establish the reason for the referral: Are the parents concerned about the child's handedness, or does the concern come from the preschool/school teachers and/or paediatrician or the child herself/himself? Second, information on the following aspects is collected to indicate possible causes or influences that have led to variable hand use. The Parent Questionnaire developed in the doctoral thesis was used as a basis and has been refined and supplemented since. Examples of respective questions are in italics:

- Heredity aspects—*Is there Left Handedness in the family?*
- Possible determining factors for pathological handedness—*Was there any birth stress?*
- Possible indications of switching handedness—*Was any pressure exerted on the child to use a certain (usually right) hand in specific activities?*
- Observations of hand use at home—*With which hand does the child brush her/his teeth?*
- The extent of practice and automation factors in relation to motor development—*Does the child practise drawing and/or writing more, the same or less than other children of the same age?*

8.3.2 Checklists on Quality of Motor Performance

The protocol sheets of the motor proficiency tests used by the test administrator each display a checklist for observing the child's quality of movement. Criteria on the checklists include the quality and efficiency of movement patterns, body symmetry and compensatory patterns such as the use of excessive pressure or associated movements of the other hand or tongue. The left and right hands are examined according to identical criteria to compare movement quality between the hands and determine if a hand is better. This qualitative information supplements the quantitative measures of accuracy and speed.

8.3.3 General Observation Protocol

As with all assessments performed in clinical practice, several factors can influence, impede or distort the results. They include, for example, socio-emotional behaviour, cognitive abilities, sensory and perceptual-motor sensitivities or dysfunctions. For example, if a child does not understand the task requirements or has problems concentrating on the task, the assessment results may be affected and possibly distorted. The aim is to provide a Differential Check by excluding possible confounding factors on the child's ability to demonstrate his/her abilities and skills.

Against this background, I compiled a general observation protocol with a checklist of criteria to observe and evaluate the child's behaviour in a standardised manner. The test administrator will complete this protocol at the end of the Handedness Profile so that the child's behaviour can be reflected on across all tests. The information obtained here is also integrated into the interpretation tool "Cluster Table" (see Sect. 8.5.2).

8.3.4 Laterality Profile

As discussed in Sect. 2.3.2, sidedness or laterality in general across the different modalities has little or ambiguous correlations with handedness (Beaton 1985; Strauss and Goldsmith 1987; Bourassa 1996). Nonetheless, footedness is the modality most closely consistent with handedness (e.g. Martin and Porac 2007; Grouios et al. 2009; Peters 1990). Also, just as degrees of handedness show great variability, the laterality of a person too seems to be pronounced to different degrees (Strauss and Goldsmith 1987). The degree of laterality seems to correlate with the degree of handedness, even though this association seems task-dependent and is not always strong.

Since the Handedness Profile differentiates degrees of handedness across various dimension, it may be more sensitive to possibly reveal a clearer relationship with degrees of laterality, as has been indicated by (Scherbel 2019—see Sect. 7.3.7). So, we can hypothesise that people with a strong degree of handedness are also more likely to have a strongly established sidedness, whilst mildly established laterality would more likely correlate with lesser degrees of handedness. In

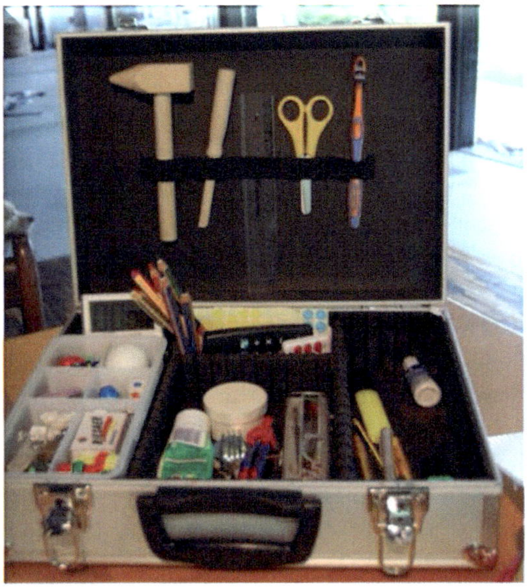

Fig. 8.2 The Handedness Profile assessment battery (Kraus 2018)

cases of unestablished and unclear handedness, information on the extent of laterality may be helpful in reaching a decision on the direction of handedness.

The HP subtests are listed in the order of analysis in the Category Profile. The standardised material for the assessment is packaged in a test case (Fig. 8.2). We will now look at the five tests in more detail and describe the procedures.

8.4 Multidimensional Subtests of the Handedness Profile *(Quantitative Data)*

8.4.1 Functional Hand Preference Test (FHPT)

Similar to the previous HP version, the Functional Hand Preference Test (FHPT) consists of 24 different everyday items that cover a variety of task features, including unimanual and bimanual; complex and simple; trained and untrained; and spontaneous and automated movements. In general, high- and low-reliability items were included (see Chap. 6) for basic assumptions and guidelines for assessing handedness. All standardised materials for the items are packed in a test kit (see Fig. 8.2).

The FHPT for hand preference is divided into two parts: it distinguishes between 12 typically ♦**trained** (i.e., practised with a particular hand, usually the right) and 12 typically ♦**untrained** items. The same differentiation is made in the proficiency tests, where the ability tests (Hammering and Tapping) are considered to be untrained, and the skill tests (Tracing and Dotting) are trained because of their high correlation with writing (see Sect. 6.2.2). This structure allows contrasting trained and untrained aspects of handedness, thereby enabling a comparison between possible sociocultural and physical environmental as well as hereditary influencing factors. For example, switching left handers typically show a left-handed preference for untrained preference and proficiency tasks and a right-handed advantage in the trained tasks. However, many factors uniquely influence the ♦**handedness status** of a person. Therefore, it is likely that the classification of trained or untrained items might not apply to an individual. For example, lighting a match has been categorised as a trained item since many parents specifically show their children how to do it for safety reasons. In this case, lighting a match would be a trained task. However, if a (young) child has not been allowed to play with matches at all because of the potential danger, s/he will have no experience, and the item would be an untrained task in this case. However, since there are 12 items that are repeatedly performed in each of the categories, one or two "incorrectly" classified items would only marginally impact the overall score.

In addition, the FHPT distinguishes between equal numbers of one-handed (unimanual) and two-handed (bimanual) activities. There are thus four subgroups with six items each: *trained unimanual items, trained bimanual items, untrained unimanual items* and *untrained bimanual items* (see Table 8.1). All items from the EHI used in the earlier studies were retained.

The child repeats each of these 24 items at least four times to obtain an ♦**internal consistency** measurement (i.e. the consistent use of the hand within the same activity). Across the whole FHPT, this means a total of at least 96 trials. This is rather demanding for younger children or those with concentration difficulties. Thus, I developed some interactive fun stories and games for this subtest to motivate children. The child is seated at the table; the administrator sits opposite. All items are presented one by one in the centre in front of the child. The hand the child uses actively is recorded. If the child swaps hands, it is also documented according to different swapping patterns. These include *ergonomic swapping* that increases the speed and efficiency of performing the task or *fatigue-related swapping* (i.e. starting always with the same hand, which then seems to tire or not cope very well and then swapping to the other hand) (Kraus 2018). When the FHPT is scored, separate laterality quotients (LQ) are calculated for each of the four subgroups as well as for the trained and untrained categories. Internal consistency is also recorded for each item and calculated as a percentage across the 24 items.

Table 8.1 Division of the 24 FHPT items into four subgroups according to task features

Untrained unimanual	Trained unimanual
1. Shake box	13. Use toothbrush[a]
2. Shoot soccer with bear	14. Eat with a spoon[a]
	15. Cut with a knife[a]
3. Insert pegs	16. Write[a] (in the air)
4. Spinning top	17. Draw[a] with a pen
5. Build tower	18. Throw a ball[a]
6. Roll dice	
Untrained bimanual	**Trained bimanual**
7. Open box[a]	19. Sew with shoelaces
8. Sweep with hand broom[a]	20. Eat with knife and fork
9. Deal cards	21. Cut with scissors
10. Open tube	22. Light a match[a]
11. Remove sticker	23. Put the key in the lock
12. Tighten screw	24. Use a screwdriver

[a] Items from the EHI

8.4.2 Midline Crossing Test (MCT)

The current MCT test is based on the same principles and parameters as the original one in my dissertation but has a simpler format. The coloured pegs and a wooden board with coloured holes that had been hand crafted in the original MCT were replaced with the current test. This consists of an A3 laminated sheet or board with a symmetrical three-coloured template on which four-knobbed Lego tiles of the same colour can be placed (see Fig. 8.3).

This modified Midline Crossing Test was easy and cheap to manufacture, and there is only one midline crossing format compared to the double formats in the PhD MCT, at the beginning of the movement sequence and at the end). The initial contralateral response from a neutral position at the beginning of a movement i.e., sequence is more likely to elicit a spontaneous midline crossing response. Midline crossing avoidance is typically revealed at the beginning of movement executions based on repeated clinical observations. Thus, allowing equal opportunity for initial ipsilateral or contralateral responses seemed fea-

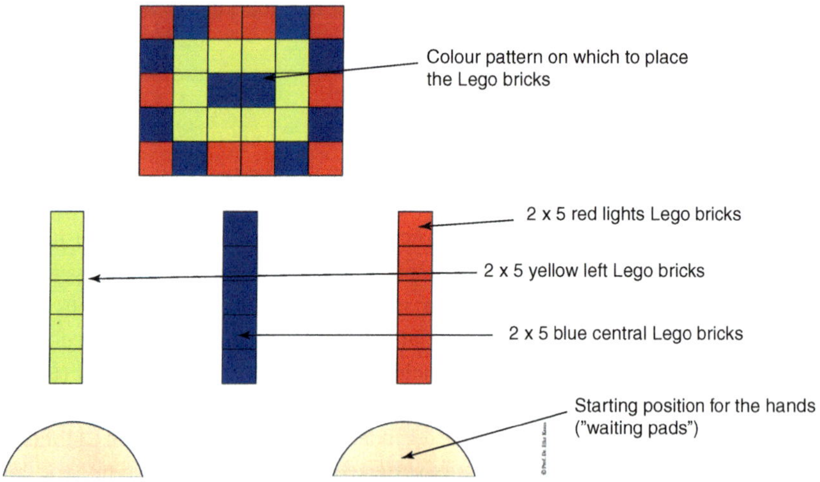

Fig. 8.3 Laminated board of the current Midline Crossing Test of the Handedness Profile (Photo by Kraus)

sible when picking up the Lego pieces. These were then placed in the centre more proximally (and not on either side, as in the PhD MCT).

The MCT allows for a total of 20 trials to cross the midline. For example, a person with explicit (high degree of) handedness and no midline crossing avoidance would be likely to perform ten ipsilateral and ten contralateral responses with the same hand. The MCT can identify the following patterns of hand use in relation to midline crossing and hand preference:

- The child does not show any midline crossing avoidance and consistently uses one hand to pick up all (or most) Lego pieces. The same hand is used to pick up the Lego pieces in the centre. This indicates well-established and explicit hand preference. The degree of handedness is displayed here: most people occasionally use the non-dominant hand to pick up pieces, especially ipsilaterally.
- The child avoids crossing the midline and shows ipsilateral responses (i.e. picks up Lego pieces on the left side with the left hand and Lego pieces on the right side with the right hand). In this case, avoiding midline crossing is likely to influence handedness development since the hand picking up the item or instrument often then proceeds to perform the action.
- If children avoid midline crossing, some will use one hand consistently to pick up the central pieces, indicating that there is some developing preference. Other children may swap hands at the centre, indicating that hand preference is still unestablished and may also display midline crossing avoidance.
- Sometimes, the child crosses over with the left hand and sometimes with the right. This indicates no avoidance of midline crossing, but that hand preference is not established. In other words, it is not the ability for contralateral reaching that impedes the development or establishment of handedness but other factors.

The test is administered according to a preset colour sequence which is called out by the administrator, and the child responds by picking up the respective Lego pieces. At the start and after each response, the child must return her/his hands to the starting position designated on the MCT board (see Fig. 9.3). Since a row of 10 Lego pieces would have been too long for the A3 board, the pieces are set up in two rounds of five pieces in a row for each colour. At the end, the contralateral responses are added as a fraction of 20 and calculated as percentages, from which a laterality quotient is obtained (R-L). The centre responses act as a control and are not added to the crossing midline LQ but are part of the overall response.

8.4.3 Trained Proficiency: Skill (Tracing and Dotting)

In addition to the two preference tests FHPT and MCT, the proficiency test for trained motor aspects consists of Tracing and Dotting tasks (Skill). The tracing task consists of a bear-shaped outline that the child traces as accurately and quickly as possible (see Fig. 8.4) these tests have largely remained the same since the PhD version.

In the dotting task, small dots are placed as quickly as possible in each of the 30 beads that make up the chain for the tracing bear. Both tasks are performed with each hand. The two tests are scored according to specified fixed criteria, and an average score is calculated to form a skill percentage for each hand with a perfect score (see Sect. 8.4.3). The time taken to perform the tests is offset against the accuracy (i.e. number of errors) and integrated into the percentage for each hand. The laterality quotient is calculated by subtracting the left percentage from the right.

The scoring of the proficiency test has also essentially remained the same as described in Chap. 7. One adjustment was made for time. A maximum score of 100% is based on tracing the bear without errors in 25 s (perfect score). For this reason, 25 s is subtracted from the time taken in the Digital Scoring Template. Times longer than 25s accumulates error points. For example, a 5-year-old child or an individual with motor problems may achieve 45% of the perfect score with the right and 17% with the left hand. Since we have already scored proficiency as a percent-

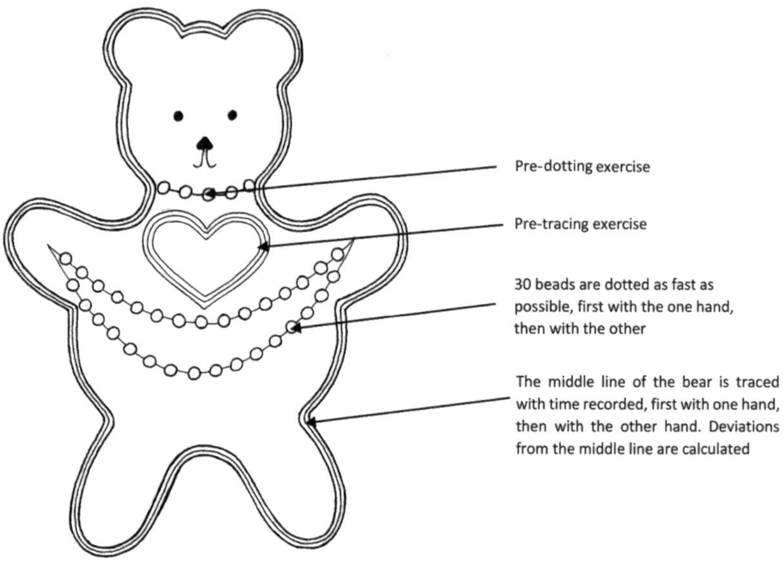

Fig. 8.4 Trained motor proficiency worksheet for Skill—Tracing and Dotting

age, we merely need to calculate the difference between right and left proficiency scores, as can be seen in Examples 1 and 2 for right handers and left handers respectively.

Examples

1. LQ-Prof = R − L = 45% − 17% = **28% better right** (but both sides perform quite **poorly**)
2. LQ-Prof = R − L = 78% − 83% = **−5% better left** (but both sides perform **well**)

Presently, there are only norms for 6-year-olds. While one can roughly extrapolate data for the other age groups, it is not very specific because of the broad categories of average, borderline and sub-average. If motor deficiencies need to be assessed more accurately other normative motor assessments should be administered additionally to obtain more detailed information. The Handedness Profile yields data on the inter-hand differences and degrees of handedness in the first place and relates this only to a broad proficiency level.

8.4.4 Untrained Proficiency: Ability (Hammering and Tapping)

Untrained motor proficiency (Ability) is captured by the Hammering and Tapping tasks. Within 15 s, the child hammers or taps as fast as possible onto a target point (0.5 cm diameter) on a piece of paper attached to a carbon paper to record the hits (see Figs. 8.5 and 8.6).

The hits within 15 s are counted, and their dispersion marked by the carbon paper is measured, thereby combining time and accuracy into the score. A percentage is then calculated in relation to the perfect (best possible) score, and a laterality quotient is calculated (R% − L%) (see Sect. 5.2.2). This test procedure is unchanged from the original Handedness Profile, but the hammer and the tapping concentric circles for scoring have since been adapted and standardised (Kraus 2018).

8.4.5 Bimanual Proficiency: Bimanual Cooperation Test (BCT)

The trained and untrained proficiency tests, Skill and Ability, are limited to unimanual performance. As explained in Chap. 3, cooperation between the hands is also an important aspect of manual dexterity. The Etch-A-Sketch board used in the PhD version was replaced by bimanual simultaneous circle drawing using two thick crayons on paper. This constitutes the new Bimanual Cooperation Test (BCT) (see Fig. 8.7).

The current BCT also demonstrates untrained proficiency with both hands, requiring a clear

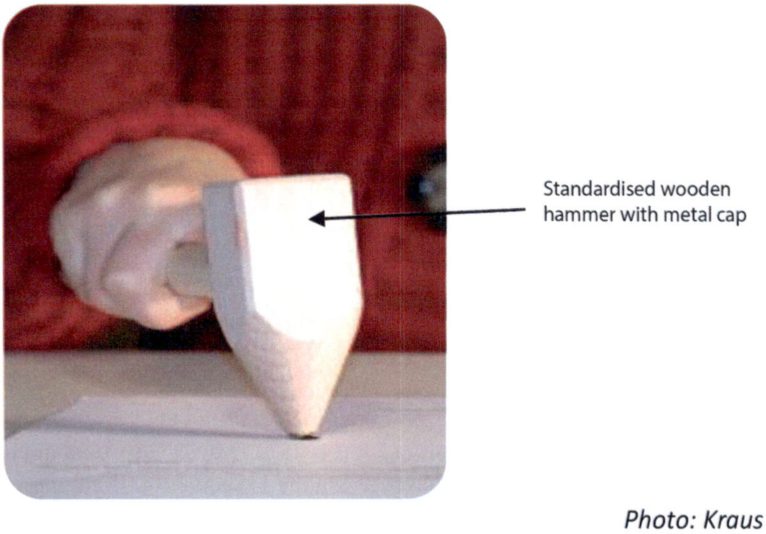

Fig. 8.5 Hammering as an untrained proficiency task (Ability) (Kraus 2018)

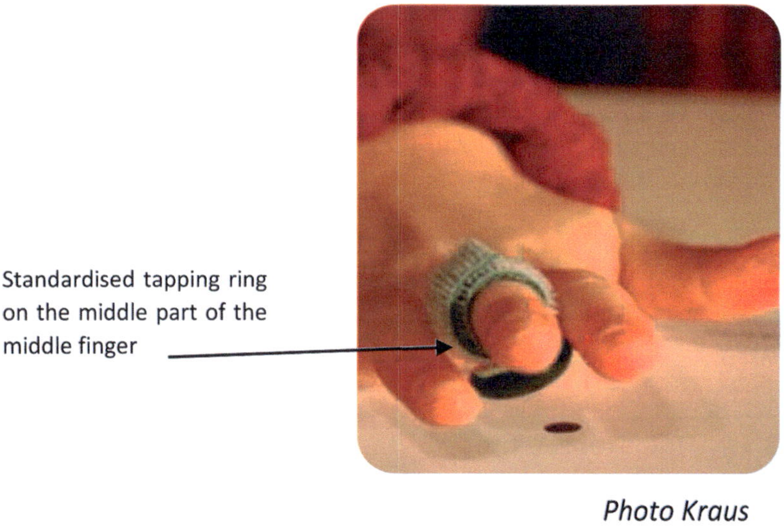

Fig. 8.6 Tapping as an untrained proficiency task (Ability) (Kraus 2018). (Photos by Kraus)

division of roles (Sect. 2.4.2). Typically, the dominant hand will lead, draw rounder circles with firmer and more consistent pressure and maintain direction, especially during parallel movement sequences (Carson et al. 1997). There are four working sheets, each with two circles approximately 8 cm in diameter assigned to one of the four directional combinations: two symmetrical (outwards and inwards) and two parallel (to the right and to the left) movement sequences. In addition, each of these directional combinations is always performed in two phases: at a slow rhythmic speed comfortable for the child and as fast as possible. Optionally, a third phase

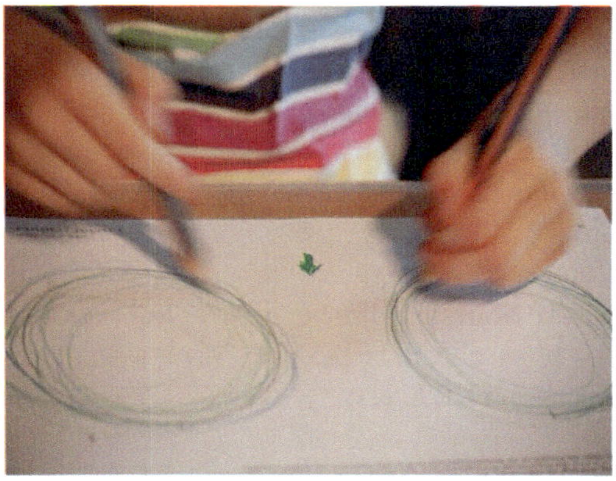

Fig. 8.7 Bimanual cooperation through simultaneous bimanual circle drawing (Kraus 2018). (Photos by Kraus)

was added: as fast as possible with eyes closed. Increasing speed and occluded visual feedback increase the demand and thereby the difference between the hands (Cattaert et al. 1999).

In the original Bimanual Coordination Test, the child could only perform 4–5 circular movements with both hands before reaching the edge of the toy. This severely limited the possibility of increasing the demand through speed. In addition, the tension of the two knobs became asymmetric and unstable with increased use. The current paper-pencil version of the Bimanual Cooperation Test enables increased speed and visual occlusion to provide amplified levels of task demands for role differentiation between the hands.

The 3-point scoring criteria for the BCT denote whether one hand is performing significantly better or faster (score 2), slightly better or faster (1) or the same (0). Similarly, the quality of the circles (roundness, pressure) is compared and scored according to the same 3-point scale. The bimanual movement patterns' general quality is also assessed to be average, borderline or sub-average. The scores of the four directional sequences are added for each hand, and the difference is calculated (LQ = R − L).

8.5 Tools for Analysis

The information collected by the Handedness Profile (HP) is diverse and extensive. If the test administrators are also therapists, they must continue their clinical reasoning after analysing and interpreting the results. This is a prerequisite for goal-directed and effective intervention. To support this complex and essential process, I developed two primary tools for **analysis** (the **Category Profile** pu and the *Cluster Table* with the **HP Stairs**), and some tools for **intervention**, two of which will be presented here (Differential Check and HP Axes).

8.5.1 Category Profile

The ♦**Category Profile** is a summary graph providing a visual overview of all laterality quotients (LQ) across the HP subtests and has already been introduced (see Sects. 7.2.4). Untrained and trained preference tasks are presented separately for both preference and proficiency, thereby comprising six HP dimensions of handedness. These are; untrained everyday preference (FHPT), trained everyday preference (FHPT), untrained proficiency (Ability), trained proficiency (Skill), midline crossing preference (MCT) and bimanual cooperation (BCT) (see Sect. 8.4). For each of the six HP dimensions, the degree of handedness corresponds to one of the eight categories based on percentiles on the right (see Sect. 8.5.1), as well as a broad rating of the proficiency level on the left side of the graph of (average, borderline and below average) (see Fig. 8.8).

The normative profiles based on the pilot study with 60 typically developed 6-year-old children were already introduced in the last chapter (see Sect. 7.2.4). Even though the number and age groups of children tested are too small for generalisation and do not cover other age groups, the data provides a very useful baseline for atypical handedness profiles. It is likely that the degree of handedness is not age-dependent but relies on a person's inherited predisposition. I hypothesise that the profiles of the eight categories will not be significantly different in adults. Finally, an overall profile score is calculated, expressing the average handedness degree.

8.5.2 Cluster Table with HP Stairs

Whilst the Category or Cat-Profile is extremely useful in summarising the quantifiable dimensions of handedness through the laterality quotients that display the degrees of inter-hand

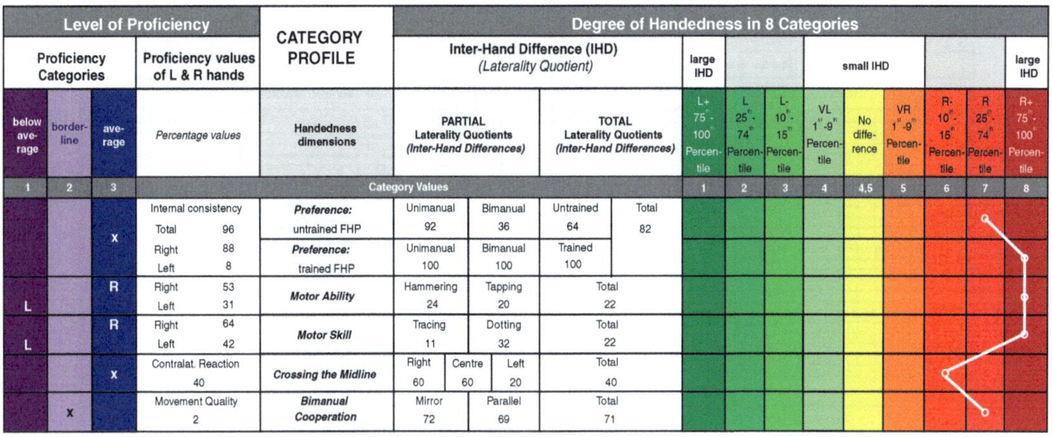

Fig. 8.8 Example of the Category Profile

differences, it cannot cover all the complexities of the handedness phenomenon. We have assumed that multidimensional handedness is a dynamic and most complex phenomenon with several determining factors. Thus, we need to consider further qualitative information that can, for example, be captured by the parent questionnaire and the structured observation checklists. Only on the basis of holistic and comprehensive information can we gain insight and clues into possible causes and influencing (determining) factors that are responsible for variable hand use.

Against this background, the ♦**Cluster Table** was developed, systematically listing information from the Cat-Profile, contextual factors from the parent (background) questionnaire, observations during testing and knowledge from the literature. The Cluster Table features criteria for ten different "types" of handedness relating to the determining factors. Each handedness type consists of 25 criteria or typical characteristics based on the literature, the Cat-Profile or the Parent Questionnaire. Handedness Profile and qualitative information. Administrators of the HP rate to what extent these criteria apply to the child they tested. The handedness type with the highest score (cluster) suggests this to be responsible for variable hand use with the highest probability (see Chap. 10 for more detail on the Handedness Typology). An example of the criteria for variable left handers is presented in Fig. 8.9.

The scores from the Cluster Table are converted to percentages to show the magnitude of the clustered criteria relating to the various handedness types, degree, motor pathology and environment and their respective variations (see Chap. 9). The three largest clusters are used as part of the explanatory model for the variable hand use of a child (see Fig. 8.10). The HP Stairs thus summarise all type of variations of the proposed typology, which are illustrated by case studies in Chap. 12.

As we have seen in Chap. 5, mixed (unestablished, variable) handedness can also be a result of certain conditions or diagnoses, such as Autism, Asperger's syndrome, intellectual disability, Schizophrenia or Down's syndrome. However, since atypical or decreased forms of lateralisation are specific to these conditions and do not directly relate to determining handedness factors, they are considered secondary and thus not part of the handedness types listed here.

Score									LEFT HANDEDNESS (explicit, moderate and mild) (D-based type)	Source		RIGHT HANDEDNESS (explicit, moderate and mild) (D-based type)	Score							
#	4	3	2	1	0	?	score						?	0	1	2	3	4	score	#
									Quotient for Left Handedness			Quotient for Right Handedness								
									VARIABLE LEFT HANDEDNESS (D-based type)			"VARIABLE RIGHT HANDEDNESS (D-based type)"								
26							0	26	**Higher LH values than RH values (but not excessively)**	see above	26	**Higher RH values than LH values (but not excessively)**							0	26
27							0	27	Ambidextrous people in close family circle	PQ	27	"Mixed" handedness in the close family circle							0	27
28							0	28	Ambidextrous people in the wider family circle		28	"Mixed" handedness in the extended family circle							0	28
29							0	29	Alternating hand use approximately half L and half R		29	Alternating hand use but more R							0	29
30							0	30	Tends to do gross motor activities R fine motor activities L		30	Performs gross and fine motor activities **more** R, but also L							0	30
31							0	31	Does untrained activities rather R trained L		31	Performs untrained and trained activities **more** R, but also L							0	31
32							0	32	**Writes consistently and better with L**		32	Writes consistently and better with R							0	32
33							0	33	Draws mostly with L, sometimes also with R (e.g. gross motor activities)		33	Always draws with R							0	33
34							0	34	Untrained preference rather R, trained preference L	FHPT	34	Untrained and trained preference **more** R							0	34
35							0	35	Internal overall consistency between 60% and 80%		35	Overall internal consistency between 70% and 85% (not above)							0	35
36							0	36	Internal consistency both hands similar use		36	Internal consistency with greater RH use, but not much							0	36
37							0	37	Skill slightly better L	Trac/Dot	37	Skill better R							0	37
38							0	38	Small IHD, skill L good, R very good for nd hand	Checklist	38	vR, R or R IHD (skill R and L average)							0	38
39							0	39	Ability slightly better R or L	Ham/Tap	39	Ability better R							0	39
40							0	40	Small IHD, ability L good, R very good for nd hand	Checklist	40	vR, R- or R IHD (skill R and L average)							0	40
41							0	41	Crosses more with R, but also with L	MCT	41	Crossed mostly with R							0	41
42							0	42	Takes centre blocks sometimes with L, sometimes with R		42	Takes central blocks mostly with R							0	42
43							0	43	Circles very similar in pressure and quality	BMK	43	Circles R better, firmer and more evenly							0	43
44							0	44	L as well as R maintain the given direction		44	R maintains direction							0	44
45							0	45	L leads in certain directions, R leads in other directions		45	R leads more consistently							0	45
46							0	46	Overall expression value of IHD around 4	Cat-Prof	46	Overall expression value of IHD between 5 and 6							0	46
47							0	47	Trained preference L; untrained preference R		47	Trained and untrained preference more R							0	47
48							0	48	Ability (Ham/Tap) better R Skill (Tra/Dot) better L		48	Ability (Ham/Tap) and Skill (Tra/Dot) a bit better R							0	48
49							0	49	Total laterality quotient between 0 and 20% L		49	Total laterality quotient between 10 and 35% R							0	49
50							0	50	Slightly higher LH values in Laterality Profile	Lat-Prof	50	Slightly higher RH values in Laterality Profile							0	50
0									Quotient for Variable Left Handedness			Quotient for Variable Right Handedness	0							
									AMBIDEXTERITY (D-based type)			DEVELOPMENTALLY DELAYED HANDEDNESS (no clear type known yet)								
51							0	51	**High scores under Variable Left Handedness**	see above	51	**No clear values for left- or right-handedness**							0	51
52							0	52	No indication of developmental delay		52	**Indication of developmental delay**							0	52
53							0	53	No early preferred hand use, both hands equally good	EFB	53	No earlier preferred hand use, atypical swapping							0	53
54							0	54	Alternating hand use within and across activities		54	Alternates hand use within and across activities							0	54
55							0	55	Writes L or R equally well, situational changes		55	Writes L or R equally poorly, tries with both hands							0	55
56							0	56	Draws L or R equally well, situational changes		56	Draws L or R equally poorly, tries with both hands							0	56
57							0	57	**Clear practice effect with both hands**		57	Avoids practising with both hands, little practising effect							0	57
58							0	58	Internal consistency below 60%	FHPT	58	Internal consistency below 60%							0	58
59							0	59	**Tendency to switch ergonomically**		59	**Tendency to atypical and compensatory swapping**							0	59
60							0	60	Similar use of both hands with internal consistency		60	Similar use of both hands with internal inconsistency							0	60
61							0	61	Skill on both sides about equally good to very good	Trac/Dot	61	Skill on **both sides atypical**							0	61
62							0	62	Quality of movement with skill on both sides good to very good	Checklist	62	Movement quality with skill on both sides show motor deficiencies							0	62
63							0	63	Ability on both sides approximately equally good to very good	Ham/Tap	63	Ability on **both sides atypical**							0	63
64							0	64	Quality of movement with skill on both sides good to very good	Checklist	64	Movement quality with ability on both sides show motor deficiencies							0	64
65							0	65	Crosses with R and with L	MCT	65	**Avoids crossing over**							0	65
66							0	66	Takes centre blocks with L or R		66	Takes centre blocks with L or R							0	66
67							0	67	No crossing avoidance in FHPT		67	Shows crossing avoidance in FHPT							0	67
68							0	68	**Circles equally well, many X**	BMK	68	**Circles equally atypcial, many ?**							0	68
69							0	69	Keeps direction with both hands		69	Changes direction with both hands							0	69
70							0	70	Quality of circles similar on both sides		70	Quality on both sides equally bad, possibly different problems							0	70
71							0	71	Good quality of movement on both sides		71	Atypical movement quality on both sides							0	71
72							0	72	Overall proficiency score between 4 and 5 with good motor skills	Cat-Prof	72	Overall score between 4 and 5 with subaverage motor skills							0	72
73							0	73	Small IHD in skill, both sides good to very good		73	Small IHD in skill, both sides show motor deficiencies							0	73
74							0	74	Small IHD in ability, both sides good to very good		74	Small IHD in ability, both sides show motor deficiencies							0	74
75							0	75	Laterality profile approximately half L and half R	Lat-Prof	75	Laterality profile approximately half L and half R							0	75
0									Quotient for Ambidexterity			Quotient for developmentally delayed Handedness	0							
									PATHOLOGICAL LEFT HANDEDNESS (M-based type)			PATHOLOGICAL RIGHT HANDEDNESS (M-based type)								
76							0	76	**Evidence of pre-, peri- or postnatal birth trauma**	PQ	76	**Evidence of pre-, peri- or postnatal birth trauma**							0	76
77							0	77	**Evidence of brain injury to the R side of the head**		77	**Evidence of brain injury on the R side of the head**							0	77
78							0	78	**Evidence of injury to the R arm/hand**		78	**Evidence of injury to L arm/hand**							0	78
79							0	79	Motor deficiencies are mentioned in the PQ		79	Motor abnormalities are mentioned in the EFB							0	79
80							0	80	Swapping tendency: starts with R and changes to L	FHPT	80	Swapping tendency: starts with L and changes to R							0	80
81							0	81	Tendency to perform untrained undemanding activities with R		81	Tendency to perform untrained undemanding activities with L							0	81
82							0	82	First hand is often R, then switches to L		82	First hand is often L, then switches							0	82
83							0	83	Tendency for compensatory switching		83	Tendency for compensatory switching							0	83
84							0	84	Shows fatigue-related switching several times, mostly to L		84	Shows fatigue-related switching several times, mostly to R							0	84
85							0	85	Skill is much better L, R is motorically deficient	Trac/Dot	85	Skill is much better R, L is motorically deficient							0	85
86							0	86	Skill is in the borderline to sub-average range with the better L hand		86	Skill is in the borderline to sub-average range with the better R hand							0	86
87							0	87	Quality is especially noticeable poor on the R side, possibly tremor	Checklist	87	Quality is especially noticeable poor on the L side, possibly tremor							0	87
88							0	88	Asymmetrical, supports/fixes mostly R		88	Asymmetrical, mostly supports/fixes L							0	88
89							0	89	Says L hand feels and performs better		89	Says R hand feels and performs better							0	89
90							0	90	Ability is much better L, motor performance on R sub-average	Ham/Tap	90	Ability is much better R, motor performance on L sub-average							0	90
91							0	91	Ability is in borderline to sub-average range with L hand, tires easily		91	Ability is in the borderline to sub-averag range with the R hand, tires easily							0	91
92							0	92	Quality is poor on the R side, possibly tremor	Checklist	92	Quality is poor on the L side, possibly tremor							0	92
93							0	93	Asymmetrical, supports/fixes mostly R		93	Asymmetrical, mostly supports/fixes L							0	93
94							0	94	Says that the L hand feels and/or performs better		94	Says R hand feels and performs better							0	94
95							0	95	Predominant use of L hand with borderline to average performance	MCT	95	Predominant use of R hand with borderline to average performance							0	95
96							0	96	Tendency to pick up stone with R and then place it in L hand		96	Tendency to pick up stone with L and then place it in R hand							0	96
97							0	97	Circles much better (pressure, shape) on L side	BMC	97	Circles much better (pressure, form) on R side							0	97
98							0	98	Movement quality better L		98	Movement quality better R							0	98
99							0	99	**Large IHD with Skill (L+)**	Cat-Prof	99	**Great IHD with Skill (R+)**							0	99
100							0	100	**Large IHD with Ability (L+)**		100	**Great IHD with Ability (R+)**							0	100
0									Quotient for pathological Left Handedness			Quotient for pathological Right Handedness	0							
									CONVERTED LEFT HANDEDNESS (E-based type)			CONVERTED RIGHT HANDEDNESS (E-based type)								
101							0	101	**Clear LH OR VLH Values**	see above	101	**Clear RH OR VRH Values**							0	101
102							0	102	**Child remembers being switched from the L to the R h**	PQ	102	**Child remembers being switched from the R to the L hand**							0	102
103							0	103	**Observation of conversion to R by parents**		103	**Observation of conversion to L by parent**							0	103
104							0	104	Retrained LH in the family (especially father)		104	**Existence of a LH role model for the child**							0	104
105							0	105	Movement of the L hand stronger during RH use		105	Movement of the R hand is stronger when LH is used							0	105
106							0	106	Partial knowledge about converted LH available		106	No knowledge of retraining available							0	106
107							0	107	Influence on R hand use at home		107	Internal motivation exists to switch from the R hand to L							0	107
108							0	108	Influence on R hand use at day care/school		108	External motivation exists to switch from the R hand to L							0	108
109							0	109	**Consequences of conversion ("often" at least 5 times)**		109	**Consequences of conversion ("often" at least 5 times)**							0	109
110							0	110	**Switching consequences ("sometimes" at least 8 times)**		110	**Switching consequences ("sometimes" at least 8 times)**							0	110
111							0	111	With high LH values: untrained preference L, trained preference R	FHPT	111	For R+ and R values: untrained preference very R, trained less R							0	111
							0		OR with high VLH values: untrained and trained preference R			OR for R- and VR values: untrained & trained preference slightly R							0	
112							0	112	R hand performs better but is borderline or sub-average	Trac/Dot	112	L hand performs better but is borderline or noticeable							0	112
113							0	113	Undecided/mixed statements which hand is better	Checklist	113	Undecided/mixed statements which hand is better.							0	113
114							0	114	The L hand is better, especially when tapping	H/K	114	The R hand is better, especially when tapping							0	114
115							0	115	The L hand feels better according to the child's statement	Checklist	115	The R hand feels better according to the child's statement							0	115
116							0	116	With high LH values: crossed always/only with L	MCT	116	With high RH values: crossed always/only with R							0	116
							0		OR with high VLH values: crossed with R or L			OR with high VRH values: crosses mainly with R							0	
117							0	117	With high LH values: better circles with L	BMC	117	At high RH values: clearly better circles with R							0	117
							0		OR with high VLH values: circles are very similar on both sides			OR at high VRH values: circles are similar on both sides							0	
118							0	118	L hand maintains direction		118	The R hand maintains direction							0	118
119							0	119	At high LH values: discrepancy between untrained & trained prefere	Cat-Prof	119	At high RH values: untrained & trained preference clearly R							0	119
							0		OR at high VLH values:trained and untrained preference R			OR at high VRH values:trained & untrained preference more R							0	
120							0	120	At high LH values: discrepancy between ability (L) & skill (R)		120	At high RH values: ability & skill clearly R							0	120
							0		OR at high VLH values: skill and ability more R			OR at high VLH values: skill & ability more R							0	
121							0	121	At high LH values: clear LH laterality profile	Lat-Prof	121	At high RH values: clear RH laterality profile							0	121
							0		OR at high VLH values: tend to have a LH laterality profile			OR at high VRH values: tend to have a RH laterality profile							0	
0									Quotient for Converted Left Handedness			Quotient for Converted Right Handedness	0							

0 does not apply
1 applies to small extent
2 partially applies
3 mostly applies
4 fully applies

PQ 0 Parent Questionnaire
FHPT 1 Functional Hand Preference Test
Trac/Dot 2 Skill (trained proficiency): Tracing and Dotting
Ham/Tap 3 Ability (untrained proficiency): Hammering and Tapping
MCT 4 Midline Crossing Test
BMC 5 Bimanual Cooperation

GOP 0 General Observations Protocoll 0
Checklist 1 Checklist of all motor tests for movement quality 1
Cat-Prof 2 Categorisation Profile 2
Lat-Prof 3 Laterality Profile 3
Cluster-T 4 Cluster Table 4
HP Stairs 5 Handedness Profile Stairs

Fig. 8.9 Example of criteria describing the degree-based handedness type (variation: *Variable Left Handedness* and *Variable Right Handedness*). If the criteria fully apply, a score of 4 is given for each hand; if they only partially apply, a score of 2 or 3 is given; if they do not apply at all, a 0

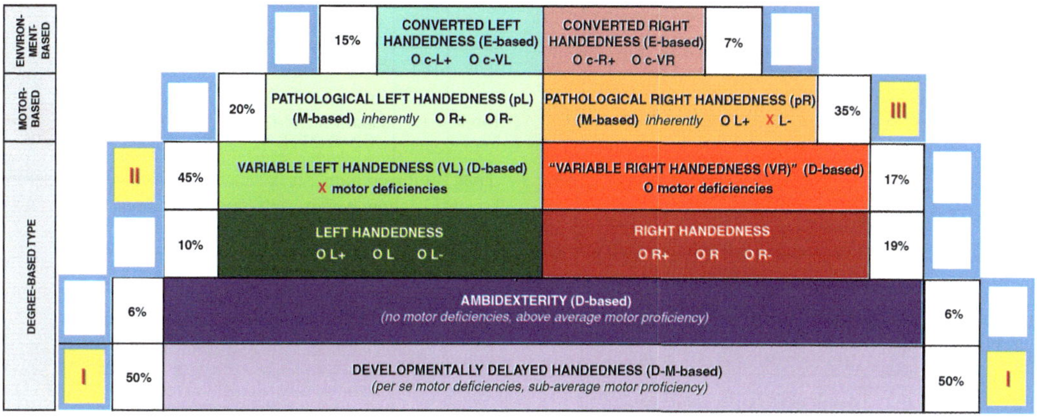

Fig. 8.10 The HP Stairs summarise the percentages of the Cluster Table according to the handedness types and variations

8.6 Tools for Intervention

8.6.1 Differential Check

The Differential Check is a short screening version of multivariate factors. It is very short and seeks to identify differential information by excluding factors that might influence the handedness status. Eight possible causes of variable handedness are identified and screened according to three of the most significant criteria for that cause or handedness type (see Fig. 8.11). In many cases, it suffices to use this screening analytic tool, so that the complex and time-consuming Cluster Table does not necessarily need to be applied.

8.6.2 HP Axes

The HP Axes graphically represent the handedness composition at multiple time intervals, and it was designed to provide a documentation tool for handedness development and formation. It broadly maps the interaction of the three determining factors of handedness: *hereditary (degree), motor (pathology)* and *environment (practice)*. It is useful in clinical practice with children to capture a handedness status at specific points in time by plotting these three factors to determine if and what changes take place over time, typically, after a period of intervention. The *degree* of handedness is taken from the Cat-Profile and plotted on the horizontal axis of the corresponding category. The *motor ability* is broadly estimated on a 6-point scale and plotted on the vertical axis, based on specific motor assessments and estimation of the administrator. Finally, the *practice effect* is rated on a 5-point scale, where the performance is compared to other typical children in the same age group. The parents estimate this in the parent questionnaire, and their ratings are transferred onto the diagram. The three plotting points can then be joined (see Fig. 8.12), thereby documenting. ♦**handedness development** or ♦**handedness formation**, for therapy particularly focussing on establishing the direction of handedness and improving the child's motor skills by increasing practice experiences.

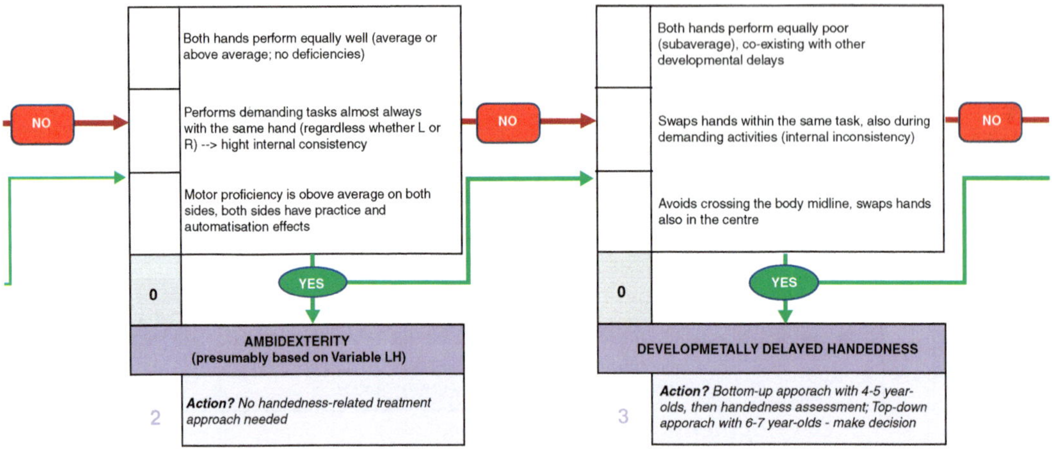

Fig. 8.11 Excerpt of the Differential Check as a screening tool for causes of variable hand use

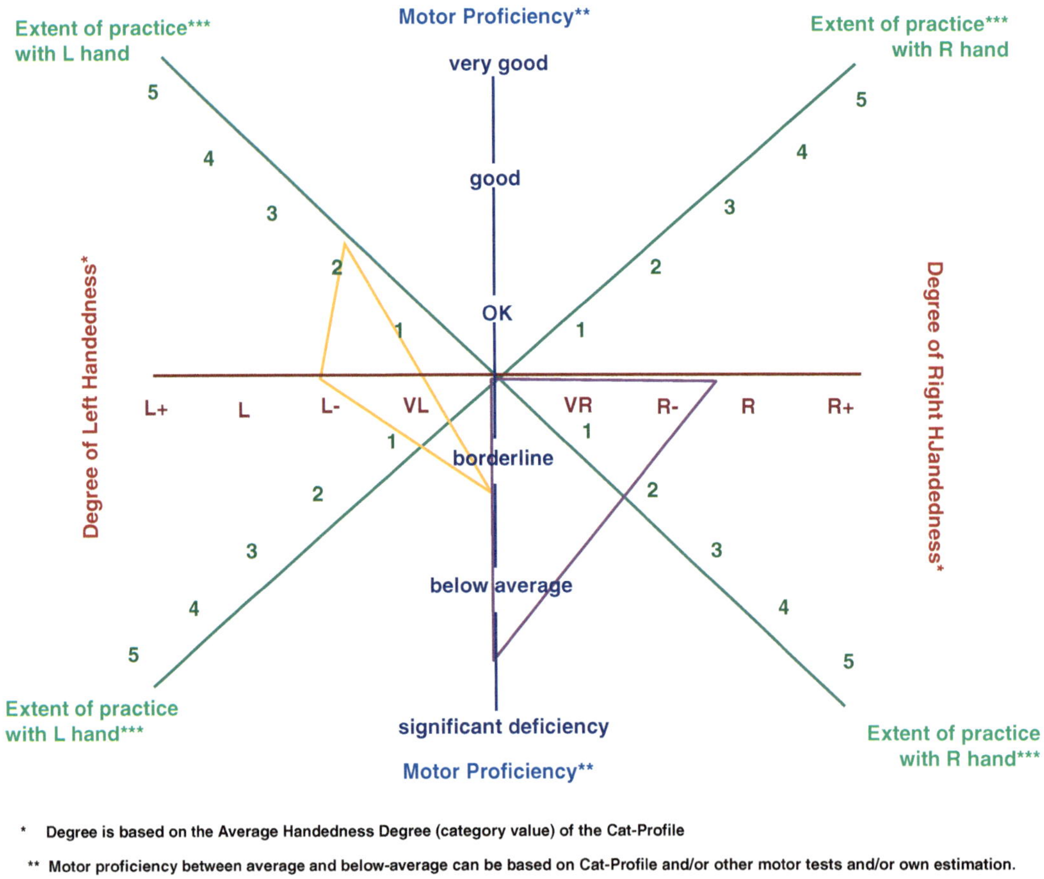

Fig. 8.12 Example of HP Axes depicting the three determining factors of handedness: hereditary (degree), motor (pathology) and environment (practice). **Yellow represents** a mild left-handed individual who tends to avoid exercise (2) and is borderline to below average in her/his motor proficiency. **Purple represents** a moderately established right-handed person who avoids graphomotor activities altogether (0) and therefore has virtually no practice effect with clearly below average motor performance

8.7 Scoring and Coding the Handedness Profile

8.7.1 Digitised Scoring Template

Using a digitised scoring template, the various laterality quotients to measure the inter-hand differences across the subtests are automated in an Excel-based soring system. The actual scoring of the tests (especially the motor tests) is first calculated by the administrator, and scores are then transferred into the template. Automated formulas then calculate all laterality quotients and produce the respective Cat-Profile (see Fig. 8.13).

8.7.2 Handedness Code

A Handedness Code was developed to assist documentation and identification of data sets by coding it to demonstrate its category, type and variation. The eight categories from the Cat-Profile (L+, L, L−, VL, VR, R, R, R+) are used to code the hereditary aspect of degree and direction of handedness (**D-based type**—see Sect. 10.2.1 in the following chapter), ending with a full stop. One of the four categories can be used for the motor pathology-determining factors (M-based type—see Sect. 10.2.11 in the following chapter): (1) **M0**—no motor deficiencies, average to good motor profi-

Fig. 8.13 Excerpt of Excel template of the scoring sheet of the Midline Crossing Test. The values entered are place holders. As soon as the scores are entered in the white fields, the quotients are calculated. A minus value always means left handed scores predominate

MIDLINE CROSSING TEST

RED	
Right: ipsilateral	
Left: contralateral	10
BLUE	
Right: centre	
Left: centre	10
YELLOW	
Right: contralateral	
Left: ipsilateral	10
Reaction Quotient (yellow + blue + red = 30)	
Right	0
Contralateral Right	0
Left	100
Contralateral Left	100
Contralateral Percentage (yellow + red = 20)*	**50**
Ipsilateral	50
Centre (which hand is used more often)	-100
Midline Crossing Quotient	**-100**
Total Reaction Quotient	**-100**

ciency; (2) **M00**—excellent, above-average motor abilities, extensive practice, very good bimanual coordination/cooperation and motor planning skills; (3) **M1**—motor problems, borderline to sub-average motor abilities; and (4) **M11**—severe motor problems, including significant motor planning problems and bimanual incoordination.

After the second full stop, the environmental factors (**E-based type**—see Sect. 10.2.8 in the following chapter) are coded as follows: (1) **E0**—no environmental influence to change handedness; environment consolidates or does not affect dominant hand; (2) **E1**—environmental influence switches the dominant hand (for writing) to non-dominant hand; and (3) **E2**—converted/switched hander reverts to dominant hand (for writing). The order of these three sub-codes depends on which one is thought to be the most determining one. So, the M-Code comes first if it appears that the poor motor abilities on the dominant side determine or result in a change in dominance; if the environment is primarily responsible for conversion of handedness, the E-Code comes first (see Fig. 8.14).

8.8 Comparing the Handedness Profile to Other Handedness Assessments

Clinical practice, including occupational therapy, needs reliable assessments for comprehensive evaluation before and after therapy to measure change and development as well as demonstrate the efficiency and effectiveness of treatment. This is also true for handedness. Some of the tests frequently used to assess handedness in research and practice were presented in Chap. 6 under Sect. 6.4. These tests usually measure either preference or performance/proficiency, making a comparison between tests difficult. Tables 8.2 and 8.3 summarise and contrast specific characteristics of tests found in the literature (with no claim to this selection being exhaustive), to the Handedness Profile (HP).

The Handedness Profile generally shows that it meets more of the criteria for a multidimensional assessment than the other handedness tests and assessments reviewed here. In particular, the features of the Handedness Profile can be summarised as a visual in Fig. 8.15.

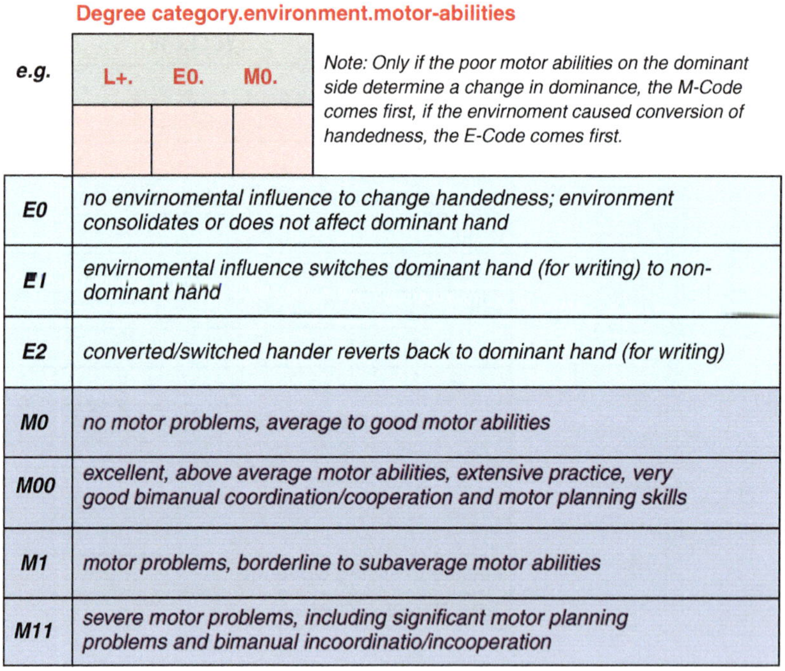

Fig. 8.14 Construction of a Handedness Code

Table 8.2 Characteristics of handedness test procedures for **preference in** research and practice, compared to the Handedness Profile

Assessment	Self/ third-party assessment	Relevant background info	Performing preference	No. of categories/ scale	Internal consistency	Preference items	Motor requirement	Developed for research	Developed for practice	Quality criteria	Standardisation
Preference											
EHI	Self/third party	-	Adapted for children	5	Partly	10	Low	Yes	Possibly	Yes	No
HAPT	–	–	Yes		Yes (3×)	14	Low	Yes	Yes	Yes	Yes
S-MH	–	Yes	Yes	2	Partly	25	Mixed	Secondary	Yes	No	No
WHCT	–	–	Yes	2 (LQ)	Yes (4×)	8	Mixed	Yes	Possibly	Yes	No
HPDT	–	–	Yes	3	Yes (3×)	8	Low	Yes	No	No	No
PHI	Third party	–	Yes		No	13	Low	Yes	No	No	No
WHQ	Adapted	–	Yes	5	Yes	33	Low	Yes	No	No	No
QHP	.	No	Yes	LQ	Yes (3)	21	Low	Yes	No	No	No
SVCU	.	No	Yes	2	No	1	Low	No	Yes	Partly	Yes
HP	.	**Yes**	**Yes**	**8**	**Yes**	**24**	**Mixed**	**Yes**	**Yes**	**Yes**	**Yes**

EHI Edinburgh Handedness Inventory (Oldfield 1971), *HAPT* Hand Preference Test (Bruckner 2011), *HP* Handedness Profile (Kraus, 2003, 2018), *HPDT* Hand Preference Demonstration Test (Soper and Satz 1984), *PHI* Preschool Handedness Inventory (Tan 1985), *QHP* Quantification of Hand preference Task (Bishop et al. 1996), *S-MH* Sattler Methode zur Austestung der Händigkeit (Sattler 2008), *SVCU* Space Visualisation Contralateral Use (Ayres 1989)

Table 8.3 Characteristics of handedness test procedures for **proficiency** in research and practice, compared to the Handedness Profile

	Type of assessment	Type of task	Number of items for each hand	Assessment of speed	Assessment of accuracy	Level of motor requirement	Items, instructions and scoring standardised	Developed for research	Developed for practice	Criteria for movement quality	Normative data
PTK/LDT	Performance	Dotting	1	Yes	Limited	High	Yes	Yes	Secondary	Yes	Yes (5–12 years)
HDT	Performance	Dotting and tracing	2 + trial	Yes	Limited	Fairly high	Yes	Yes	Yes	Yes	Yes (6–70 years)
MAcc	Performance	Tracing	1	Yes	Yes	High	Yes	Secondary	Yes	Yes	Yes (4–11 years)
PP	No	Move pegs	2 × 25	Yes	No	Medium	Yes	Yes	Yes	Yes	Yes (5–16 years)
ZNT	No	Neurol. movement sequence	6 areas	Partially	Partially	Low	Yes	Yes	Yes	Yes	Yes (5–16 years)
FT	No	Finger tapping	No. of taps in sec	Yes	No	Medium	Partly	Yes	No	No	No
PMT	No	Move pegs	30× per hand	Yes	No	Medium	Partly	Yes	No	No	No
BCD	No	4	4 directions	No	Partly	Medium	Yes	Yes	No	No	No
BMC	No	Copying bilat. movements	10	No	No	Medium	Partly	Yes	Yes	Yes	Yes (4–11 years)
HP	Performance	Dotting and tracing	**4+ trials**	**Yes**	**Yes**	**High**	**Yes**	**Yes**	**Yes**	**Yes**	**Yes (6 years)**

BCD Bimanual circle drawing (Carson et al. 1997), *BMC* Bilateral Motor Coordination (Ayres 1989), *FT* finger tapping (Peters 1990), *HDT* Hand Dominance Test (Steingrüber and Linert 2010), *HP* Handedness Profile (Kraus, 2003, 2018), PTK/LDT dominance Test (Schilling 1974, 2009), *MAcc* Motor Accuracy Test (Ayres 1989), *PMT* Peg-Moving Task (Annett 1992), *PP* Purdue Pegboard (Tiffin 1948), WatHand Cabinet Test (Bryden et al. 2007), *WHQ* Waterloo Handedness Questionnaire (Cavill & Bryden 2003), *ZNT* Zurich Neural Motor Test (Largo et al. 2007)

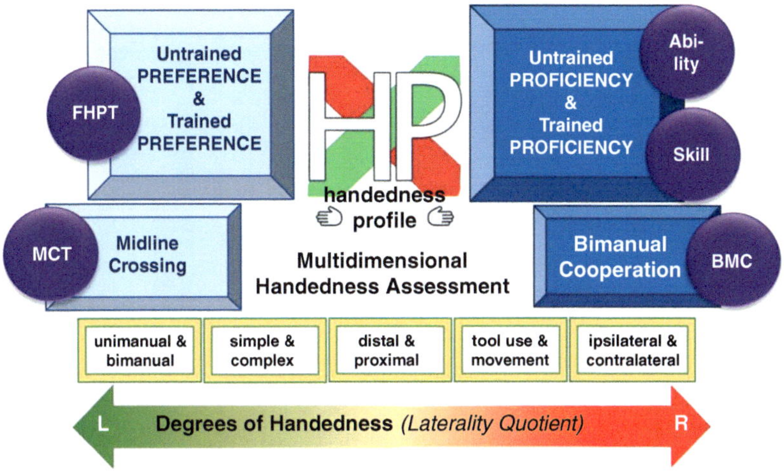

Fig. 8.15 Overview of the multidimensional features of the Handedness Profile 2018. The blue boxes represent handedness dimensions, the purple circles the subtests and the yellow boxes the range of different task features. *FHPT* Functional Hand Preference Test, *MCT* Midline Crossing Test (preference), *Ability* Average of Hammering and Tapping, *Skill* Average of Tracing and Dotting, *BMC* Bimanual Cooperation Test based on simultaneous bimanual circle drawing

8.9 Evaluation of the Handedness Profile by Trained Practitioners

Between 2018 and 2021, 115 practitioners that were fully trained on the Handedness Profile participated in a practicability study on the Handedness Profile.

8.9.1 Summary of Closed Questions

A 4-point Likert scale was used for some closed questions to rate the overall estimation of the Handedness Profile, how it can be implemented and its perceived usefulness and suitability in clinical practice. In addition, the structure and organisation of the Handedness Profile were rated, as well as the scoring procedure and the tools for interpretation (see Fig. 8.16).[2]

8.9.2 Perceived Benefits and Advantages of the Handedness Profile

Here are some comments that practitioners find positive about the Handedness Profile. I have clustered the responses to form categories.[3]

8.9.3 Multidimensional Assessment, Comprehensiveness

- *It is very comprehensive and gives a good overview—the application works very well.* (*HPA*022222/11.50.36)
- *Many aspects are taken into account in the test, and find comprehensive diagnostics useful.* (*HPA060120/15.16.53*).
- *Very comprehensive, many aspects are considered it is well researched and founded in science.* (*HPA*060320/12.45.12)

[2]Note: The questions were not compulsory, since participants had different levels of competencies using the HP and only answered those questions where they could draw on their own experiences. Thus, the number of answers varies across the questions.

[3]These findings were translated from German using deepL.

Fig. 8.16 Results of an evaluation of trained practitioners using the Handedness Profile (N = between 91 and 103)

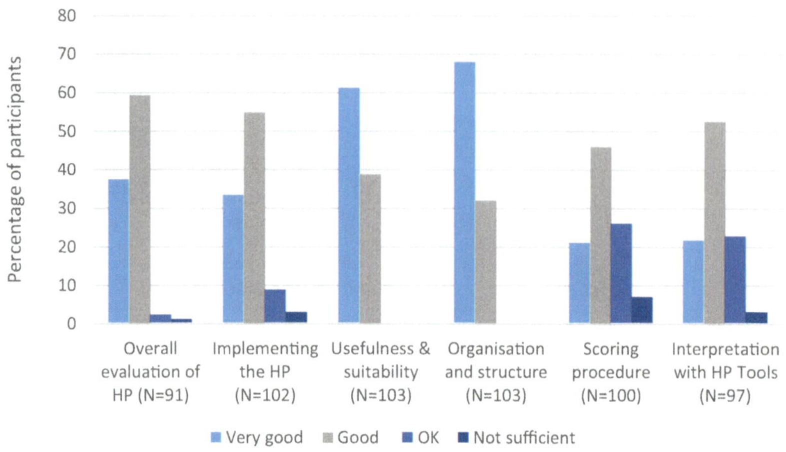

- *The HP is very well thought out and provides broad and detailed results.* (*HPA*121518/23.03.07)
- *I find the complexity, and consideration of several functions/skills in the test phase as well as the classification of the handedness types excellent.* (*HPA*010219/9.09.11)
- *Good basis to get a grasp on handedness.* (*HPA*112018/19.03.00)
- *I find the diversity of the aspects examined very convincing. The execution of the individual items requires some practice, but then the assessment is very practicable. (TN* 200222/17.06.42)
- *I think it's great that all aspects of the handedness are addressed, so not only preference and consistency, but above all tapping tasks and bimanual cooperation.* (*HPA*020619/8.26.05)
- *The best and most meaningful handedness assessment on the market. I don't want to miss it anymore. So far, I have always come to a valid conclusion about a child with unestablished or mixed handedness using the Handedness Profile. Thank you!!!! (HPA121218/6.43.10)*
- *Overall, the Handedness Profile is very meaningful. The differentiation of the individual areas, such as bimanual coordination and midline crossing are particularly useful.* (*HPA*111918/21.32.07)
- *It covers many aspects of handedness, but does not claim that there is "the" answer. Further aspects of the environment are taken into account in the interpretation.* (*HPA*122018/16.03.26)
- *I like the differentiation performance/preference and especially the last item. I hated that at first, and now it's often very revealing. (HPA060120/16.29.25)*
- *I appreciate the differentiation of individual areas and the wide range of applicability with regard to age. It is the best assessment for me so far in terms of handedness and implementation, even if it is time-consuming, because it is so clear and structured. (HPA191118/21.32.07)*
- *I love performing the Functional Hand Preference Test and Crossing the Middle of the Body. I also like the variety in the sequences. (HPA060120/20.28.17)*

Basis for Clinical Reasoning, Analysis and Interpretation

- *[The HP] structures clinical reasoning, [it provides] a comprehensive view to better bring about and justify decisions.* (*HPA*060520/9.59.50)
- *The Category Profile is clear, although motor skills and alternating behaviour are still sometimes open to interpretation* (*HPA*122718/17.04.52)
- *I love it that the HP results in both a quantitative statement and scope for subjective observation. (HPA060320/13.33.34)*
- *It really helps understand the switching behaviour and determine the writing hand. (HPA092121/15.45.31)*

- *Provides a good overview of un/trained exercises in the FHPT also for a short check of handedness, good diagnostics for each age group, Diff-Check I find good, especially to clarify whether the test is necessary. (HPA060420/11.20.01)*

Structure and Construct of the Assessment
- *Clear structures that can be learned easily and comprehensively.* (*HPA*052520/20.38.52)
- *I like the structured construction, the different aspects that are taken into account and the graphical representation of the results. (HPA123018/8.59.01)*
- *It is standardised and has very clear structures, and it is manageable in terms of the time taken for implementation. (HPA011719/22.14.46)*
- *It has a clear structure and is a compact system in itself.* (*HPA*122018/16.03.26)
- *It is well structured, and the data makes sense. (HPA060420/11.20.01)*

Administration, Implementation, Practicability
- *Implementation of the subtests is great.* (*HPA*122718/17.04.52)
- *The implementation is very nicely structured and the resulting overall picture of the child in all fine motor and coordinative areas is very good.* (*HPA*060220/19.04.27)
- *It is great that the suitcase comes with all materials included and that the protocol sheets are very clearly designed.* (*HPA*050822/13.30.41)

8.9.4 Appropriateness for Children

- *The HP is very varied and child-friendly, so that the children remain motivated and concentrated.* (*HPA*123018/22.50.48)
- *The HP is child-friendly, they usually have great fun.* (*HPA*123118/10.23.47)
- *The children join in enthusiastically!* (*HPA*080619/9.35.46)
- *The first part is the most practical, which most children do quite well in one piece. As soon as they see the pen, they get more restless …. (HPA121918/7.51.03)*
- *The children are very well motivated. The implementation, presentation and explanation are easy. The testing is usually carried out smoothly, only Tapping with the fingers is often difficult [for children], as the Velcro tape sometimes slips. Especially primary school children enjoy the test.* (*HPA*121718/7.39.48)
- *Despite the length of the test, the children participate very well, as it is very child-friendly. (HPA060120/16.29.25)*
- *It is fun for children and young people. (HPA060420/11.20.01)*
- *It is child-friendly and clearly structured. (HPA*050822/13.30.41)

Suitability for Feedback to Parents and Other Professionals
- *The scope of the tests convinces parents and doctors of the reliability of the test. Input* via *Excel mask.* (*HPA*11518/21.31.20)
- *The results of the HP lend themselves to be communicated well to parents.* (*HPA*121518/23.03.07)
- *Clients usually find Category Profile exciting, they usually get into a good conversation about further steps.* (*HPA*112018/19.03.00)
- *The vivid Category Profile is a very good basis to discuss [results] with parents as well as other caregivers or doctors/other professions.* (*HPA*123118/10.23.47)
- *All subtests show the aspects of handedness very well, so when parents watch the assessment they understand well what it is about.* (*HPA*080619/9.35.46)
- *It is very everyday and easy to explain to parents.* (*HPA*080619/9.35.46)
- *The Handedness Profile presents a clearly structured template with measured values that facilitate consultation. (TN* 200222/17.06.42)
- *It is a professional instrument, especially in parent discussions and with doctors. It is standardised and provides clear structures. Time constraints are manageable. (HPA011719/22.14.46)*
- *The decision tree is good if reversion is necessary - also for parent discussions. (HPA060420/11.20.01)*

Usefulness of Digitisation

- *I really like the Digital Scoring Template and the graphical presentation of all the values [of the laterality quotients].* (HPA052520/20.38.52)
- *I find the Digital Scoring Template mask very good.* (HPA010219/9.09.11)
- *I really like the Excel Digital Scoring Template! (HPA060120/15.16.53).*
- *The Digital Scoring Template really facilitates the evaluation. (HPA122018/16.03.26)*
- *There is a clearly structured Digital Scoring Template with all the values summarised that facilitate consultation. (HPA022022/17.06.42)*
- *I find the diversity of the aspects examined very convincing. The execution of the individual items requires some practice, but then the test is very practical. (HPA022022/17.06.42)*
- *It is great to have the Digital Scoring Template for faster evaluation.* (HPA050822/13.30.41)

Participants mostly agree that the Handedness Profile is a well-structured, comprehensive, child-friendly assessment that not only assists in understanding mixed handedness but also helps communicate the results clearly to other professionals and parents.

8.9.5 Perceived Challenges and Recommendations Using the Handedness Profile

Here are some of the critical appraisals from practitioners about the Handedness Profile. I again clustered the responses to form categories.

Administration and Implementation of Items

- *It is difficult to trace [the bear], as many children press so hard that the pen is flattened after using it only a few times. (HPA121718/7.39.48)*
- *The testing procedure is exhausting for some of our patients with DCD and takes too long time. (HPA121918/7.58.28)*
- *HP is carried out by me only in "urgent" cases due to the long duration of the scoring. Maybe it is possible to score everything with the [digital] Ergo Pen (teddy bear, hammering, tapping)* via *computer. (HPA123118/10.23.47)*
- *Bear tracing is very easily and quickly administered, but takes an incredibly long time to score therefore impractical. Crossing the midline could be clearer if the "crossing radius" was larger, and additional tasks (*e.g. *with tools). Bimanual circle drawing is a very good and important task, but in the scoring it is unfortunately very subjective and sometimes difficult to observe. (HPA020619/8.26.05)*
- *I find the bimanual cooperation too detailed. For the preschool children it is exhausting and think you could shorten it. (HPA060120/15.16.53)*
- *Short version would be helpful. (HPA060520/11.37.07)*
- *It should be much easier to use, score and interpret. (HPA061220/12.20.17)*
- *Idea: make new revisions of protocol sheets regularly available to trained participants in the newsletter. (HPA02421/19.38.19)*
- *A short version for preschool children and children with difficulty concentrating. (HPA092121/15.45.31)*

Analysis and Interpretation

- *Interpretation is usually still tricky for me because I have not used the assessment often. Maybe more examples for correct interpretation? (HPA112018/19.03.00)*
- *We need normative data for all different age groups, this is important and make the proficiency dimension more specific. (HPA123018/22.50.48)*
- *More research and support in this area using the Handedness Profile is necessary, sharing cases and feedback. (HPA123118/10.23.47)*
- *I would like to have more elaborate background knowledge on handedness and occupations in everyday life, how the environment influences left handers, about everyday objects for left and right handers, retraining consequences, physiological backgrounds,* etc. *so that I am fit in counselling, which is so important to parents and educators. This should be part of the training of the Handedness Profile. (HPA011719/22.14.46)*
- *It is a very extensive instrument, unfortunately very time-consuming also in the evaluation, often unfortunately very unclear results,*

sometimes wish me clearer results (but maybe this is exactly the sticking point with unclear handedness and there can be no reliable results ...). (HPA060220/18.33.06)

- *It would be great if the "staircase" could provide an even clearer interpretation aid and be automated. This is certainly mathematically a huge challenge and perhaps impossible with the abundance of possibilities. (HPA060320/13.33.34)*

Scoring and Calculation

- *I find it too complicated to use and evaluate. (HPA120818/9.51.34)*
- *The evaluation would have to be simplified, this takes too long in everyday practice. (HPA121118/18.55.03)*
- *Please do not make the scoring even more complicated with more tools like another diagram, stairs,* etc. *There is no time for this in everyday life. (HPA121418/3.58.06)*
- *I am very interested in an affordable digitised version of the test, which will make the scoring so much easier. (HPA121518/21.31.20)*
- *Scoring the bear is cumbersome and time-consuming. Maybe you could use a pen with a sensor or similar, which transmits the data directly to the PC. In addition, I find it difficult and very subjective to make statements about the bimanual circles, often do not know what exactly I should enter there. (HPA121618/18.11.20)*
- *The HP needs to be fully digitised so that the scoring can be facilitated and time reduced. (HPA122018/16.03.26)*
- *I would love to have a "short version" or screening that is not so time-consuming. (HPA122218/14.54.59)*
- *An automated Cluster Table would be great! (HPA012519/15.46.58)*
- *The evaluation is very time-consuming! The interpretation is difficult because (in my opinion) too little attention is paid to it in training. Otherwise a very good profile and very complex! I'm glad to be able to do it. (HPA02.1219/10.39.16)*
- *Scoring of the testing is very time-consuming, and I am looking forward to the full digitisation. I am scared of the new Digital Scoring Template that I got to know last year at the Refresher—simply too little time in everyday life for it. Also, there is also no time to discuss everything with the parents and if I wrote everything in the reports, they would be very long, which again takes time. A template for a report would be great. I have already had several critical questions from doctors, particularly concerning variable Left handers. Maybe a short explanation on the scoring sheet? (HPA080519/6.49.01)*
- *The planned app would certainly make scoring a lot easier and faster. (HPA060120/14.20.59)*
- *I am looking forward to the digitised, time-saving evaluation. (HPA060120/16.29.25)*
- *Evaluation of tapping and hammering is very difficult and often leads to different results, the evaluation of trailing and bimanual cooperation is very time-consuming. (HPA060120/20.28.17)*
- *I would be very happy about an automatic test evaluation. (HPA060220/10.33.29)*
- *I think digitisation makes a lot of sense. (HPA060220/13.09.50)*
- *We need software for the entire scoring and analysis. As it is, it is too complicated for everyday life. (HPA060220/19.04.27)*
- *Improve the scoring! (HPA061820/0.13.53)*
- *Digitalisation would be very helpful. (HPA062720/20.43.38)*
- *Provide overview for results of individual subtests as an app for faster evaluation of the results. Excel has many sources of error ... (HPA02421/19.38.19)*
- *Provide digital scoring also of the items "Dotting, tracing, tapping ... to reduce the time required for evaluation. (HPA053020/17.24.49)*

The biggest challenge reported on the Handedness Profile is that it is too time-consuming for some practitioners, particularly regarding the scoring and interpretation procedures. These challenges can be addressed through complete digitisation of the Handedness Profile.

8.10 Concluding Remarks

We have seen that the current Handedness Profile systematically examines various dimensions of handedness by providing a standardised multidimensional assessment. In addition, it captures relevant contextual factors such as medical history, background information and *Left Handedness* in the family. However, the Handedness Profile goes beyond a mere assessment and assists the therapy process by providing graphical overviews as tools for analysis and interpretation that combine all quantitative and qualitative data and offer a differentiated system for analysis. In addition, the scoring is partially supported digitally, and handedness codes can be constructed to systemise cases. When comparing the Handedness Profile with other assessments, we see that it incorporates more dimensions. Trained administrators generally evaluate the Handedness Profile positively, although they find the manual scoring and analysis very time-consuming.

The Handedness Typology brings together the data yielded by Handedness Profile and its tools. This is particularly helpful for interpretation and clinical decision-making regarding specific and effective interventions. Chapter 9 shows how the handedness types were constructed as a basis for interpreting the Handedness Profile.

References

Annett M (1992) Five tests of hand skill. Cortex 28(4):583–600

Ayres AJ (1989) Sensory integration and praxis tests. Los Angeles: Western Psychological Services

Beaton A (1985) Left side, right side. A review of laterality research. Batsford Academic and Educational, London

Bishop DVM, Ross VA, Daniels MS, Bright P (1996) The measurement of hand preference: A validation study comparing three groups of right-handers. British journal of psychology 87(2):269–285

Bourassa DC (1996) Handedness and eye-dominance: a meta-analysis of their relationship. Laterality 1(1):5–34

Bruckner J, Deimann P, Kastner-Koller U (2011a) HAPT 4-6. Handpräferenztest für 4-6-jährige Kinder. Göttingen: Hogrefe

Bryden PJ, Roy EA, Spence J (2007) An observational method of assessing handedness in children and adults. Developmental Neuropsychology 32(3):825–846

Carson RG, Thomas J, Summer JJ, Walters MR, Semjen A, Summers J, Cattaert D (1997) The dynamics of bimanual circle drawing. Q J Exp Psychol Sect A 50A(3):664–683

Cattaert D, Semjen A, Summers JJ (1999) Simulating a neural cross-talk model for between-hand interference during bimanual circle drawing. Biol Cybern 81(4):343–358

Cavill S, Bryden P (2003) Development of handedness: comparison of questionnaire and performance-based measures of preference. Brain and cognition 53(2):149–151

Grouios G, Hatzitaki V, Kollias N, Koidou I (2009) Investigating the stabilising and mobilising features of footedness. Laterality 14(4):362–380

Kraus E (2003) The handedness profile. The development of a normative profile to determine the extent of handedness in children. Doctoral thesis. La Trobe University, Melbourne, Australia

Kraus E (2018) Manual zum Händigkeitsprofil. Manual for assessment

Kraus E (Hg.) (2019) Zwischen Links-& Rechtshändigkeit. Theorie, Diagnostik & Therapie bei Kindern mit wechselndem Handgebrauch. Springer, Berlin

Largo RH, Rousson V, Caflisch JA, Jenni OG (2007) Zürich Neuromotor Assessment. Zürich: AWE Verlag

Martin WLB, Porac C (2007) Patterns of handedness and footedness in switched and nonswitched Brazilian left-handers: cultural effects on the development of lateral preferences. Dev Neuropsychol 31(2):159–179

Peters M (1990) Neuropsychological identification of motor problems: can we learn something from the feet and legs that hands and arms will not tell us? Neuropsychol Rev 1(2):165–183

Sattler JB (2008) Händigkeitsabklärung SMH nach der Sattler-Methodik. Donauwörth: Auer Verlag

Scherbel M (2019) Der Zusammenhang von Lateralitätsmerkmalen & dem Ausprägungsgrad der Händigkeit bei Erwachsenen. BSc. Fresenius University of Applied Sciences, Munich

Schilling FS (2009) PTK - LDT Material - Punktiertest und Leistungs- Dominanztest für Kinder (5-12 Jahre). Dortmund: Verlag Modernes Lernen

Soper HV, Satz P (1984) Pathological left-handedness and ambiguous handedness: A new explanatory model. Neuropsychologia 22(4):511–515

Strauss E, Goldsmith SM (1987) Lateral preferences and performance on non-verbal laterality tests in a normal population. Cortex 23(3):495–503

Tan LE (1985) Laterality and motor skills in four-year-olds. Child Development 119–124

Tiffin J, Asher EJ (1948) The Purdue Pegboard: norms and studies of reliability and validity. Journal of applied psychology 32(3):234

Proposing an Architecture for a Handedness Typology

9

Contents

It is more than evident that the way in which we characterise hand preference is influenced by the nature of the questions we ask. The multifactorial approach to hand preference may offer an avenue to explore and resolve the discrepancies that have often been noted between hand preference and hand performance by offering some clues about the types of tasks for which one should expect large performance differences.... and those where the differences should be relatively minor. (Steenhuis & Bryden 1989: 301)

9.1 Introduction

Clinical practice with children focussing on handedness needs a clear foundation based on research findings to ensure relevant, specific, evidence-based diagnostics and treatment approaches (or the development thereof). So how can the wealth of diverse knowledge on handedness be merged to form a theoretical underpinning for practitioners in an understandable, comprehensive and systematic way? This challenge has confronted me continuously over the years. In this chapter, I attempt to "bring it all together" from the earlier chapters to lay the foundations for a Handedness Typology—a necessary reference for analysing and interpreting the results of atypical variable hand use in clinical practice.

The chapter consists of six parts. (1) I propose a defining description of *multidimensional* handedness with six dimensions drawing on Chaps. 1–8. (2) I then relate the multiple dimensions of handedness (including preference, proficiency,

E. Kraus, *Beyond Left and Right Handedness*, https://doi.org/10.1007/978-3-031-24389-9_9

direction and degree) to the co-determinants discussed in Chaps. 1 and 3, respectively. The latter include *multivariate* factors such as hereditary and polygenetic influences, development cascades, as well as the environmental and pathological impact on handedness. (3) Subsequently, distinct subgroups of handedness from the literature are identified. (4) I then construct handedness types and variations based on the three co-determinants and the subgroups of handedness, drawing on Chaps. 4–8. (5) Finally, the proposed handedness variations are related to the handedness categories. Together, these parts make up the architecture of the Handedness Typology.

9.2 Defining Six Dimensions of Handedness

As discussed, the definitions of handedness lack uniformity and often do not consider important related aspects. In an attempt to combine knowledge from the literature and my own research, I propose the following **defining description of multidimensional handedness**.[1]

> *Handedness is a polygenetic, multidimensional phenomenon that develops predominantly during the first six years of life and continues to be formed throughout life, influenced by multivariate factors. It is co-defined by individual motor learning ability with four defining and two compound dimensions.* ***Hand preference*** *reveals how often a hand is used compared to the other.* ***Hand proficiency*** *indicates how well the hands perform motorically and which is the better hand. The* ***direction of handedness*** *specifies whether handedness is left or right, whilst the* ***degree of handedness*** *discloses how strongly handedness is displayed. Two compound dimensions complement these defining dimensions. The* ***function-based dimension*** *incorporates aspects related to individual manual performance, whilst the* ***task-related dimension*** *comprises task characteristics that externally influence hand use.*

[1] See Glossary for more detailed definitions.

Figure 9.1 visualises the described multidimensionality of handedness.

So ***PREFERENCE (I)*** and ***PROFICIENCY (II)*** are the two dimensions that define handedness in terms of its *substance*: how often the hands are used to *perform* movement and tasks and how good the hands are at executing these. In addition, the ***DIRECTION (III)*** and ***DEGREE (IV)*** can be considered dimensions defining handedness in terms of how it is presented, indicating whether a person is left or right handed, and to what extent this is the case.

The ***FUNCTION (V)*** dimension refers to the individual performing manual actions. It differentiates the tasks according to several dual characteristics that differ in their extent of lateralisation (the first always being more lateralised and the second less): distal and proximal; unimanual and bimanual; skilled and unskilled, as well as trained and untrained. In addition, repeated execution through practice forms automated movements, habits and routines within the context of meaningfulness and experiences and are subject to motivational factors. This dimension is unique to every person.

The ***TASK (VI)*** dimension includes external influences on hand use and hand function externally, including the following: type of task needs to be performed; required tools and other demands; ipslateral or contralateral placement of an item; exposure to items; and the extent of item availability. This dimension is more related to environmental factors and represents the external demands for performance. The function and task dimensions are referred to as the compound dimensions since they consist of several subdimensions that form unique constellations in every individual.

We will now explore how these six dimensions relate to the co-determinants of handedness discussed in Chap. 3.

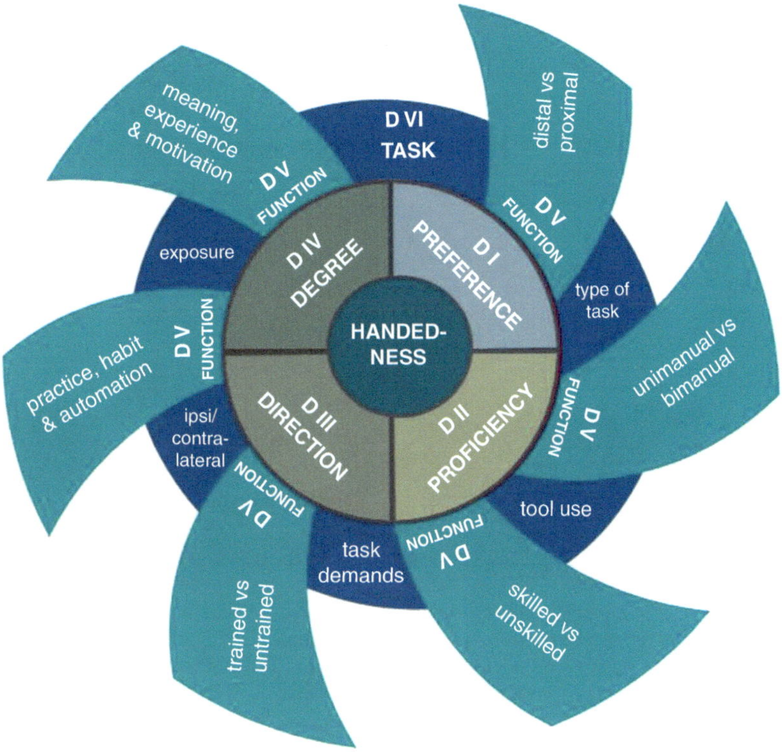

Fig. 9.1 *Six Dimensions of Handedness.* The four defining dimensions, Preference, Proficiency, Direction and Degree of Handedness, are depicted in the centre circle. The two compound dimensions, Function-based and Task-related Dimensions, are portrayed on the outside as a dynamic wheel, which is not attached to a particular defining dimension but affects all of them

9.3 Combining Multidimensional Handedness with Multivariate Co-Determinants

The proposed handedness dimensions do not exist in a vacuum but are dynamically intertwined with reciprocal influences, particularly those that determine handedness. As we saw in Chap. 3, there are four major clusters, the so-called ♦**co-determinants of handedness**: *Inheritance*, *Development*, *Environmental* factors and pathological *Motor impact*. However, for the purpose of a practice-based approach, *Development* is a very diffuse co-determinant: in some ways it is part of *Inheritance*, it is very difficult to separate it from *Motor impact,* and it is also intricately linked to *Environmental influences*. For this reason, *Development* does not constitute a separate co-determinant but is an important part of the other three co-determinants (see Fig. 9.2).

If we now add the six dimensions of handedness to the co-determinants to demonstrate their interrelationship and the complex reciprocal and dynamic processes underpinning manual action become more tangible, as Fig. 9.2 illustrates.

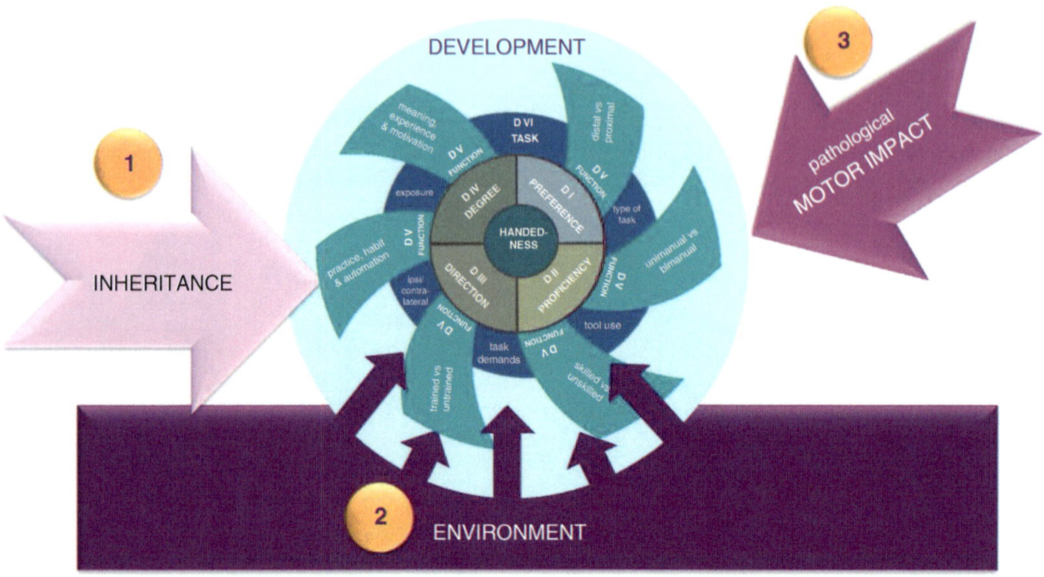

Fig. 9.2 Combining handedness dimensions and co-determinants. In Chap. 3, (Fig. 3.3) four co-determinants using the same visuals were identified. In this chapter, I propose only **three** co-determinants: Inheritance, Environment and Motor Impact, with Development being an integral part of the other three. In addition, the six dimensions of handedness are integrated

9.4 Identifying Distinct Handedness Groups from the Literature

Based on the literature (Chaps. 2–5) and my research (Chaps. 7 and 8), the co-determinants are responsible for both ♦**handedness development** and ♦**handedness formation**. This has led to the identification of subgroups of handedness in the literature (particularly Chaps. 4 and 5). I have clustered these subgroups in the following way.

- Firstly, the varying degree of handedness has prompted studies to differentiate between left and right handers, even if arbitrarily. In particular, **left and right handers with either strong, moderate or mild degrees** of handedness have been identified (see Sects. 4.2 and 4.3). Furthermore, both degree and direction have been found to be inherited and have polygenetic origins, even though the impact of the inheritance is only about 25%. So we can conclude that the different groups of left and right handers based on degrees of handedness are particularly related to the *Inheritance Co-Determinant*, making up a specific group[2] of handedness.
- Secondly, there is a group of **converted left** (and more rarely right) **handers**, who learned to write with their non-dominant hand (see Sect. 4.5). The right-biassed physical and socio-cultural environments are mainly responsible for such handedness conversion, i.e. particularly the *Environment Co-Determinant*. Moreover, switching handwriting may affect manual asymmetry in other activities and tasks (see Sect. 3.4.2), making this group of individuals share similar challenges, even though their degree of handedness will affect the extent of the conversion.
- Thirdly, in some cases, early brain insult before, at or after birth affects the inherently dominant cortex, leading to substantially better proficiency of the non-dominant hand (see Sect. 3.5). Here the pathological *Motor Impact Co-Determinant*

[2] In Chap. 10, these groups of handedness will be defined in more detail as handedness types with their subgroups or Variations.

is particularly responsible, and it may affect the left and right cortices, resulting in **pathological left and right handers**. However, since the incidence of right handers has been widely found to be considerably higher than left handers, *pathological Left Handedness* is more common. Pathological handedness has been clearly differentiated from familial handedness and can be considered a separate handedness group.

In addition, two distinct subgroups of mixed handedness can be found in the literature, **ambidextrous** and **unestablished handedness** (see Chap. 5). *Ambidextrous handers* are very rare with the unusual ability to use both hands for writing and other complex manual tasks equally well with an exceptional level of proficiency (see Sect. 5.4). This distinct feature makes them a specific subgroup of handers. In contrast, *unestablished handers* also show virtually no difference between the hands, but both sides perform exceptionally poorly. This group particularly consists of children where lateralisation and specialisation of the hemispheres and manual tasks have not yet taken place sufficiently to reveal a preferred and/or more proficient hand. Certain conditions and disorders may also result in reduced lateralisation and unestablished handedness (see Sect. 5.6). Typically, these children also have suffered from complications around birth and other well-known risk factors. They almost always present with a motor deficiency that usually affects both sides even if the type of deficit differs between the sides. This group of individuals thus also comprise a separate group.

9.5 Constructing Handedness Types and Variations Based on the Three Co-Determinants of Handedness

In a first step, I propose three **handedness types,** directly derived from the three co-determinants[3] of handedness, since they are based on the same content. In particular,

- the *Co-Determinant Inheritance* is responsible for polygenetic and epigenetic factors that determine both the direction and the degree of handedness particularly. For the purpose of constructing handedness types, this Co-Determinant corresponds to the **♦Degree- and Direction (D)-based Handedness Type**.
- Similarly, the *Co-Determinant Environment* parallels the **♦Environment (E)-based Handedness Type** and encompasses those types of handedness where the handedness direction has been changed due to physical and socio-cultural (right)-biassed influences.
- *Co-Determinant pathological Motor Impact* directly corresponds with the **♦Motor-Impact (M)-Based Handedness Type** and incorporates those types of handedness where an early brain insult is responsible for a less proficient dominant hand, resulting in the non-dominant hand becoming more proficient (see **♦handedness reshaping**).

In the second step, I allocated the handedness subgroups found in the literature to the three handedness types, referring to them as **♦handedness variations**. These ten variations make up the foundation of the **♦Handedness Typology** as seen in Fig. 9.3.

To generate the necessary information for the different handedness variations, assessments need to collect both quantitative[4] and qualitative[5] data in order to cover the various dimensions of handedness and incorporate the multivariate factors, as exemplified in the Handedness Profile (Chaps. 7 and 8).

[3] Having clarified the intricate relationship between handedness co-determinants and types, I will only refer to handedness types in the forthcoming parts of the book.

[4] *Quantitative* data are typically based on *continuous measures* (e.g. based on laterality quotients) and particularly capture the *degree* and *direction* of multidimensional handedness.

[5] *Qualitative* data are particularly important to the Environment-based and the Motor-Impact-based handedness types, requiring information on risk and development factors, and possible pressures or influences causing switched handedness.

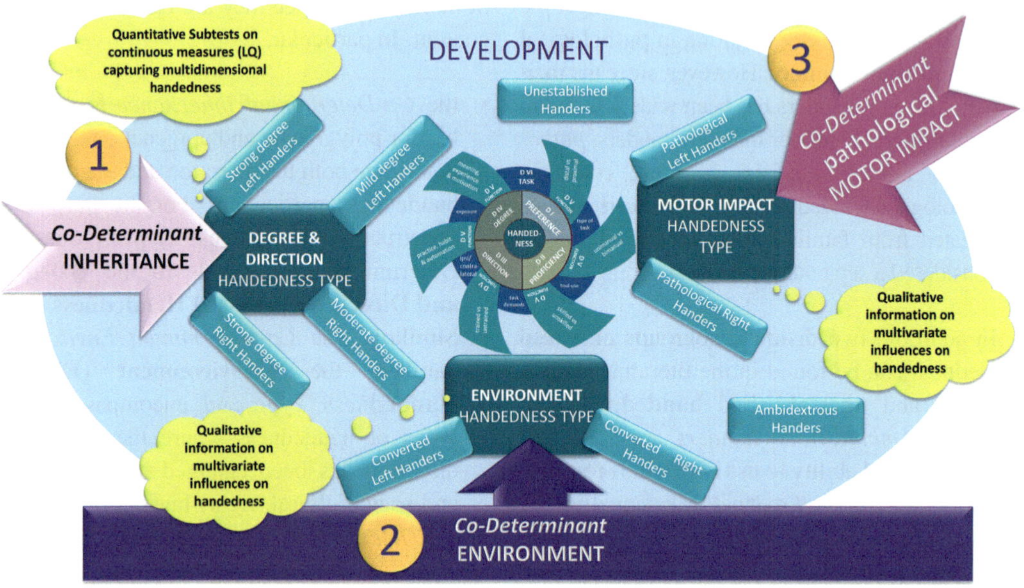

Fig. 9.3 Basic architecture for the Handedness Typology. Each of the Co-determinants directly corresponds to a handedness type (dark green boxes). The subgroups of handedness identified in the literature are assigned to the various handedness types (light green) and are considered to be Variations of the Handedness Types. The yellow clouds indicate the assessment of multidimensional and multivariate handedness, using both quantitative and qualitative data to ensure sufficient information for the three Handedness Types

9.6 Specifying the Variations of the Handedness Types

Let us now look more specifically at how the variations of the types are related to both degrees of handedness and motor abilities. Figure 9.4 provides an overview of these relationships.

More specifically, the ***Degree-based (D-based) Type*** consists of six variations *Left Handedness (LH), Variable Left Handedness (VLH), Variable Right Handedness (VRH), Right Handedness (RH), Ambidextrous Handedness (AH)* and *Developmentally Delayed Handedness (DDH)*. The distinction between mild left and *Variable Left Handedness* may not always be clear. Therefore, VLH extends upward into the L− category. In addition, *Variable Right Handedness* may extend into the category of VLH, since it may include switched left handers with a low handedness degree.

Furthermore, for the purpose of the Typology, the categories explicit (L+/R+), moderate (L/R) and mild (L−/R−) have been collapsed into one variation each, namely ***Left Handedness*** (***LH***) and ***Right Handedness*** (***RH***), since the handedness direction is unambiguous even though there are differences in degree of handedness. (see Sect. 10.2.1). Importantly, these two variations make up the *typical* presentation of handedness, where the variations correspond directly with the categories.

In contrast, the variations ***Variable Left Handedness*** (***VLH***) and ***Variable Right Handedness*** (***VRH***) do not display unambiguous handedness direction and are thus considered atypical and in need for a separate variation. In addition, ***Ambidextrous Handedness*** (***AH***) as well as ***Developmentally Delayed Handedness*** (***DDH***) are also **atypical**. They are part of the D-based Type, since they fall into the middle of the continuum of the laterality quotients, which form the basis for the 8 categories (see Sect. 10.2.1 for more detail).

The ***Environment-based (E-based) Type*** comprises the variations ***converted Left Handedness (c-LH)*** and ***converted Right Handedness (c-RH).*** Both variations are also

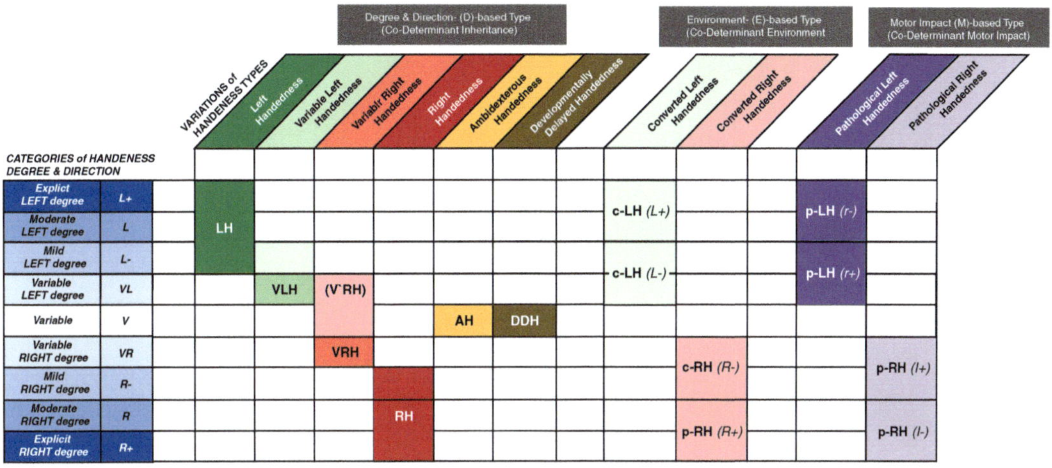

Fig. 9.4 Overview of handedness types, their variations and categories of handedness. The three **handedness types** are shown at the top in the grey boxes with their **handedness variations** in the coloured parallelograms below. The handedness types are always abbreviated with an H (Handedness) at the end. On the left side of the diagram, the **Handedness Categories** of handedness are displayed in the 8 categories of direction and degree as defined in the Handedness Profile. The Handedness Categories are abbreviated only with L, R and V in addition with + or –

likely to be influenced by the inherent degree of handedness (L+, L−, R+ or R−). For example, the variation *converted Left Handedness* may be coupled with an inherently strong degree (category L+) or mild degree (category L−) of handedness (see Sect. 10.2.8 for more detail).

Finally, the ***Motor-Impact-based (M-based) Type*** consists of two variations, ***pathological Left Handedness (p-LH)*** and ***pathological Right Handedness (p-RH).*** They are also likely to be influenced by the inherent degree of handedness (L+, L−, R+ or R−). For example, the variation *pathological Left Handedness* may be coupled with an inherently strong degree (category L+) or mild degree (category L−) of handedness (see Sect. 10.2.11 for more detail).

9.7 Concluding Remarks

In this chapter, the literature's most important and relevant information for a practice-based approach to handedness has been drawn together and used—in combination with my own research—as a basis for constructing a Handedness Typology. I first defined handedness according to six dimensions to structure its well-cited multidimensionality before combining these dimensions with the co-determinants of handedness. I then identified subgroups of handedness from the literature and proposed three types of handedness that correspond directly to the co-determinants. Subsequently, I linked the handedness subgroups to the three handedness types and further subdivide these into variations. The variations are to the handedness categories based on a multidimensional and multivariate handedness assessment, the Handedness Profile. Together, these aspects make up the basic architecture for the Handedness Typology, which aims to provide practitioners with a systematic structure for assessing and understanding the phenomenon. It could also be useful as a framework for research and teaching. The next chapter will describe how the Handedness Typology can be used for interpretation by detailing each of the handedness variations.

Reference

Steenhuis RE, Bryden MP (1989) Different dimensions of hand preference that relate to skilled and unskilled activities. Cortex 25(2):289–304. https://doi.org/10.1016/S0010-9452(89)80044-9

10 Interpreting Handedness Profiles Using the Handedness Typology

Contents

The Handedness Profile and its features were linked to the body of literature reviewed initially, enabling the proposed construction of a conceptual framework for the analysis of variable handedness and the description of possible handedness types. Knowledge of the types of handedness may, in turn, facilitate the final part of the clinical decision-making process related to treatment implementation and evaluation. (Kraus 2003: 252)

10.1 Introduction

As we have seen over the last chapters, the need to understand variable hand use inevitably leads us to the necessity to assess, differentiate and analyse the handedness dimensions and determine the factors involved. This allows us to plan and implement specific treatment strategies to address mixed handedness. The idea of dividing handedness into distinct types was already conceived in my doctoral thesis (as can be seen in the above quote from the final concluding remarks), based on various handedness groups documented in the literature. Since then, my research and many documented cases from clinical practice have confirmed different handedness types, allowing me to expand and differentiate a system over the years and to construct a basic architecture for a Handedness Typology in Chap. 9. In particular, the terminology has been refined within the Handedness Typology (see Glossary). By using co-determinants of handedness as a foundation for the three handedness types, I built a framework to systematically attach the various handedness subgroups, i.e. **variations**, to the handedness types (Chap. 9). Using the multidimensional data from the subtests of the Handedness Profile and tools for analysis such as the Category Profile and the Cluster Table (see Chap. 8), sufficient data is generated to differentiate between the ten handedness variations.

In this chapter, the three handedness types and their variations are presented in detail. This provides practitioners with a framework to understand and interpret the results from the Handedness Profile. The Handedness Typology is particularly

E. Kraus, *Beyond Left and Right Handedness*, https://doi.org/10.1007/978-3-031-24389-9_10

relevant and important in complex cases with children presenting with the so-called mixed handedness[1] (i.e. atypical variable use). Specifically, the relationship between the handedness type and degrees, as well as handedness type and motor abilities, is discussed, informed by many cases from my clinical experience. Each of the respective variations of the handedness types are described in relation to relevant literature and criteria used in the Cluster Table (the HP Analysis Tool—see Sect. 8.5.2) that summarises the specific quantitative and qualitative data. Finally, a prototypical[2] Category Profile is presented for each variation.

10.2 Handedness Categories, Types and Variations

10.2.1 Interpreting Degree-Based Handedness Type (Inheritance) with D-Based Variations

Description of D-Based Handedness Type

As discussed in Chap. 9, there are six variations of the D-based type. Compared to the E-based and M-based types where the variations are "mirror" images of one another, the variations of D-based type are more complex. As can be seen in Fig. 10.1, the variations *Left Handedness* and *Right Handedness* are typical and probably displayed by the majority of individuals. The variations *Variable Left Handedness* and *Variable Right Handedness*, on the other hand, are rarer and frequently involve using of the non-dominant hand, making the direction of handedness not unambiguously clear. This makes these two variations **atypical**. Similarly, *Ambidextrous Handedness* is very rare (and thus atypical), but not associated with problems. Conversely, *Developmentally Delayed Handedness* is atypical, since handedness development has not sufficiently occurred to display clear manual lateralisation and specialisation, and it is usually associated with motor problems.

The Relationship Between Degrees of Handedness and the D-Based Handedness Type

All handedness variations are closely related to degrees of handedness. In the Handedness Profile, the degrees are quantified with laterality quotients using a continuous measure and then assigned to one of eight categories based on the Category Profile of the Handedness Profile. In the case of the D-based handedness type, degrees define its variations.

The Relationship Between Motor Abilities and the D-Based Handedness Type

Based on my clinical practice experience, particularly with the D-based variations, the inherent motor abilities have to be considered not just as proficiency, a dimension of handedness, but also as an influencing factor on handedness (see Sect. 6.5.1). In the case of the D-based type, there are several possible relationships between motor ability and handedness:

- The typical variations of *Left Handedness* and *Right Handedness* may coexist **with or without motor deficits**. If there are motor problems, it is likely that there is **no causal relationship in either direction** between handedness and motor abilities.
- In the case of genuine *Variable Left Handedness* and *Variable Right Handedness*,[3] there would be

[1] The term "mixed" handedness designates a fabricated category of handedness of "residual" handers that have not been classified in a category. I will refer to the "atypical variable hand use" as a more neutral term denoting that the handedness category and variation are unclear. I will use "mixed" handedness only in reference to society and research communities, where it is used as a particular label.

[2] *Prototypical* in this context means exemplary and generalised, where the category profiles refer to relevant research results displaying a specific *tendency* of a pattern. Real case examples would reveal individual category profiles displaying definite similarities with the corresponding prototypical profiles but still being unique (see Chap. 12 for four case studies illustrating the typology). In particular, I differentiate between prototypical and real profiles by referring to left or *Right handedness* in prototypical profiles and left or right *handers* in real profiles.

[3] "Genuine" refers to the definition of natural variable

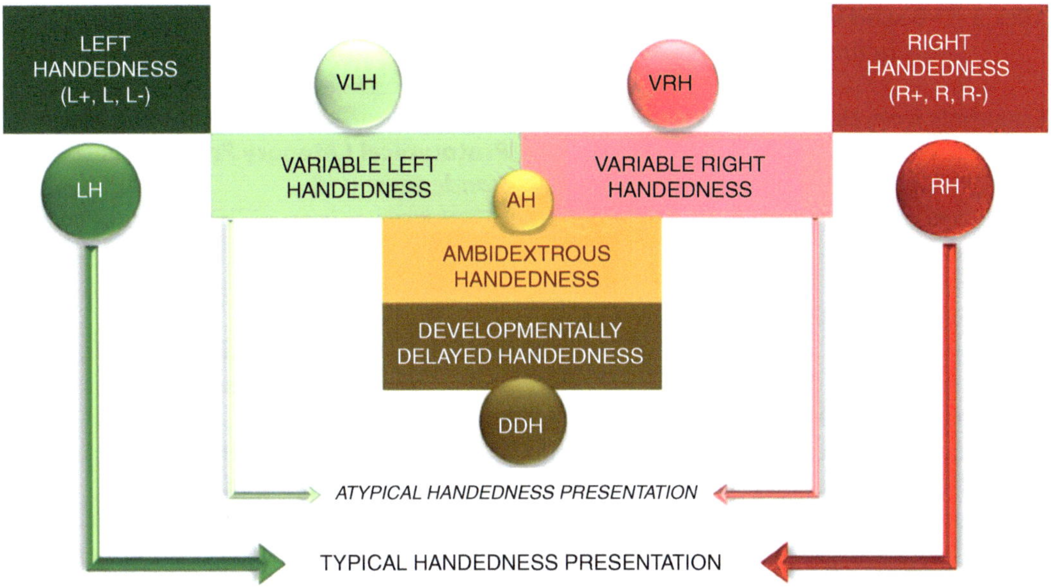

Fig. 10.1 Handedness D-based type with its six variations. The D-based variations are *Left Handedness* and *Right Handedness*, both including explicit, moderate and mild degrees and making up typical handedness presentations; *Variable Left Handedness* and *Variable Right Handedness*; *Ambidextrous Handedness*; and *Developmentally Delayed Handedness*

no motor deficits by definition, and thus sub-average motor abilities cannot influence handedness. However, if motor skills are particularly good on both sides, this may increase the variability of hand use. Similarly, variable *Left* or *Right Handedness* could contribute to acquiring higher motor skills on both sides. So, there may be a **possible bidirectional causal relationship** between handedness and motor skill **if manual performance is above average**.

- The variation *Ambidextrous Handedness* shows extremely small or no apparent differences between the hands, with **both sides showing exceptional dexterity**. In this case, extraordinary motor skills (and practice) result in both hands being equally dextrous even in handwriting and other highly complex tasks, which in turn improves motor proficiency. Consequently, there may be a **bidirectional causal relationship between excellent motor abilities and mild degrees of handedness**.
- The atypical manual variability seen in the variation *Developmentally Delayed Handedness* is usually related to developmental disorders. Lateralisation of the hemispheres has not (yet) taken place sufficiently to display clear manual asymmetries in preference and/or proficiency. This variation is typically associated with general sub-average motor skills, particularly fine motor skills on both sides, resulting in both hands showing an equal extent of poor motor abilities. When a child attempts a demanding fine motor task, it tries with the one hand, fails, then tries with the other hand, fails, etc. Learning of dextral task is thus impeded. There is thus a **bidirectional causal relationship between sub-average motor abilities and mild degrees of handedness**.

We now look at each of the six variations of the D-based handedness type in more detail.

handedness that exists solely based on very mild degrees of handedness and lateralisation.

10.2.2 D-Based Variation *Left Handedness* (*LH*)

Essentials from the Literature on *Left Handedness* (*LH*)

Substantiating evidence from the literature for some of the criteria is summarised in Table 10.1. The other criteria are based on results of the Handedness Profile, observations and background information. Criterion refers to features in Fig. 10.2.

Features of *Left Handedness* (*LH*)

The characteristics are shown in the form of criteria in Fig. 10.2. As already mentioned, the categories of explicit, moderate and mild degrees of *Left Handedness* (*LH*) have been combined into one variation since they unambiguously demonstrate *Left Handedness* and show differences only in degree but not in direction. This variation is the counterpart to the D-based variation *Right Handedness* (*R*) (see 10.1.4, Variation 4).

Prototypical Category Profile of *Left Handedness* (*LH*)

A prototypical Category Profile of this variation is shown in Fig. 10.3.

10.2.3 D-Based Variation *Variable Left Handedness* (*VLH*)

Essentials from the Literature on *Variable Left Handedness* (*VLH*)

Substantiating evidence from the literature for some of the criteria is summarised in Table 10.2. The other criteria are based on the results of the Handedness Profile, observations and back-

Table 10.1 Summary of relevant literature on explicit, moderate and mild *Left Handedness*

Summary	Sources	Criterion
Although the genetic or epigenetic basis of handedness is not yet fully understood, there is some genetic predisposition to *Left Handedness*	Ocklenburg et al. (2014)	1, 2, 3
Multiple genetic aspects contribute to the inheritance of handedness. The number of genetic loci involved has been estimated to be at least 30–40	McManus et al. (2013)	1, 2, 3
The androgen receptor gene on the X chromosome, among others, influences the direction of handedness	Arning et al. (2015)	1, 2, 3
The degree of handedness is inherited. Thus, different degrees of handedness should be defined and categorised	Annett (1978, 2002); Arning et al. (2013, 2015)	1 and 2
If both parents are left handed: child 26% *LH*; if one parent is left handed: child 20% left handed. If both parents are right handed: child 10% left handed	McManus et al. (2010)	1 and 3
Maternal *Left Handedness* has a stronger effect on the inheritance of *Left Handedness* than paternal *Left Handedness*	Annett (1978)	3
Lateralised motor behaviour can be observed very early. For example, foetuses as young as 15–18 weeks show preferred thumb sucking of a hand	Hepper et al. (2005)	4
The head position after birth and the ATNR correlate with later handedness	Corbetta and Thelen (2002)	4
According to studies, there are more male left handers: ♀:♂ = 4:5	McManus et al. (1988)	Male/ female
Writing is an activity that makes particularly high demands on people and is correspondingly highly lateralised	Gruber (2016)	5 and 6
Left handers are more skilled with their right hand than right handers with their left hand (small difference in performance between the hands)	Bryden et al. (2007); McManus et al. (1988); Hill and Khanem (2009)	11–13, 21
Evidence shows that the more pronounced a left- or right-handed person is, the further and more often s/he? crosses the centre of the body with the dominant hand	Carlier et al. (2006)	15
Evidence shows that unobtrusive, mature left and right handers generally lead with the dominant hand during **bimanual circle drawing**, generating more rounder circles with firmer pressure	Volman et al. (2002)	17 and 19

	LEFT HANDEDNESS (explicit, moderate and mild) (D-based type)
1	Left-handed in the close family circle
2	Left-handed in the wider family circle
3	Mother is left-handed
4	Early L hand use (longer than 3 months)
5	**Always writes with L**
6	**Always draws with L**
7	Preferred visual and drawing direction: from R to L
8	Large/larger IHD (L+,L) in preference
9	Int. consistency over 60%, both hands greater LH use
10	Skill slightly better L, good quality of movement
11	Skill RH is slightly weaker, above average for ndH
12	Ability better L, good quality of movement
13	Ability RH is slightly weaker, above average for ndH
14	Clearly finds performance of motor tests better with the L hand
15	Crosses mostly or always with L only
16	Takes lego pieces in centres only with L
17	Circles better on L, pressure is firmer and more even
18	L maintains direction more than the R
19	L leads (somewhat) when drawing circles
20	Overall category profile score of IHD between 1 and 3
21	Larger IHD (L-, L), performance especially L good
22	Large IHD (L and L+) in preference
23	All values are on the leftside
24	Total laterality quotient between 30 and 100% L (preference)
25	Significantly higher LH values in Laterality Profile

Fig. 10.2 Criteria for *Left Handedness*. *ndH* non-dominant hand; *IHD* inter-hand differences; *RH* right hand; *LH* left hand. Bold criteria indicate that these are particularly important for this variation

ground information. Criterion refers to features in Fig. 10.4.

Characteristics of *Variable Left Handedness* (*VLH*)

The characteristics are shown in the form of criteria in Fig. 10.4.

Prototypical Category Profile of *Variable Left Handedness* (*VLH*)

A typical exemplary categorisation profile of this variation is shown in Fig. 10.5. In this profile, the overall profile score indicates a right-handed category.[4] However, since individuals in this variation perform handwriting unambiguously with their left hand despite the right-biassed environment, we can assume that they are left handed with a very mild handedness degree. Importantly, the profile score of the Category Profile does not necessarily correspond to the handedness variation. For example, the profile score of the eight categories may average on the right side even if the variation is *Variable Left Handedness*. For this reason, it is important to differentiate between ♦**handedness categories** and ♦**handedness variations**.

A prototypical Category Profile of this variation is shown in Fig. 10.5.

[4]Incidentally, it is possible to obtain a laterality quotient of 0% for one or more tests. This indicates that there is no difference between the hands for that test. In this case, there would be a profile (category) score of 4.5.

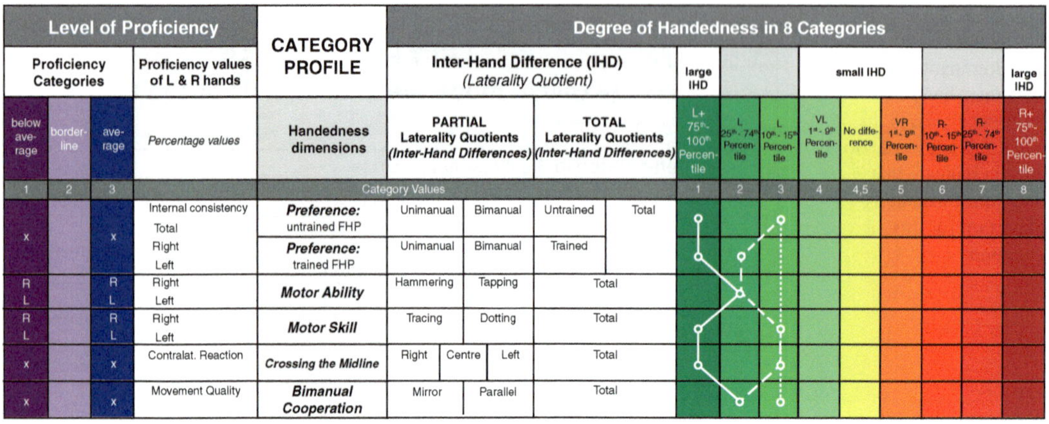

Fig. 10.3 Prototypical Category Profile of *Left Handedness* (*LH*), with or without motor deficits. **Degree of handedness for preference and proficiency:** L+: explicit (solid white line), with a profile score (Total **profile score**: The sum of the categories, numbered 1–8, is divided by 6 (number of subtests of the Handedness Profile).) of degree of about 1.33 (e.g. 1 + 1 + 2 + 1 + 2 = 8:6 = 1.33); L: moderate (dashed white line), with a total degree of about 2.50 (e.g. 3 + 2 + 2 + 3 + 2 = 15:6 = 2.50); L−: mild (dotted white line), with a total degree of about 3.00 (e.g. 3 + 3 + 3 + 3 + 3 = 18:6 = 3.00). The average total profile score for this is about 2.28 (e.g. 1.33 + 2.50 + 3.00 = 6.83:3 = 2.28). **Proficiency level**: explicit, moderate or mild *Left Handedness* can exist *with* motor deficiencies (below-average proficiency scores) or *without* motor deficiencies (average or above-average proficiency scores). *FHP* functional hand preference

Table 10.2 Summary of relevant literature on *Variable Left Handedness*

Summary	Sources	Criterion
Different degrees of handedness should be defined and categorised	Peters and Murphy (1992)	27 and 28
Writing is an activity that makes particularly high demands on people and is correspondingly highly lateralised	Gruber (2016)	32
Left-handed people have more variable hand patterns than right-handed people. They use their non-dominant right hand much more often than right-handers use their non-dominant left hand	Annett (1994); Bryden et al. (2007)	29, 30, 31
There are different groups of left handers, "strongly pronounced" and "less pronounced". The less pronounced left handers do gross motor activities predominantly on the right and write with the left. This group otherwise does *not* display any problems	Peters (1990); Peters and Murphy (1992)	30, 31
Left handers often develop their preference later than right handers	Scharoun and Bryden (2014)	35, 36
Evidence shows that the more strongly established left or right handers are, the further and more often they cross the centre of the body with the dominant hand	Carlier et al. (2006)	41, 42
Left handers tend to have more variable hand patterns than right handers. They use their non-dominant right hand more often than right handers use their non-dominant left hand	Annett (2004); Bryden et al. (2007)	34, 35, 36

VARIABLE LEFT HANDEDNESS (D-based type)	
26	**Higher LH values than RH values**
27	Mixed handedness in close family circle
28	Mixed handedness in the wider family circle
29	Alternating hand use approximately half L and half R
30	Tends to do gross motor activities R and fine motor activities L
31	Does untrained activities rather R and trained L
32	**Writes consistently and better with L**
33	Draws mostly with L, sometimes also with R (e.g. gross motor activities)
34	Untrained preference rather R, trained preference L
35	Internal overall consistency between 60 and 80%
36	Internal consistency with both hands similar use
37	Skill slightly better L
38	Small IHD, Skill L good, R very good for nd-H
39	Ability slightly better R or L
40	Small IHD, Skill L good, R very good for nd hand
41	May cross over more with R, but may also cross over also with L
42	Takes centre lego pieces sometimes with L, sometimes with R
43	Both circles are very similar in pressure and quality
44	L as well as R maintain the given direction
45	L leads in certain directions, R leads in other directions
46	Overall profile score of IHD around 4
47	Trained preference L; untrained preference R
48	Ability (Ham/Tap) better R; Skill (Tra/Dot) better L
49	Total laterality quotient between 0 and 20% L
50	Slightly higher LH values in Laterality Profile

Fig. 10.4 Criteria for *Variable Left Handedness*. *ndH* non-dominant hand; *IHD* inter-hand differences; *RH* right hand; *LH* left hand. Bold criteria indicate that these are particularly important for this variation

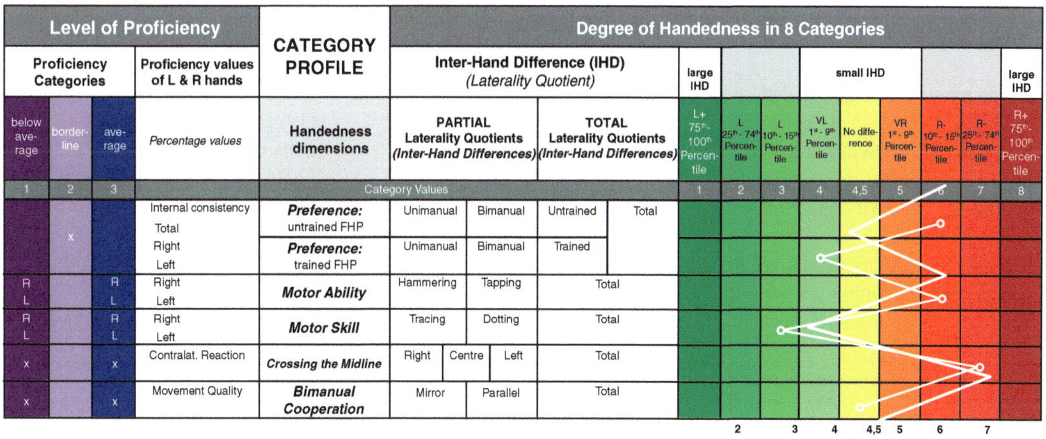

Fig. 10.5 Prototypical Category Profile of *Variable Left Handedness* (*VLH*) with or without motor deficits. **Degree of handedness for preference and proficiency:** The solid white line shows an average profile score of about 5.08 (e.g. 6 + 4 + 6 + 3 + 7 + 4.5 = 20.5:6 = 5.08). **Proficiency level:** *Variable Left Handedness* can exist with motor deficiencies (below-average proficiency scores) or without motor deficiencies (average or above-average proficiency scores). *FHP* functional hand preference

10.2.4 D-Based Variation *Right Handedness (RH)*

Essentials from the Literature on *Right Handedness* (*RH*)

Substantiating evidence from the literature for some of the criteria is summarised in Table 10.3. The other criteria are based on the results of the Handedness Profile, observations and background information. Criterion refers to features in Fig. 10.6.

Characteristics of Explicit to Mild *Right Handedness* (*RH*)

The characteristics are shown in the form of criteria in Fig. 10.6. The explicit, moderate and mild handedness categories of the variation *Right Handedness* (*RH*) do not show differences in direction. Only moderate differences are seen in the degree between categories, so they will be combined into one category. This variation is the counterpart to the D-based variation *Left Handedness* (*LH*). However, they are more strongly lateralised than left handers.

Prototypical Category Profile of *Right Handedness* (*RH*)

A prototypical Category Profile of this variation is shown in Fig. 10.7.

10.2.5 D-Based Variation *Variable Right Handedness* (*VRH*)

Essentials from the Literature on *Variable Right Handedness* (*VRH*)

Substantiating evidence from the literature for some of the criteria is summarised in Table 10.4.

Table 10.3 Summary of relevant literature on explicit, moderate and mild *Right Handedness* (*RH*)

Summary	Sources	Criterion
Although the genetic or epigenetic basis of handedness is not yet fully understood, there is some genetic predisposition to *Right Handedness*	Annett (1985); Ocklenburg et al. (2014)	1, 2, 3
Multiple genetic aspects contribute to the inheritance of handedness. The number of genetic loci involved is estimated to be at least 30–40	McManus et al. (2013)	1, 2, 3
The androgen receptor gene on the X chromosome, among others, influences the direction of handedness	Arning et al. (2013, 2015)	1, 2, 3
The degree of handedness is inherited, and different degrees of handedness should be defined and categorised	Arning et al. (2013); Peters and Murphy (1992)	1, 2
If both parents are right handed, the child's chance of also being right handed increases	McManus and Bryden (1992)	1, 3
Right handers often develop their preference earlier than left handers	Scharoun and Bryden (2014)	8, 9
Writing is the activity most influenced by cultural values	Porac and Lee Berdel Martin (2007)	5,6
Writing is an activity that makes particularly high demands on people and is correspondingly highly lateralised	Gruber (2016)	5, 6
There are different groups of right handers, strongly pronounced and less pronounced	Peters and Murphy (1992)	General
Right-handed people usually have less variable action patterns than left-handed people and predominantly use their dominant hand	Annett (2004); Bryden et al. (2007)	9, 23, 24
Evidence shows that the more pronounced a left- or right-handed person is, the further and more often s/he? crosses the centre of the body with the dominant hand	Carlier et al. (2006)	15
Evidence shows that typically developed, left and right handers generally lead with the dominant hand during **bimanual circle drawing** and generate rounder circles with firmer pressure	Volman et al. (2002)	17, 18, 19
Right handers are less proficient with their left hand than left handers with their right hand (greater difference in performance between the hands)	Bryden et al. (2007); Hill and Khanem (2009)	21, 22

Fig. 10.6 Criteria for the variation *Right Handedness* (*RH*). *ndH* non-dominant hand; *IHD* inter-hand differences; *RH* right hand; *LH* left hand. Bold criteria indicate that these are particularly important for this variation

	RIGHT HANDEDNESS (explicit, moderate and mild) (D-based type)
1	Only right-handed people in the close family circle
2	Only right-handed people in the wider family circle
3	No conversion/switching known in close or extended family circle
4	Early R hand use (longer than 3 months)
5	Always writes with R
6	Always draws with R
7	Preferred visual and drawing direction: from L to R
8	Large/larger IHD (R+,R) in preference
9	Internal consistency over 60%, both hands greater RH use
10	Skill clearly better R, good quality of movement
11	Skill LH is clearly weaker, average for ndH
12	Ability clearly better R, good quality of movement
13	Ability LH is clearly weaker, average for ndH
14	Clearly finds performance of motor tests better with the R hand
15	Always crosses the midline with R only
16	Takes central blocks only with R
17	R circles better, firmer and more evenly
18	R maintains direction
19	R leads (somewhat) when painting circles
20	Total Profile Score IHD between 6 and 8
21	Larger IHD (R), performance especially R good
22	Large IHD (R+) in preference
23	All values are on the right
24	Total laterality quotient between 50 and 100% R (preference)
25	Significantly higher RH values in lateralisation profile

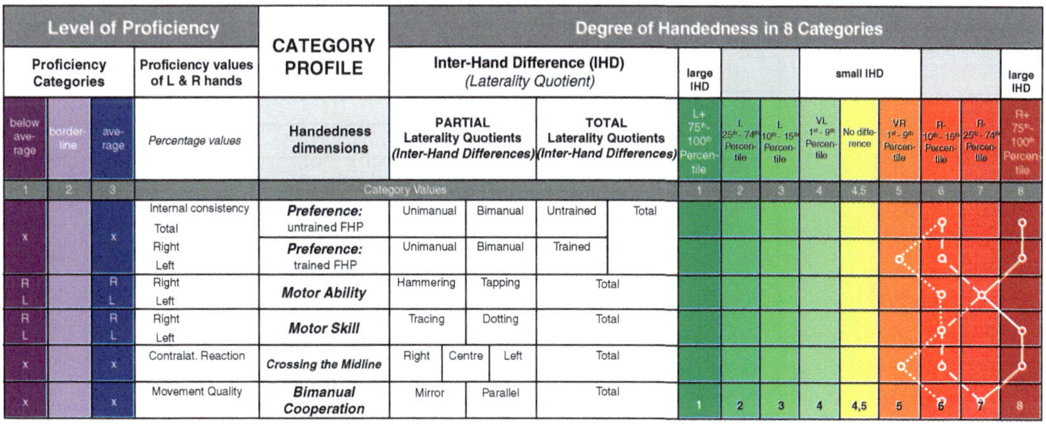

Fig. 10.7 Prototypical Category Profile of *Right Handedness* (*RH*) with or without motor deficits. **Degree of handedness for preference and proficiency:** R+: explicit (solid white line), with a profile score of degree of about 7.67 (e.g. 8 + 8 + 7 + 8 + 8 + 7 = 46:6 = 7.67); R: moderate (dashed white line), with a Category Profile score of about 6.33 (e.g. 6 + 6 + 7 + 6 + 6 + 7 = 38:6 = 6.33); R−: mild (dotted white line), with a total degree of about 5.67 (e.g. 6 + 5 + 6 + 6 + 5 + 6 = 34:6 = 5.67). The average total profile score for this variation is about 6.56 (e.g. 7.67 + 6.33 + 5.67 = 6.56.). **Proficiency level**: explicit, moderate or mild *Right Handedness* can exist *with* motor deficiencies (below-average proficiency scores) or *without* motor deficiencies (average or above-average proficiency scores). *FHP* functional hand preference

Table 10.4 Summary of relevant literature on *Variable Right Handedness*

Summary	Sources	Criterion
The degree of handedness is hereditary. Thus, different degrees of handedness should be defined and categorised	Arning et al. (2013); Peters and Murphy (1992)	27, 28
There are different groups of right handers, strongly pronounced and less pronounced	Peters (1990); Peters and Murphy (1992)	27, 28
Writing is an activity that makes exceptionally high demands on people and is correspondingly highly lateralised	Gruber (2016)	32, 33
Evidence shows that the more pronounced a left- or right-handed person is, the further and more often he/she crosses the centre of the body with the dominant hand	Carlier et al. (2006)	41, 42
Evidence shows that typically developed left and right handers generally lead with the dominant hand during **bimanual circle drawing** and generate rounder circles with firmer pressure	Volman et al. (2002)	43, 44, 45
Right handers are less proficient with their left hand than left handers with their right hand (greater difference in performance between the hands)	Bryden et al. (2007)	26

	"VARIABLE RIGHT HANDEDNESS (D-based type)"
26	**Higher RH values than LH values**
27	more R than L handers as well as mixed handers in the close family circle
28	more R than L handers as well as mixed handers in the wider family circle
29	Alternating hand use but predominantly R
30	Performs gross and fine motor activities more R
31	Performs untrained and trained activities more R
32	Writes consistently and better with R
33	Always draws with R
34	Untrained and trained preference more R
35	Overall internal consistency between 70 and 90%
36	Internal consistency with greater RH use
37	Skill significantly better R
38	vR, R or R IHD, skill R and L average
39	Ability significantly better R
40	vR, R - or R IHD, skill R and L average
41	Crossed always/ only with R
42	Takes central lego pieces mostly/only with R
43	Circles R better, firmer and more even
44	R maintains direction more than left
45	R leads (somewhat) consistently
46	Overall profile score of IHD between 5 and 6
47	Trained and untrained preference R
48	Ability (Ham/Tap) and Skill (Tra/Dot) better R
49	Total laterality quotient between 20 and 50% R
50	Slightly higher RH values in Laterality Profile

Fig. 10.8 Criteria for *Variable Right Handedness*. *ndH* non-dominant hand; *IHD* inter-hand differences; *RH* right hand; *LH* left hand. Bold criteria indicate that these are particularly important for this variation

The other criteria are based on the results of the Handedness Profile, observations and background information. Criterion refers to features in Fig. 10.8.

Characteristics of *Variable Right Handedness* (*VRH*)

The characteristics are shown in the form of criteria in Fig. 10.1.

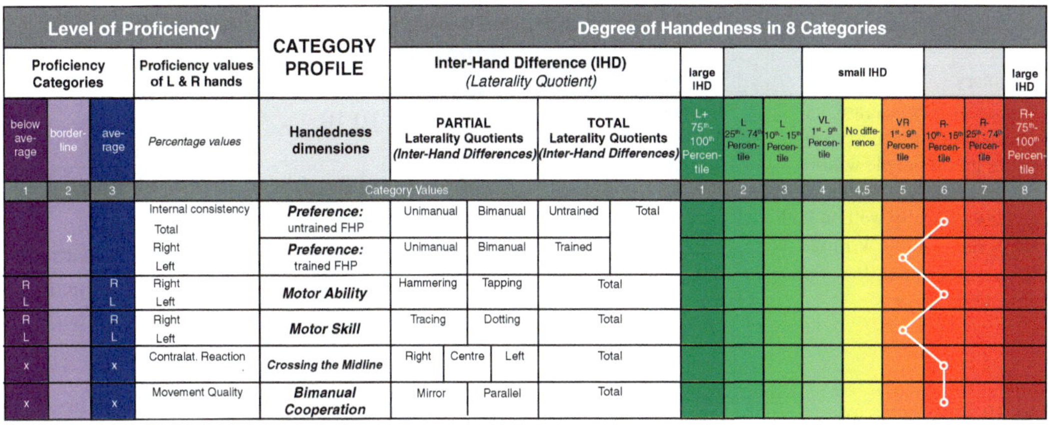

Fig. 10.9 Prototypical Category Profile of *Variable Right Handedness* (*VRH*) with or without motor deficits. **Degree of handedness for preference and proficiency:** The solid white line shows an average profile score of about 5.67 (e.g. 6 + 5 + 6 + 5 + 6 + 6 = 34:6 = 5.67). **Proficiency level**: *Variable Right Handedness* can exist *with* motor deficiencies (below-average proficiency scores) or *without* motor deficiencies (average or above-average proficiency scores). *FHP* functional hand preference

These criteria are based on the literature. However, since right handers are significantly stronger lateralised than left handers (see Sect. 4.3), variable right handers are not the mirror image of variable left handers. In fact, as we discussed earlier, variable left handers often perform more tasks on average with their right hand than with their left. They also do not differ significantly from the mild right handers. It can be suspected that these two categories forming the bottom 25% of right handers contain a substantial number of converted variable left handers. These are likely to have good motor skills and may have switched from an early age, possibly without even being aware of it. Thus, many left handers with mild degrees of handedness are likely to end up in the variation of variable (or mild) *Right Handedness*. This means that we need to consider these two variations of variable and mild *Right Handedness* to be somewhat "fabricated" (a bit like "mixed" handedness), since they presumably comprise a diverse group of handers.

Prototypical Category Profile of *Variable Right Handedness* (*VRH*)

A prototypical Category Profile of this variation is shown in Fig. 10.9. In this profile, the overall profile score indicates *Variable Right Handedness*.

10.2.6 D-Based Variation *Ambidextrous Handedness* (*AH*)

Essentials from the Literature on Ambidexterity

Substantiating evidence from the literature for some of the criteria is summarised in Table 10.5. The other criteria are based on the results of the Handedness Profile, observations and background information. Criterion refers to features in Fig. 10.10.

Table 10.5 Summary of relevant literature on ambidexterity

Summary	Sources	Criterion
Ambidexterity is a rare phenomenon that describes motor gifted people who perform highly complex activities equally well on both sides, for example writing	Hildreth (1949)	55, 56
It is estimated that 1% of people are ambidextrous	Elneel et al. (2008)	55, 56, 61, 64

Characteristics of *Ambidextrous Handedness*

The characteristics are shown in the form of criteria in Fig. 10.10.

Prototypical Profile of *Ambidextrous Handedness*

A prototypical Category Profile of this variation is shown in Fig. 10.11. It can be assumed that *Variable Left Handedness*, together with an

AMBIDEXTERITY (D-based type)	
51	**High scores under Variable Left Handedness**
52	No indication of developmental delay
53	No early preferred hand use, both hands equally good
54	Alternating hand use within and across activities
55	Writes L or R equally well, situational changes
56	Draws L or R equally well, situational changes
57	**Clear practice effect with both hands**
58	Internal consistency below 60%
59	**Tendency to switch ergonomically**
60	Similar use of both hands with some internal consistency
61	Skill on both sides about equally exceptionally good
62	Quality of movement with Skill on both sides very good
63	Ability on both sides approximately equally exceptional
64	Quality of movement with Ability on both sides equally exceptional
65	Crosses with R and with L
66	Takes centre blocks with L or R
67	No crossing avoidance in FHPT
68	**Circles equally well, many X (denoting no difference between hands)**
69	Can maintain direction with both hands
70	Quality of circles similar on both sides
71	Very good quality of movement on both sides
72	Overall proficiency score between 4 and 5 with good motor skills
73	Small IHD in Skill, both sides very good
74	Small IHD in Ability, both sides very good
75	Laterality Profile approximately half L and half R

Fig. 10.10 Criteria for *Ambidextrous Handedness*. *ndH* non-dominant hand; *IHD* inter-hand differences; *RH* right hand; *LH* left hand. Bold criteria indicate that these are particularly important for this variation

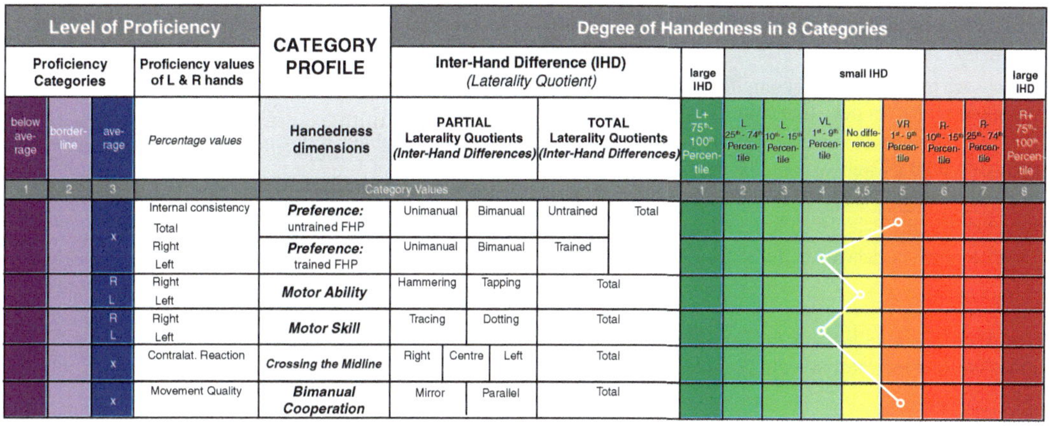

Fig. 10.11 Prototypical Category Profile of *Ambidextrous Handedness*. **Degree of handedness for preference and proficiency:** R+: explicit (solid white line), with a profile score of degree of about 4.00 (e.g. 5 + 3 + 4,5 + 3 + 4.5 + 4 = 24:6 = 4.00). *Ambidextrous Handedness* is characterised by both hands being equally good (and usually above average), and therefore it presents *without* motor deficiencies in the prototypical profile. *FHP* functional hand preference

above-average motor ability of both hands and a significant practice factor, underlies *Ambidextrous Handedness*.

10.2.7 D-Based Variation *Developmentally Delayed Handedness* (*DDH*)

Essentials from the Literature on Developmental Delay Affecting Handedness

Substantiating evidence from the literature for some of the criteria is summarised in Table 10.6. The other criteria are based on the results of the Handedness Profile, observations and background information. Criterion refers to features in Fig. 10.12.

Characteristics of *Developmentally Delayed Handedness* (*DDH*)

The characteristics are shown in the form of criteria in Fig. 10.12.

Prototypical Profile of *Developmentally Delayed Handedness* (*DDH*)

A prototypical Category Profile of this variation is shown in Fig. 10.13. In the case of *Developmentally Delayed Handedness*, both hands are equally clumsy, and motor deficiencies are evident bilaterally. As a result, there may be very small or no inter-hand differences. Typically, these children also show low internal consistency and avoid midline crossing, two indicators for developmental delay (see Sect. 3.6).

10.2.8 Interpreting Environment-Based Handedness Type with E-Based Variations

Description of E-Based Handedness Type

The Environment-based (E-based) handedness type draws from the environment co-determinant and shows a causal relationship between the sociocultural and physical environments and handedness formation. It presents in two variations: *converted Left Handedness* and (less likely) *converted Right Handedness*. As discussed in Chap. 4, switching the dominant hand particularly refers to handwriting. *Converted Left Handedness* is much more common because of the right-oriented and right-biassed physical and sociocultural environments that predominate most societies the world over. In particular, left-

Table 10.6 Summary of relevant literature on developmental delay and handedness

Summary	Sources	Criterion
If there are pregnancy, birth complications or premature birth, these children are at increased risk for developmental disabilities	de Moura et al. (2010)	52
In motor-based developmental disorders, motor clumsiness could be heritable, body or spatial awareness could be impaired, or control and coordination of movements could be impaired	Krombholz (2005)	52
Developmentally delayed children alternate hand use within an activity	Bishop (1990)	58, 59
Developmentally delayed children tend to avoid crossing the centre of the body	Cermak and Ayres (1984); Eason and Surburg (1993)	65–67
The development of handedness can also be considered a developmental milestone and indicates neurological maturity	Surburg (1999); Woodard and Surburg (1999)	52
Bimanual coordination with role differentiation is a development indicator	Babik (2014)	68–71
Children with inconsistent hand use are often developmentally delayed	Bishop (1990)	58, 59

	DEVELOPMENTALLY DELAYED HANDEDNESS
51	**No clear profile scores for left-or right-handedness**
52	**Indication of developmental delay**
53	No early observed preferred hand use, continual swapping of hands during tasks
54	Alternates hand use within and across activities
55	Writes L or R equally poorly, tries with either hand
56	Draws L or R equally poorly, tries with either hand
57	Avoids practising with both hands, little practising effect
58	Internal consistency below 60%
59	**Tendency to uncertain and compensatory switching**
60	Similar use of both hands with internal inconsistency
61	Skill on both sides poor, maybe in different ways
62	Movement quality during Skill on both sides show motor deficiencies
63	Ability on both sides poor, maybe in different ways
64	Movement quality with Ability on both sides show motor deficiencies
65	**Avoids crossing over**
66	Takes centre lego pieces with L or R
67	Shows crossing avoidace in FHPT
68	**Circles equally poor many? (denotes alternating leads)**
69	Unable to maintain direction with both hands
70	Quality on both sides equally poor, possibly different problems
71	Poor States that both hands are equally difficult
72	Overall profile score between 4 and 5 with subaverage motor skills
73	Small IHD in Skill, both sides show motor deficiencies
74	Small IHD in Ability, both sides show motor deficiencies
75	Laterality Profile approximately half L and half R

Fig. 10.12 Criteria for *Developmentally Delayed Handedness*

handed children with a low degree of handedness are more at risk of being switched. Unfortunately, many parents, educators, paediatricians, practitioners and educators are not well informed about the dangers and risks of converted handedness. *Converted Right Handedness* can also occur in

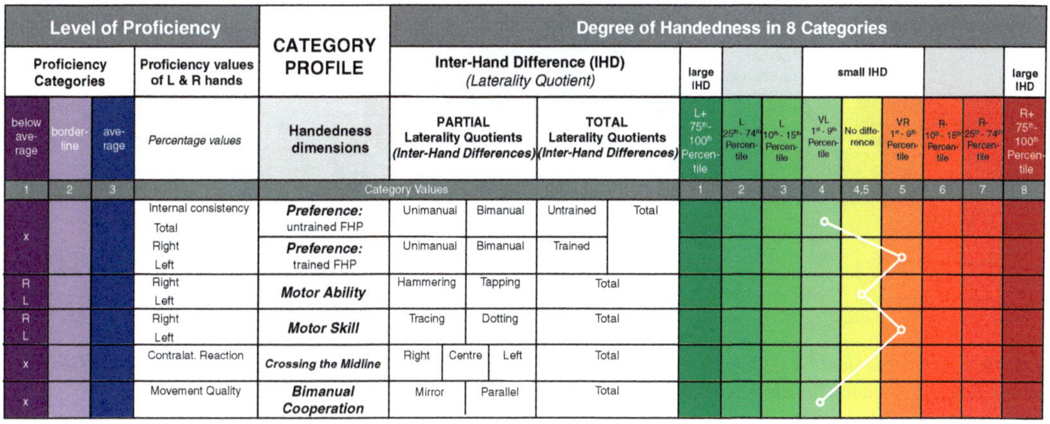

Fig. 10.13 Prototypical Category Profile of *Developmentally Delayed Handedness*. **Degree of handedness for preference and proficiency:** *DDH* (solid white line) has a profile score of degree of about 4.17 (e.g. 4 + 5 + 4.5 + 5 + 4.5 + 4 = 25:6 = 4.17). *Developmentally Delayed Handedness* is characterised by both hands being equally poor (and both below average), and therefore motor deficiencies are part of this prototypical profile. *FHP* functional hand preference

rarer cases, usually because of some incentive to use the non-dominant left hand for writing. For example, a 6-year-old boy wants to be like his older left-handed brother that he adores. There could also be extrinsic motivation leading to *converted Right Handedness*, such as an incorrect handedness assessment and subsequent training of the non-dominant left hand.

The Relationship Between Degrees of Handedness and the E-Based Handedness Type

The degree of handedness is likely to affect the variability of *converted Left* or *Right Handedness*. For example, a left hander with a strong handedness degree would typically perform trained activities, including writing with the right hand, but continue to perform other untrained and spontaneous activities with the left. In contrast, a converted left hander with a mild or variable degree of handedness would be more likely to perform the majority of tasks with the right and thereby typically show a Category Profile that may resemble that of *Variable Right Handedness*. The rarer variation of *converted Right Handedness* has been shown in clinical practice to exhibit a different profile than *converted Left Handedness*, particularly if the handedness is explicit. For example, a converted right hander with a strong degree of handedness would presumably perform the vast majority of activities with the right hand and only use the left hand for writing or other specific high-skill activities being switched. In contrast, a right hander with a milder degree of handedness shows a somewhat more variable Category Profile, but most actions and tasks would remain on the right side. The two variations are thus not mirror images of each other (see Fig. 10.14 for a summary).

The Relationship Between Motor Abilities and the E-Based Handedness Type

Generally, a tendency can be observed in clinical practice, indicating that inherent motor abilities are likely to affect the "success"[5] of being switched. The better the motor abilities, the "easier" it seems to be to adjust to writing with the non-dominant hand, and the less severe the switching repercussions. However, it does not mean that handedness conversion does not come at a cost, even in proficient switched handers.

[5] "Success" merely refers to the switched hander continuing to write with their right non-dominant hand. It does not mean that there are no conversion problems—these might indeed be severe in many "successfully" switched left handers.

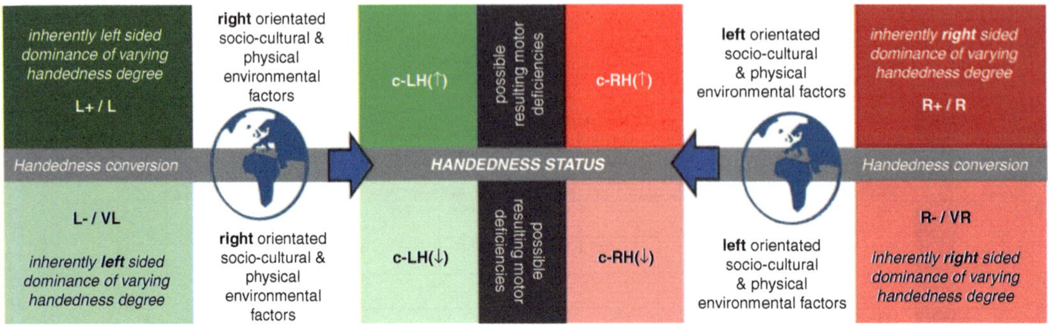

Fig. 10.14 Environment-based handedness type with E-based variations *converted Left Handedness* (*c-LH*) and *converted Right Handedness* (*c-RH*)

The association between motor abilities and the E-based handedness type is usually a **unidirectional causal relationship, with the conversion negatively impacting motor performance**. Interestingly, there is evidence that converted left handers have fewer **♦switching repercussions** if they play sports or a musical instrument (see Sect. 11.3.5). In particular, it is hypothesised that these complex bilateral activities intensify interhemispheric interaction and build up the corpus callosum (see Sects. 2.2.2 and 2.4.2). This enables new neurophysiological interhemispheric connections, thereby facilitating adjustment to demanding processes. A further hypothesis states that people with good motor proficiency and plasticity of the brain are more likely to cope with the neurophysiological impact that switching may cause (see Marcori et al. 2019; Andersen and Siebner 2018). Conversely, switched handers with average or below-average motor skills and less efficient brain plasticity are more likely to develop motor problems as a result of converted handedness (for writing). It means that motor dysfunction could result from switching, supporting a causal relationship between handedness formation and proficiency (see Sect. 3.3).

10.2.9 E-Based Variation *Converted Left Handedness (c-LH)*

Essentials from the Literature on *Converted Left Handedness* (*c-LH*)

Substantiating evidence from the literature for some of the criteria is summarised in Table 10.7. The other criteria are based on the results of the Handedness Profile, observations and background information. The criterion refers to features in Fig. 10.15.

Characteristics of *Converted Left Handedness* (*c-LH*)

The characteristics are shown in the form of criteria in Fig. 10.16.

Prototypical Category Profile of *Converted Left Handedness* (*c-LH*)

A prototypical Category Profile of this variation is shown in Fig. 10.16.

Table 10.7 Summary of relevant literature on *converted Left Handedness* (*c-LH*)

Summary	Sources—examples	Criterion
In addition to the polygenetic causes of handedness, physical and sociocultural environmental influences exist	Ida and Bryden (1996); Ida and Mandal (2003)	
It is generally assumed that sociocultural pressures to switch handedness have decreased over the past decades and that conversions tend to occur less frequently	Porac (1996)	102, 103, 107, 108
Researchers nevertheless suspect that even today there are hidden or subtle attempts to switch handedness. These may manifest themselves, for example, in rewards, moral pressure or negative expressions when using the left hand	Sattler and Klußmann (2014)	
Some studies demonstrate that the mother's influence in the first year of life can stimulate a left or right preference, especially in children with a low-degree handedness	Michel and Harkins (1988)	102, 107
Writing is the activity most influenced by cultural values	Porac and Lee Berdel Martin (2007)	General
A high degree of conformity in a society or a cultural devaluation of *Left Handedness* can lead left-handed children using their non-dominant right hand more often for certain activities	DeAgostini et al. (1997); Dahmen and Fagard (2005)	103, 108
Sociocultural retraining can be found, for example, in Japan, China or Turkey	Hatta and Kawakami (1995); Koeda and Takeshita (1988); Kushner (2013); Perelle and Ehrman (1994)	103, 108
Study results show that many switched left handers write with their right hand but continue to perform other activities primarily with their left hand	Siebner et al. (2002); Klöppel et al. (2007); Porac (2009)	119, 120
Converted left handers have a comparable hand performance as non-converted left or right handers, so their motor performance is not necessarily worse	Porac (2009)	112
Less pronounced left handers are more likely to be "successfully" retrained, whereby the success is related only to the fact that they continued to write with their right hand only	Porac and Searlman (2002); Searleman and Porac (2001, 2003)	107, 108
There is evidence that converted handedness can result in switching repercussions, for example, stuttering (1), learning difficulties (2), dyslexia and dysgraphia (3), physical and psychological well-being (4) or concentration disorders (5)	(1) Orton and Travis (1929); Travis (1934); Kushner (2012); (2) Rett et al. (1973); Benton et al. (1965); Kushner (2012); (3) Masud and Ajmal (2012); Denny and O'Sullivan (2007); Sovák (1968); (4) Lin and Tsuang (2018); Porac and Searlman (2002); Siengthai et al. (2008); (5) Hawkyard et al. (2014); Sattler and Klußmann (2014); Siengthai et al. (2008)	109, 110
With practice, the non-dominant hand can learn to write simple sequences as legibly as the preferred hand. There are no differences in motor aspects such as control, strength or positioning between the hands with appropriate practice	Teixeria and Paroli (2000); Galobardes et al. (1999); Klöppel et al. (2007); Walker and Henneberg (2007)	112, 113
Other studies, however, indicate that handedness conversion is associated with increased activation of brain areas and thus increased effort	Klöppel et al. (2007)	112, 113

Fig. 10.15 Criteria for *converted Left Handedness* (*c-LH*) *ndH* non-dominant hand; *IHD* inter-hand differences; *RH* right hand; *LH* left hand. Bold criteria indicate that these are particularly important for this variation

	CONVERTED LEFT HANDEDNESS (E-based type)
101	**Clear LH OR VLH values**
102	**Child remembers being switched from the L to the R hand**
103	**Observation of conversion to R by parent**
104	Switched LH in the family (especially father)
105	Movement of the L hand stronger during RH use
106	Partial knowledge about converted LH by child and family
107	Influence to use the R hand at home
108	Influence to use the R hand use at day care/kindergarten/school
109	**Consequences of conversion ("often" 5+ times)**
110	**Switching consequences ("sometimes" 8+ times)**
111	with high LH values: untrained preference L, trained preference R
	OR with high VLH values: untrained and trained preference R
112	R hand performs better but is borderline or sub-average
113	Undecided/mixed statements by child on which hand is better.
114	The L hand is better, especially when tapping
115	The L hand feels better according to the child's statement
116	With high LH values: crosses mostly or always/only with L
	OR with high VLH values: crossed with R or L
117	With high LH values: better circles with L
	OR with high VLH values: circles are very similar on both sides
118	L hand maintains direction more thant the R during bimanual circle drawing
119	At high LH values: discrepancy between untrained & trained preference
	OR at high VLH values:trained and untrained preference R
120	At high LH values: discrepancy between Ability (L) & Skill (R)
	OR at high VLH values: Skill and Ability more R
121	At high LH values: clear LH Laterality Profile
	OR at high VLH values: tend to have a LH Laterality Profile

10.2.10 E-Based Variation *Converted Right Handedness* (*c-RH*)

Essentials from the Literature on *Converted Right Handedness* (*c-RH*)

Substantiating evidence from the literature for some of the criteria is summarised in Table 10.8. The other criteria are based on the results of the Handedness Profile, observations and background information. The criterion refers to features in Fig. 10.17.

Characteristics of *Converted Right Handedness* (*c-RH*)

The characteristics are shown in the form of criteria in Fig. 10.17.

Prototypical Category Profile of *Converted Right Handedness* (*c-RH*)

A prototypical Category Profile of this variation is shown in Fig. 10.18.

10.2.11 Interpreting Motor-Based Handedness Type and Variations

Description of the M-Based Handedness Type

Due to cortical damage before, at or after birth, the dominant hemisphere is (more) impaired and the infant will have greater success using the non-dominant hand for demanding activities. This

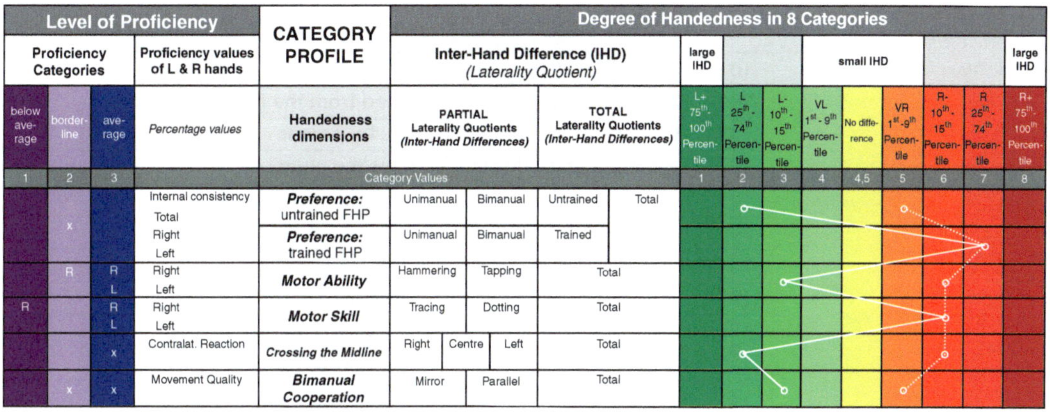

Fig. 10.16 Prototypical Category Profile of *converted Left Handedness* (*c-LH*). The E-based prototypical Category Profile of *converted Left Handedness* with or without resulting motor dysfunction may present differently depending on the degrees of handedness. If the degree of the inherent dominant left hand is high, *converted Left Handedness* is likely to show a clear difference between trained and untrained aspects (see dotted line), with a total profile score of about 3.83 (e.g. 2 + 7 + 3 + 6 + 2 + 3 = 23:6 = 3.83), with a possible resulting sub-average proficiency score under the proficiency level. If the degree of the inherent dominant left hand is low as is the case with mild or variable left handers, *converted Left Handedness* is likely to shift the profile to the right for all trained and untrained aspects (see solid line), with a total profile score of about 5.83 (e.g. 5 + 7 + 6 + 6 + 6 + 5 = 35 :6 = 5.83), again with a possible resulting sub-average proficiency score under the proficiency level. It is also possible that a motor dysfunction exists independently of handedness. *FHP* functional hand preference

Table 10.8 Summary of relevant literature on *converted Right Handedness* (*c-RH*)

Summary	Sources—examples	Criterion
Switched right handers are much rarer than switched left handers	Sattler and Klußmann (2014)	General
The conversion to the left then happens for particular reasons of interest and mostly in adulthood	Sattler (2011)	General
Studies demonstrate that the mother's influence in the first year of life can stimulate a left or right preference, especially in children with low degrees of handedness	Michel and Harkins (1988)	108
There is evidence that converting handedness can result in switching consequences, for example stuttering (1), learning difficulties (2), dyslexia and dysgraphia (3), physical and psychological well-being (4) or concentration disorders (5)	(1) Orton and Travis (1929); Travis (1934); Kushner (2012); (2) Rett et al. (1973); Benton et al. (1965); Kushner (2012); (3) Masud and Ajmal (2012); Denny and O'Sullivan (2007); Sovák (1968); (4) Lin and Tsuang (2018); Porac and Searlman (2002); Siengthai et al. (2008); (5) Hawkyard et al. (2014); Sattler and Klußmann (2014); Siengthai et al. (2008)	109, 110
The non-dominant hand can learn to write simple sequences as legibly as the preferred hand with practice. There are no differences in motor aspects such as control, strength or positioning between the hands with appropriate practice	Teixeria and Paroli (2000); Galobardes et al. (1999); Klöppel et al. (2007); Walker and Henneberg (2007)	112

Fig. 10.17 Criteria for *converted Right Handedness* (*c-RH*)

	CONVERTED RIGHT HANDEDNESS (E-based type)
101	**Clear RH or VRH values**
102	**Child remembers being switched from the R to the L hand**
103	**Observation of conversion to L by parent**
104	**Existence of a LH role model for the child**
105	Movement of the R hand is stronger when LH is used
106	No knowledge or recollection of being switched
107	Internal motivation exists to switch from the R hand to L
108	External motivation exists to switch from the R hand to L
109	**Consequences of conversion ("often" 5+ times)**
110	**Switching consequences ("sometimes" 8+ times)**
111	For R+ and R values: untrained preference very R, trained less R
	OR for R- and VR values: untrained & trained preference slightly R
112	L hand performs better but is borderline or is notably poorer
113	Undecided/mixed statements by child which hand is better.
114	The R hand is better, especially when tapping
115	The R hand feels better according to the child's statement
116	With high RH values: crossed always/only with R
	OR with high VRH values: crosses mainly with R
117	At high RH values: clearly better circles with R
	OR at high VRH values: circles are similar on both sides
118	The R hand maintains direction more than the L
119	At high RH values: untrained & trained preference clearly R
	OR at high VRH values:trained & untrained preference more R
120	At high RH values: Ability & Skill clearly R
	OR at high VLH values: Skill & Ability more R
121	At high RH values: clear RH Laterality Profile
	OR at high VRH values: tend to have a RH Laterality Profile

leads to increased practice and automation with the non-dominant hand. The two variations of M-based handedness type are thus *Pathological Left* and *Right Handedness*, whereby the probability of *pathological Left Handedness* is much greater (see Sect. 4.4).

The Relationship Between Degrees of Handedness and the M-Based Handedness Type

Pathological Handedness overlays the genetically determined degree of handedness. For example, an individual with a right-handed predisposition suffered left cortical insult affecting dominant right-hand function. If the degree of *Right Handedness* is explicit or moderate, the inherent right hand would likely be preferred in spontaneous and undemanding activities. However, more complex and demanding tasks would probably be performed with the better but non-dominant left hand. The mirror image would be true for pathological right handers. In other words, if the degree is high (explicit to moderate handedness), the dominant hand is likely to be used more frequently in easy tasks, resulting in a milder pathological handedness. If the degree is low (mild to variable handedness), the dominant hand will probably be used less frequently, resulting in a stronger pathological handedness. This pattern would apply to *pathological Right Handedness* as well as *pathological Left Handedness* (see Fig. 10.19 for summary).

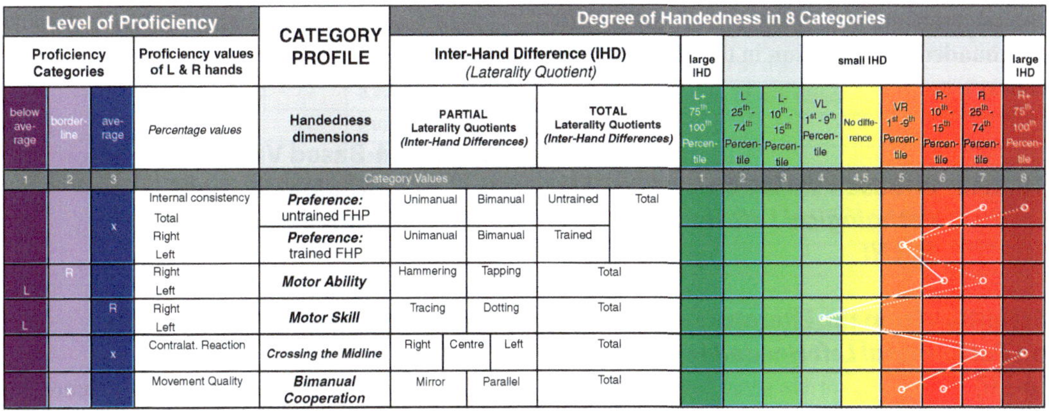

Fig. 10.18 Prototypical Category Profile of *converted Right Handedness*. The E-based prototypical Category Profile of *converted Right Handedness* with or without resulting motor dysfunction may present differently depending on the degrees of handedness. If the degree of the inherent dominant right hand is high, *Converted Right Handedness* is likely to show a clear difference between trained and untrained aspects (see dotted line) probably only in regard to the targeted left-handed activities, with a total profile score of about 5.67 (e.g. 7 + 5 + 6 + 4 + 7 + 5 = 34:6 = 5.67), with a possible resulting sub-average proficiency score under the proficiency level. If the degree of the inherent dominant right hand is low as is the case with mild or variable right handers, *converted Right Handedness* is unlikely to show a different prototypical profile and will be likely to be slightly more shifted to the left (see solid line), with a total profile score of about 6.33 (e.g. 8 + 5 + 7 + 4 + 8 + 6 = 38:6 = 6.33), again with a possible resulting sub-average proficiency score under the proficiency level. It is also possible that a motor dysfunction exists independently of handedness but will probably be exaccerbated through the conversion. *FHP* functional hand preference

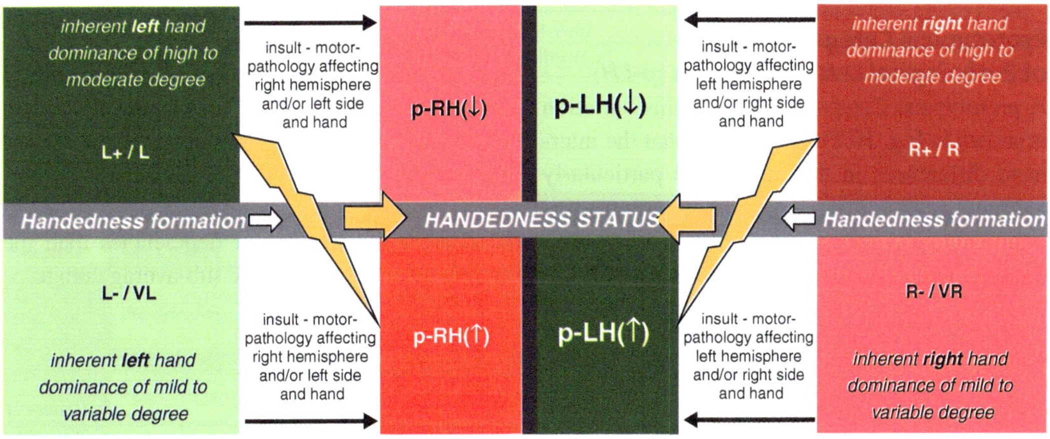

Fig. 10.19 Motor function-based handedness type with the variation *pathological Left Handedness* and *pathological Right Handedness*

The Relationship Between Motor Abilities and the M-Based Handedness Type

Since pathological handedness is defined in relation to early risk factors and brain insult, it is a motor deficit on the inherently dominant side that causes a change in handedness direction, resulting in the non-dominant hand becoming more proficient compared to the dominant one. Therefore, by definition, there is a **unidirectional**

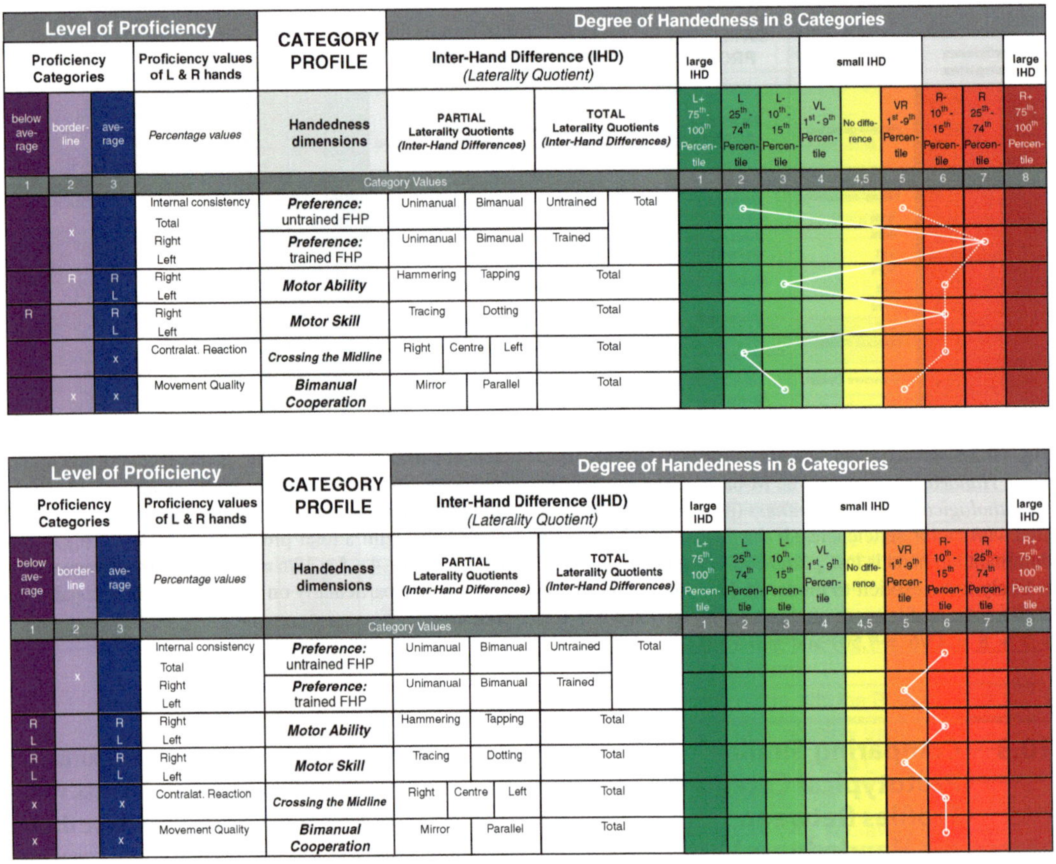

Fig. 10.24 Comparing similar Category Profiles of *Converted Variable Left Handedness* (above, dotted line) and *Variable Right Handedness* (below)

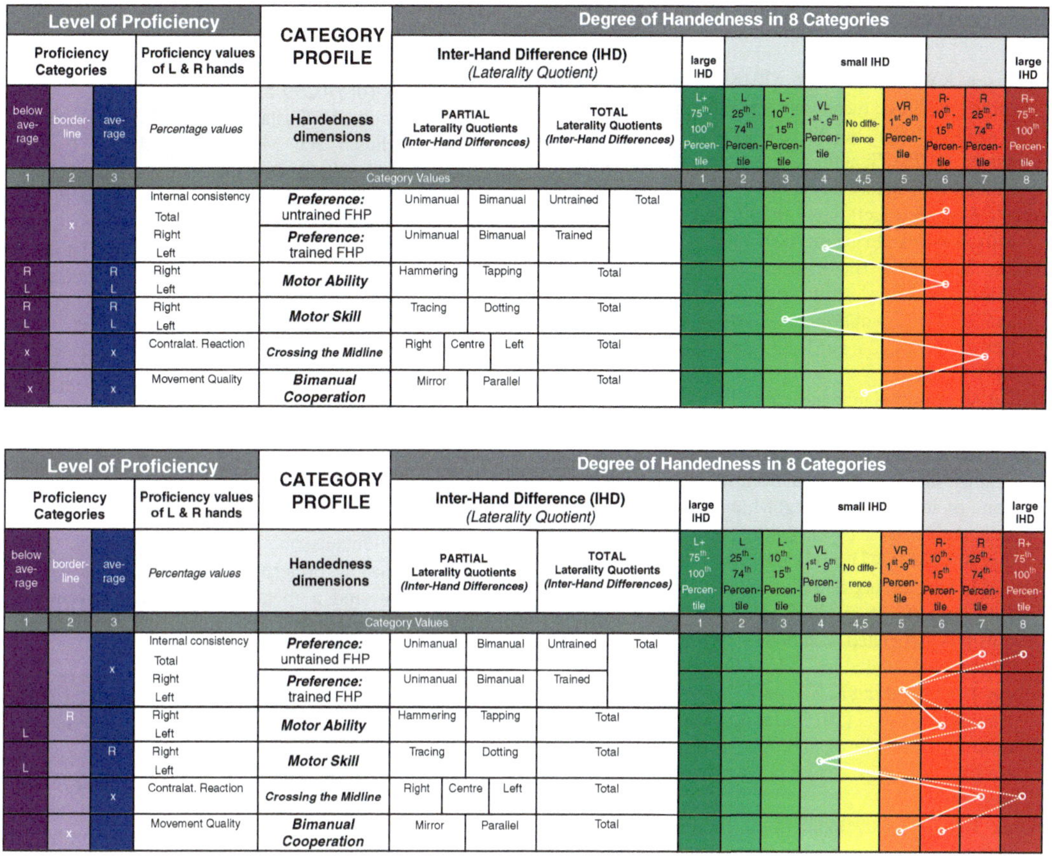

Fig. 10.25 Comparing similar Category Profiles of *Variable Left Handedness* (above) and *Converted Right Handedness* (below)

10.4 Concluding Remarks

This chapter describes the variations of the three handedness types based on the co-determinants: *inheritance*, *environment* and *motor impact*. The degree (D)-based, motor (M)-based and environment (E)-based variations of the Handedness Typology show distinct differences between them, particularly if data includes both the multivariate qualitative and multidimensional quantitative information. In occupational therapy practice, they have shown to provide a useful structure for systematically classifying handedness according to respective criteria. In particular, the variations allow practitioners to compare individual handedness profiles with prototypical ones for orientation when assessing children with unestablished and variable hand use. Practitioners report that the Handedness Typology has substantially increased their ability to understand atypical handedness and, in most "challenging" handedness cases, provided enough information to make decisions on subsequent intervention.

This chapter concludes the second part of the book on assessment and analyses of handedness, building a bridge between theory and practice. We now want to examine to what extent the Handedness Profile and the Handedness Typology are practicable and useful for implementation. In order to link subsequent clinical reasoning for intervention to the real cases presented, I will first describe some of the general principles and ideas for treating atypical handedness in the following chapter.

References

Andersen KW, Siebner HR (2018) Mapping dexterity and handedness: recent insights and future challenges. Curr Opin Behav Sci 20:123–129
Annett M (1978) Genetic and nongenetic influences on handedness. Behav Genet 8(3):227–249
Annett M (1985) Left, right, hand, and brain. The right shift theory. L. Erlbaum Associates, London
Annett M (1994) Handedness as a continuous variable with dextral shift: sex, generation, and family handedness in subgroups of left- and right-handers. Behav Genet 24(1):51–63. https://doi.org/10.1007/BF01067928
Annett M (2002) Handedness and brain asymmetry. The right shift theory. Psychology Press, Hove
Annett M (2004) Hand preference observed in large healthy samples: classification, norms and interpretations of increased non-right-handedness by the right shift theory. Br J Psychol 95(3):339–353. https://doi.org/10.1348/0007126041528130
Arning L, Ocklenburg S, Schulz S, Ness V, Gerding WM, Hengstler JG et al (2013) PCSK6 VNTR polymorphism is associated with degree of handedness but not direction of handedness. PLoS One 8(6):e67251
Arning L, Ocklenburg S, Schulz S, Ness V, Gerding WM, Hengstler JG et al (2015) Handedness and the X chromosome: the role of androgen receptor CAG-repeat length. Sci Rep 5(1):655. https://doi.org/10.1038/srep08325
Babik I (2014) Development of handedness for role-differentiated bimanual manipulation of objects in relation to the development of hand-use preferences for acquisition. Dissertation. The University of North Carolina at Greensboro, Greensboro
Benton CD, McCann JW, Larsen M (1965) Dyslexia and dominance: SLACK Incorporated Thorofare, NJ (2). J Pediatr Ophthalmol Strabismus (3)
Bishop DVM (1990) Handedness and developmental disorders. Mac Keith Press; J.B. Lippincott, Oxford (Clinics in developmental medicine, 110)
Bryden PJ, Roy EA, Rohr LE, Egilo S (2007) Task demands affect manual asymmetries in pegboard performance. Laterality 12(4):364–377. https://doi.org/10.1080/13576500701356244
Carlier M, Doyen A-L, Lamard C (2006) Midline crossing: developmental trend from 3 to 10 years of age in a preferential card-reaching task. Brain Cogn 61(3):255–261. https://doi.org/10.1016/j.bandc.2006.01.007
Cermak SA, Ayres AJ (1984) Crossing the body midline in learning-disabled and normal children. Am J Occup Ther 38(1):35–39. https://doi.org/10.5014/ajot.38.1.35
Corbetta D, Thelen E (2002) Behavioral fluctuations and the development of manual asymmetries in infancy: contributions of the dynamic systems approach. Handb Neuropsychol 8(1):311–330
Coren S, Searleman A (1990) Birth stress and left-handedness the rare trait marker model. Adv Psychol 67:3–32
Dahmen R, Fagard J (2005) The effect of explicit cultural bias on lateral preferences in Tunisia. Cortex 41(6):805–815. https://doi.org/10.1016/s0010-9452(08)70299-5
de Moura, Danilo R.; Costa, Jaderson C.; Santos, Iná S.; Barros, Aluísio JD; Matijasevich, Alicia; Halpern, Ricardo et al. (2010): Risk factors for suspected developmental delay at age 2 years in a Brazilian birth cohort. Paediatr Perinat Epidemiol 24 (3), 211–221
DeAgostini M, Khamis AH, Ahui AM, Dellatolas G (1997) Environmental influences in hand preference: an African point of view. Brain Cogn 35(2):151–167. https://doi.org/10.1006/brcg.1997.0935
Denny K, O'Sullivan V (2007) The economic consequences of being left-handed some sinister results. J Human Resources 42(2):353–374
Domellöf E, Rönnqvist L, Titran M, Esseily R, Fagard J (2009) Atypical functional lateralization in children with fetal alcohol syndrome. Dev Psychobiol 51(8):696–705
Domellöf E, Johansson A-M, Rönnqvist L (2011) Handedness in preterm born children: a systematic review and a meta-analysis. Neuropsychologia 49(9):2299–2310. https://doi.org/10.1016/j.neuropsychologia.2011.04.033
Eason BL, Surburg PR (1993) Effects of midline crossing on reaction time and movement time with adolescents classified as mildly mentally retarded. Adapt Phys Act Q 10(3):269–280
Elneel FHF, Carter F, Tang B, Cuschieri A (2008) Extent of innate dexterity and ambidexterity across handedness and gender: implications for training in laparoscopic surgery. Surg Endosc 22(1):31–37. https://doi.org/10.1007/s00464-007-9533-0
Galobardes B, Bernstein MS, Morabia A (1999) The association between switching hand preference and the declining prevalence of left-handedness with age. Am J Public Health 89(12):1873–1875. https://doi.org/10.2105/ajph.89.12.1873
Gruber R (2016) Making it right? Social norms, hand writing and cognitive skills. Paper presented at the Beiträge zur Jahrestagung des Vereins für Socialpolitik 2016: Demographischer Wandel
Hatta T, Kawakami A (1995) Patterns of handedness in modern Japanese: a cohort effect shown by re-administration of the H.N. Handedness Inventory after 20 years. Can J Exp Psychol 49(4):505–512. https://doi.org/10.1037/1196-1961.49.4.505
Hawkyard R, Dempsey I, Arthur-Kelly M (2014) The handwriting experiences of left-handed primary school students in a digital age. Australian data and critique. Aust J Educ 58(2):123–138
Hepper PG, Wells DL, Lynch C (2005) Prenatal thumb sucking is related to postnatal handedness. Neuropsychologia 43(3):313–315. https://doi.org/10.1016/j.neuropsychologia.2004.08.009
Hildreth G (1949) The development and training of hand dominance; characteristics of handedness. J Genet Psychol 75(2):197–220. https://doi.org/10.1080/08856559.1949.10533517

Hill EL, Khanem F (2009) The development of hand preference in children: the effect of task demands and links with manual dexterity. Brain Cogn 71(2):99–107. https://doi.org/10.1016/j.bandc.2009.04.006

Ida Y, Bryden MP (1996) A comparison of hand preference in Japan and Canada. Can J Exp Psychol 50(2):234

Ida Y, Mandal M (2003) Cultural difference in side bias: Evidence from Japan and India. Laterality: Asymmetries of Body, Brain and Cognition, 8(2):121–33

Kim H, Yi S, Son EI, Kim J (2001) Evidence for the pathological right-handedness hypothesis. Neuropsychology 15(4):510

Klöppel S, Vongerichten A, van Eimeren T, Frackowiak RSJ, Siebner HR (2007) Can left-handedness be switched? Insights from an early switch of handwriting. J Neurosci 27(29):7847–7853. https://doi.org/10.1523/JNEUROSCI.1299-07.2007

Koeda T, Takeshita K (1988) Relationship between corrected handedness and dysgraphia. No To Hattatsu 20(3):191–194

Kraus E (2003) The handedness profile. The development of a normative profile to determine the extent of handedness in children. Doctoral thesis. La Trobe University, Melbourne, Australia

Krombholz H (2005) Motorische Entwicklungsstörungen. In: Enzyklopädie der Psychologie 5

Kushner HI (2012) Retraining left-handers and the aetiology of stuttering: the rise and fall of an intriguing theory. Laterality 17(6):673–693

Kushner HI (2013) Why are there (almost) no left-handers in China? Endeavour 37(2):71–81. https://doi.org/10.1016/j.endeavour.2012.12.003

Liederman, J. (1983): Mechanisms underlying instability in the development of hand preference. In: Gerald Young, Carl M. Corter, Sidney J. Segalowitz & Sandra E. Trehub (Hg.): Manual specialization and the developing brain: an overview: Academic New York, S. 71–90

Lin H-L, Tsuang H-C (2018) Handedness and attention deficit/hyperactivity disorder symptoms in college students. Psychiatry Q 89(1):103–110. https://doi.org/10.1007/s11126-017-9517-8

Marcori AJ, Monteiro PHM, Okazaki VHA (2019) Changing handedness: what can we learn from preference shift studies? Neurosci Biobehav Rev 107:313–319

Masud Y, Ajmal MA (2012) Left-handed people in a right-handed world: a phenomenological study. Pak J Social Clin Psychol 10(1):49–60

McManus C, Bryden MP (1992) The genetics of handedness, cerebral dominance and lateralisation

McManus IC, Sik G, Cole DR, Mellon AF, Wong J, Kloss J (1988) The development of handedness in children. Br J Dev Psychol 6(3):257–273. https://doi.org/10.1111/j.2044-835X.1988.tb01099.x

McManus C, Nicholls M, Vallortigara G (2010) The right hand and the left hand of history. Laterality 15(1–2):1–3. https://doi.org/10.1080/13576500903201818

McManus IC, Davison A, Armour JAL (2013) The evolution of human handedness. Ann N Y Acad Sci 1288(1):48

Michel GF, Harkins DA (1988) Evidence for a maternal effect on infant hand-use preferences. Dev Psychobiol 21:535–541

Ocklenburg S, Beste C, Arning L (2014) Handedness genetics: considering the phenotype. Front Psychol 5(9):221. https://doi.org/10.3389/fpsyg.2014.01300

Orton ST, Travis LE (1929) Studies in stuttering: IV. Studies of action currents in stutterers. Arch Neurol Psychiatr 21:61–68

Perelle IB, Ehrman L (1994) An international study of human handedness: the data. Behav Genet 24(3):217–227. https://doi.org/10.1007/BF01067189

Peters M (1990) Subclassification of non-pathological left-handers poses problems for theories of handedness. Neuropsychologia 28(3):279–289. https://doi.org/10.1016/0028-3932(90)90021-f

Peters M, Murphy K (1992) Cluster analysis reveals at least three, and possibly five distinct handedness groups. Neuropsychologia 30(4):373–380. https://doi.org/10.1016/0028-3932(92)90110-8

Porac C (1996) Attempts to switch the writing hand: relationships to age and side of hand preference. Laterality 1(1):35–44. https://doi.org/10.1080/713754205

Porac C (2009) Hand preference and skilled hand performance among individuals with successful rightward conversions of the writing hand. Laterality 14(2):105–121. https://doi.org/10.1080/13576500802299418

Porac C, Lee Berdel Martin W (2007) A cross-cultural comparison of pressures to switch left-hand writing: Brazil versus Canada. Laterality 12(3):273–291. https://doi.org/10.1080/13576500701269462

Porac C, Searlman A (2002) The effects of hand preference side and hand preference switch history on measures of psychological and physical well-being and cognitive performance in a sample. Neuropsychologia 40(12):2074–2083

Ramadhani MK, Koomen I, Grobbee DE, van Donselaar CA, van Marceline Furth A, Uiterwaal CSPM (2006) Increased occurrence of left-handedness after severe childhood bacterial meningitis: support for the pathological left-handedness hypothesis. Neuropsychologia 44(12):2526–2532. https://doi.org/10.1016/j.neuropsychologia.2006.03.026

Rett A, Kohlmann T, Strauch G (1973) Linkshänder: Analyse einer Minderheit [Left-handers: Analysis of a minority]. Jugend & Volk

Sattler JB (2011) Der umgeschulte Linkshänder oder der Knoten im Gehirn. Auer.

Sattler JB, Klußmann A (2014) Leitlinie Händigkeit. - Bedeutung & Untersuchung / 002/017 - S1. Unter Mitarbeit von DGAUM. AWMF, zuletzt aktualisiert am 06.2020

Satz P (1972) Pathological Left-Handedness. An Explanatory Model. [Place of publication not identified]: Distributed by ERIC Clearinghouse

Satz P, Orsini DL, Saslow E, Henry R (1985) The pathological left-handedness syndrome. Brain Cogn 4(1):27–46

Table 1 Synoptic summary of Part II

SYNOPSIS OF CHAPTERS IN PART II

	Chapter 6	Chapter 7	Chapter 8	Chapter 9	Chapter 10
Title	***Assessing handedness***	***Constructing a multidimensional assessment: the Handedness Profile 2003***	***Developing the Handedness Profile 2018***	***Proposing an Architecture for a Handedness Typology***	***Interpreting Handedness Profiles using the Handedness Typology***
What was done	Reviewed literature on handedness assessments	Summarised studies and construction process	Presented the development, evaluation and validation of current HP	Devloped a Conceptual Framework to understand different groups of handedness	Illustrated in detail the 10 variations of the Cluster Table and prototypical category profiles
Type of work	LITERATURE REVIEW	RESEARCH	RESEARCH AND PRACTICE	THEORY AND CONCEPTUALISATION	APPLICATION OF THEORY TO PRACTICE
Goals and Objectives	To establish a scientific foundation for assessment	To construct a **multidimensional** handedness assessment, the **Handedness Profile** (HP)	To expand and develop the HP 2018 with **multivariate** data	To propose a Handedness Typology based on **multidimensional** and multivariate handedness	To **interpret** and differentiate between the **10 Handedness Variations**
Outcome	Overview, influences, recommendations from the literature	5 multi-dimensional Subtests based on **quantitative** data of **8 HP categories** of handedness degrees and direction	10 handedness variations based on **quantitative** and **qualitative data** for the most likely reasons for variable hand use	Definition of multidimen-sional Handedness, 3 Handedness Types and 10 Handedness Variations	Detailed description of all ten handedness variation
Type of outcome	ASSESSMENT (review)	ASSESSMENT & Basic ANALYSIS (construction)	Advanced ANALYSIS (development)	CONCEPTUAL FRAMEWORK	INTERPRETATION
Specific Tools and Products	**GUIDELINES for assessing handedness in practice**	**TOOL 1: Category Profile of the Handedness Dimen-sions** (for basic analysis)	**TOOL 2: Cluster Table for a Handedness Typology** (for advanced analysis)	**Handedness Typology**	**Prototypical handedness profiles** for each handedness variation
Purpose of HP Tools		**TOOL 1:** to quantify an average of degree and direction of handedness	**TOOL 2:** to rate and cluster the 25 criteria for each variations, and to visually summarises and ranks the results of the Cluster Table with the HP Stairs	None	See Chapter 7, 8 and 9

Part III

Intervention and Case Studies: Implications for Practice

Looking back on the developments around the Handedness Profile and the Handedness Typology, I admit that I neither had the intention nor the vision to develop the Handedness Profile to its current form after finishing my PhD in 2003. Instead, this was prompted by occupational therapist colleagues, also working with children with unestablished handedness and feeling perplexed by their ambiguous hand use. They urged me to share my knowledge and ideas on assessing, analysing and treating handedness, which I was more than happy to do. However, I was seriously challenged when attempting to convey the complexity, immensity and diversity around handedness to practitioners, who were most interested in the practicalities rather than research and theory. Thus, to help impart intricate postulates and findings from the literature, I increasingly resorted to visual summaries, diagrams and tables.

Most importantly, intervention with children with variable hand use has been the starting point of my journey and remains the main motivation for developing instruments that can be implemented. We need to better understand how the development of handedness can be enhanced and facilitated once the baseline of a child's performance is clearly defined. Using multidimensional instruments such as the Handedness Profile enables us to generate the data we need both for clinical decision-making as well as researching processes around manual lateralisation. So focussing on clinical practice and documenting handedness cases in accordance with the Handedness Typology by using the Handedness Profile and its tools is the logical next step. In this third part of the book, we look at some real cases, mainly from my own clinical experience, of children with atypical handedness and the appropriate interventions.

impedes the child's everyday function and participation. Years of practice in the field have shown that particular handedness variations require specific intervention strategies. The atypical handedness variations most frequently presenting to occupational therapy include: ♦***Variable Left Handedness*** with motor deficits; children with ♦***Developmentally Delayed Handedness***; ♦***Pathological Left* or *Right Handedness*** and ♦***Converted (Left) Handedness***. The intervention ideas were tailored to these variations and originated mainly from occupational therapy. They are meant to provide broad guidelines and suggestions to therapists and educators working in this field.

11.2 Contextualising Guidelines for Intervention

Before we turn to the intervention strategies, it is useful to contextualise intervention in terms of a ♦**client-centred approach** as well as **bottom-up vs top-down approaches**, typically used in occupational therapy.

11.2.1 Client-Centred Approach

The client-centred approach has its roots in person-centred psychotherapy. It follows the philosophy that humans are intrinsically motivated, innately striving for self-actualisation within the reality they perceive (Gillon 2007). According to Carl Rogers (Schmid 2002), the following three attitudes are fundamental to a therapeutic relationship between therapist and client group: (1) congruence or genuineness, (2) accurate empathic understanding and (3) unconditional positive esteem. Client-centred occupational therapy enables a balanced partnership between the therapist and the client (child, patient or group such as a family). It aims to empower clients to function and engage in various roles and environments (Sumsion 2000).

In paediatric occupational therapy, we often work with client groups, addressing both the child and his/her parents or caregivers and the child's educators and teachers. "Client" is used in this context synonymously with "person" and differs from the term "patient" in that the latter implies a particular hierarchical gradient between a person seeking help (the patient) and an expert providing help (e.g. therapist, expert, doctor). In the conventional paramedical setting, the child has a problem, and it is the general expectation that it is the therapist's responsibility to solve the problem. Using a client-centred approach, the hierarchical dynamic changes to a partnership at eye level based on the assumption that the clients are experts of their everyday life and thus best able to solve the problems themselves. The therapist merely facilitates the process. This makes excellent sense for professions such as occupational therapy with its expertise of understanding and enabling occupation. Acknowleding that the child and his/her parents are the experts of their everyday life, enables collaborative work at eye-level. The clients (child and parents) know and understand the complex multimodal reciprocal influences of their everyday life best, and professionals working with them are well advised to try and capture this understanding (see also Kraus et al. 2015). In this regard, the therapist takes on the role of an empowering educator and requires specific communication and interactional skills. The needs, expectations and treatment goals are reached together with the client group. The ultimate aim of the client-centred approach is to enable the child and parents to make decisions related to the child's personal goals, whereby the therapist plays an accepting and supportive role (Mortenson and Dyck 2006).

Relating the principle of client-centeredness to the field of handedness in paediatric occupational therapy, we can say that children are the experts on their hand use since only they have subjective perception and perspective on what it feels like when they engage in manual activities. Honouring the expertise on all sides, the therapist, child and caregivers work constructively together in an equal partnership and take joint responsibility for the treatment process. As a result, the client group is empowered to identify and solve related problems, which significantly increases the motivation and compliance of the client group and positively influences the sustainability of the process (Law et al. 1995). While such active cooperation in partnership is not always possible, especially when parents lack personal resources (Kraus et al.

2015), this approach has proven very successful in clinical practice with mixed- handed children.

11.2.2 Bottom-Up and Top-Down Approaches

The so-called ♦**bottom-up approaches** imply that intervention focuses on the level of the child's basic functions, offering repeated targeted sensory-motor experiences that enhance developmental processes (e.g. Weinstock-Zlotnick and Hinojosa 2004). Sensory integration (Ayres 1972; May-Benson and Koomar 2010) is an example of a bottom-up intervention. Significantly, these approaches' effectiveness will depend on whether the presumed body function deficits are indeed co-responsible for the delayed handedness development. Therefore, the therapist needs to identify, specify and then decide which body functions should be targeted in therapy. For example, in therapy, a bottom-up approach would be to stimulate and support the development of lateralisation of sensory-motor skills by using a broad sensory-motor intervention programme.

The hierarchically based bottom-up approaches assume that basic functional components such as motor control and concentration are essential for more complex activities such as reading or riding a bike. Whilst this assumption is based on well-known developmental processes and specific body functions that make up more complex tasks and activities, we should be careful not to conclude that this approach automatically impacts the child's participation in everyday life and the problems s/he might experience my alternative[1]. Many other aspects influencing participation, particularly personal and environmental factors, could also be responsible for successful participation (see Mandich et al. 2001).

A ♦**top-down approach** is typically rooted in a cognitive-behavioural context, starting at and focussing on the participation level of the child's everyday life. This has been found to be very effective, particularly if knowledge transfer, empowerment, active problem-solving and decision-making are part of the strategies used. For example, the CO-OP approach (Cognitive Orientation to Daily Occupational Performance) is a good example (Mandich et al. 2001). Children are enabled to identify their own goals and reflect on their implementation to solve problems cognitively and actively—and have fun doing it!

11.2.3 Communication and Education

Against the background of client-centred and top-down approaches, good communication flow and transparency between all parties involved is essential. This means that the client group (i.e. parents or caregivers and child) and teachers are informed about the results of the handedness assessment. Furthermore, they should and receive all relevant information and understand the probable reasons for the atypical variable hand use so that they can participate and be co-responsible during the intervention phase. In addition, therapists need to bridge the gap between specialist knowledge base around handedness and its relevance to everyday life. Creating transparency and knowledge is an important prerequisite if changing specific manual and behavioural patterns are to be successful and the collaboration effective.

The suggested intervention strategies in this chapter are based on four of the variations with their general prototypical category profiles presented in the previous chapter. These generalised profiles suffice when we want to establish principles of treatment and guidelines. However, the complexity and uniqueness of reciprocal influences and co-existing factors warrant an individualised treatment approach in real cases to make intervention effective—this will be demonstrated in the following chapter. The strategies and ideas in this chapter are predominantly based on the experience and expertise of practitioners[2] and my own practice. To date, there is little evidence-based research to substantiate these approaches with mixed handed in children. The following ideas on intervention are both bottom-up and top.

[1]Participation is defined in the International Classification of Functioning, Disability and Health (ICF) as the **"involvement in a life situation"** (Noonan et al. 2009).

[2]In particular, Ursula Nagele, a teacher and motopedagogical expert, has substantially contributed to Chaps. 11 and 12 (see Kraus & Nagele-Hiedl 2019).

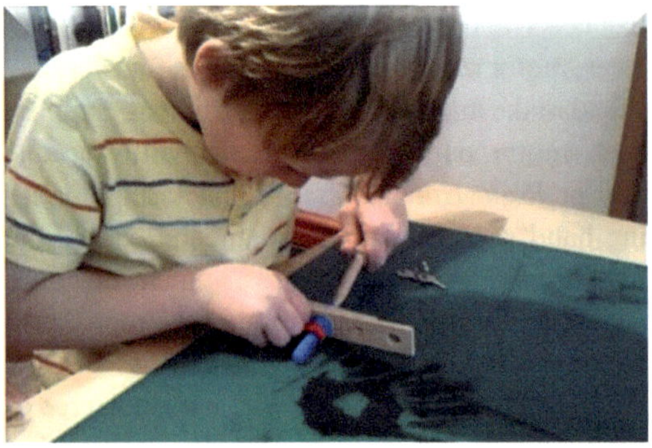

Fig. 11.2 Division of roles between the hands using a screwdriver to turn a bolt into a nut

Although variable left handers typically use either hand for many less demanding activities and often use the right hand for some demanding activities such as cutting with scissors, writing is performed consistently and unambiguously with the left hand, despite the right-biassed environment. This pattern is particularly confusing to parents and teachers if there is a lack of knowledge about degrees of handedness. Such variable left handers are often switched to the right, because they seem to be doing more activities with the right hand. Therapists should recognise this risk and very definitely confirm that the child should continue to draw and write with the left hand.

Overall, there are three parts guiding handedness-related intervention with variable left handers:

1. Fine motor and writing skills are trained **solely with the left hand**.
2. Demanding activities are identified together with the child to see which need proficiency training. Here a decision needs to be made for a consistent hand, but it does not matter whether this is the right or the left hand. The main goal is to increase the **internal consistency** of the more demanding tasks.
3. Activities performed **arbitrarily** with either left or right hand with satisfactory performance are not targeted since the everyday function of the child is not affected. These are often less demanding activities.

The challenge with Variable Handedness is the interference of **motor problems** with the low degree of handedness. Frequently the two hands show different strengths and weaknesses that need to be understood. For example, the left hand may have better proprioceptive abilities but shows a tremor. Conversely, the right hand is more steady but has poor proprioceptive skills, often compensating with increased pressure and muscle tension (see Sect. 12.3). These differences could also contribute to the child's variable hand use.

11.5 *Developmentally Delayed Handedness* (D-Based Variation)

Developmentally Delayed Handedness is assigned to the D-based handedness type because of its unestablished direction and underdeveloped degree of handedness. As per definition, there are accompanying motor deficiencies with this variation (see Sect. 10.2.1). Intervention approaches for this variation can be divided into bottom-up or top-down, depending on how much time is left before the child starts school and needs a final decision for the writing hand (see Figs. 11.3 and 11.4).

11.5.1 Bottom-Up Approach

Up to 3 years, it is typical for children to alternate hand use across activities (see Sect. 1.3). Particularly in right handers, the handedness direction emerges between the second and third years of life; left handers take longer. Generally, handedness intervention is indicated if the handedness direction is not clear from the age of four. At this point, the decision for the writing hand is not yet imminent, so intervention should focus on two aspects: neutralising the environment and developing sensory-motor skills using a bottom-up approach.

Neutralising the socio-cultural and physical environments: Parents, caregivers and teachers need to be educated to avoid social pressure or subtle suggestion to use one side, usually the right. Instead, they should help to reduce the right-biassed influence and create neutralised physical and social environments where both hands have equal chances to be used. Neutralising

11.6 Pathological *Left* or *Right Handedness* (M-Based Variation)

Pathological left or right handers (*p-LH* and p-RH) have a significant motor deficit on their inherently dominant side. Consequently, they develop better motor skills and proficiency on their non-dominant side, leading to ♦**reshaping** their handedness to the non-dominant side (see Sect. 3.5). Pathological left handers (originally right handed by predisposition) often show soft neurological signs, particularly on the right, such as tremor, unrefined release and grasping, or significantly worse incoordination than the left hand. The Categorisation Profile typically illustrates this by very large inter-hand differences, with the right hand often being in the borderline or sub-average range. Pathological right handers (originally left handed by disposition) mirror the *p-LH* profile but they are much rarer (see Sect. 4.4).

As we saw in Chap. 10, the original degree of handedness could play an essential role in atypical variable hand use of pathological left and right handers (see Sect. 10.2.11). Although handedness in these cases has been reshaped from very early in their development, it is unclear if and to what extent ♦**conversion repercussions** may occur. Compared to the E-based variation Converted Handedness, where preferred neurophysiological pathways were already established before switching, the lateralisation processes must still develop in *pathological Left Handedness*.

Be that as it may: whenever there is spontaneous hand use on the affected side, it should be supported since it would activate the areas of the inherently dominant cortex. Together with the child and parents, activities that this hand can perform should be identified. The child is then encouraged (but never forced or bribed) to perform these tasks with the inherently dominant hand as often as possible. It is rather unlikely that the child will want to use the motor-deficient hand for highly demanding tasks such as writing.

The option to write on a laptop or computer keyboard is a great opportunity for pathological left and right handers since they circumvent having to write with one hand. Typing is not only much easier motorically, but it is a bimanual task where both hands can be used, even if the affected hand is only involved with a finger or thumb. In order to implement the keyboard alternative, close work with teachers is required. At least one visit to the classroom is necessary, where the therapist works together with the teachers to establish alternative writing methods for the child. Educating classmates may also be important, especially when a child is teased for being different or envied using a keyboard (see Fig. 11.7).

In addition, therapy with pathological handers should also focus on fine motor skills and bimanually differentiated tasks as discussed in Sects. 11.3 and 11.4).

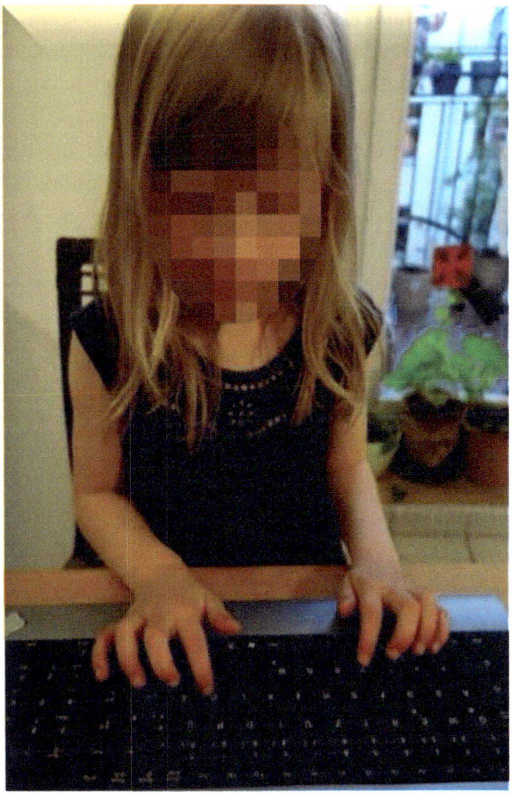

Fig. 11.7 Using a keyboard for both hands instead of writing with one hand can be an effective alternative for pathological handers

11.7 Reverting *Converted Left Handedness* (E-Based Variation)

Whilst conversions can take place in both directions, we will focus here on *converted Left Handedness* since this is most common (see Sect. 4.5). ♦**Handedness reversion** means that after converting the non-dominant hand for writing, the dominant hand is retrained (or trained) for writing. As a prerequisite for reversion training, it is important to establish if handedness conversion did indeed occur in the first place. Such evidence may be based on a child's recollection of switching, observations and reports of parents and teachers, or early photos and videos showing a clear preference for the left hand. However, obtaining clear evidence is not always possible because switching may have occurred very early on without the child or parents recollecting it, or there may be a denial that it happened.

Nevertheless, the possibility of *Left Handedness* in children with alternating hand use should not be underestimated since it is especially left handers that display high variability in manual tasks. Thus, a Leon-Left experimental programme or the Stamina Test with both hands may be an option. If the results indicate *Left Handedness*, they can also be considered evidence.

Once evidence for *converted Left Handedness* has been established, the next question is whether to revert to the left dominant hand for writing. To make this decision, it is necessary to answer the following questions.

1. Is the child motivated to revert his/her writing hand?
2. Is there full support for this at home environment and at school?
3. Is the performance of the dominant hand average or above average, at least compared to the other hand?
4. Is there a relatively stress-free and writing-free period (at least 8 weeks), in which daily writing exercises with the hand can be done?
5. Is regular occupational therapy and follow-up possible during and after the retraining?

A decision tree in Fig. 11.8 provides an overview of favourable conditions or prerequisites for successful handedness reversion in the form of questions. These factors need to be considered together. If most questions are answered with YES, reversion could be indicated; if the answer is NO, the child would probably continue to write with the non-dominant hand. However, it is important to note that these conditions do not necessariy carry the same weight, so the final decision has to be based on the therapists professional reasoning taking all relevant factors into account.

11.7.1 Reverting to the Inherently Dominant Hand

There is evidence that reverting to the dominant for writing may reduce or even reverse switching repercussions in converted left and right handers (e.g. Kushner 2012; Randolph 2007; Neumann

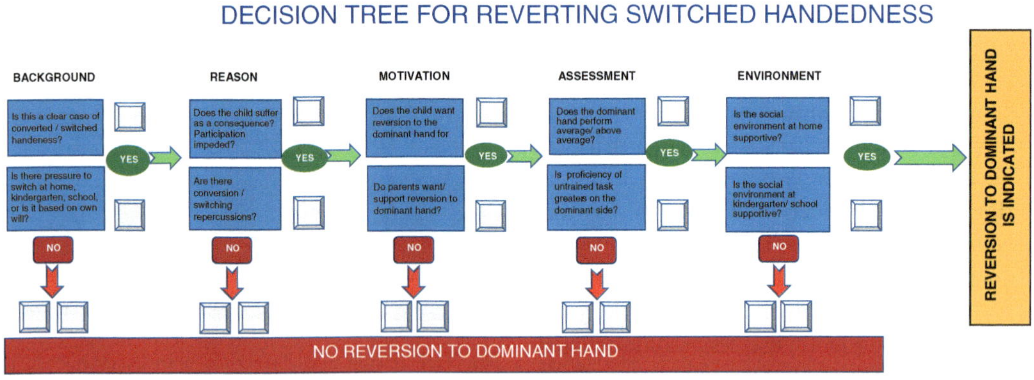

Fig. 11.8 Decision tree for reversion to the dominant hand (Kraus 2018a, b)

2014; Sattler 2000). Reversion should thus always be considered because of the potential to minimise or eliminate switching repercussions (see Sect. 4.5.5). However, there is also evidence that reversion may exacerbate existing problems in real life, especially if the conditions described in the decision tree are not met (Kraus 2009; Sattler 2000). The different outcomes for this may have to do with the differences in hemispheric lateralisation following handedness conversion, as has been shown in MRI studies (Klöppel et al. 2007; Grabowska et al. 2012; Siebner et al. 2002), but implications at a behavioural level are not well researched. Nevertheless, it seems plausible that a non-converted left hander would differ from a converted left hander, even if all other factors such as handedness degree, motor skill and habits were comparable. Therefore, for clinical and educational practice, we, together with the child, parents or caregivers, need to work on the behavioural level and establish whether the conditions for a handedness reversion are favourable. If they are unfavourable at that point, handedness reversion should not implemented.

In particular, if there is evidence of distress and severe problems related to switching repercussions, reversion may make a significant change. However, these affirmed conditions should always include the child's and caregivers' motivation and support. Even if all the other conditions are favourable but the child lacks motivation, reversion training is likely to fail. In this regard, Nagele-Hiedl has specified some criteria that can aid or hinder successful reversion in addition to the conditional questions (Kraus and Nagele-Hiedl 2019). They include the following:

- Background information and diagnosis—*results of the Handedness Profile, the extent of handedness conversion, type of handedness repercussions*
- Child's life situation—*point in time of conversion and possible reversion, general health and resilience, social and familial situation and support at home and at school*
- Reactions of client group—*relief, resistance, motivation, indifference*
- Expectations—*pessimistic, unrealistic, passive attitude*
- Emotional stability—*ability to critically reflect, willpower, assertiveness*
- Therapy—*competencies and experience of the therapist, assistive devices, collaboration and cooperation with all parties involved*

When all of these aspects have been considered and the decision is made that reversion is indicated, we can orientate ourselves using the five phases based on Willikonsky 2016 with some additions:

1. The client's intrinsic motivation for reversion is determined in the **analysis phase**.
2. This is followed by the **orientation phase.** In addition to writing, other activities are identified and deliberately performed in everyday life with the left hand. This is very individual and should be tailored according to the child's handedness degree and her/his specific life situations. Subsequently, the therapist creates a training programme with the child and provides information about the reversion process to the child, parents and teachers.
3. The **activation phase** consists of fine motor exercises such as tracing and in-hand manipulation activities with the dominant hand (see Fig. 11.9). This phase prepares the hand for writing.
4. The **stabilisation phase** focuses on handwriting by slowly increasing the intensity in terms of time, frequency, complexity and endurance.
5. The final **automation or transfer phase** consists of repetitive writing exercises to automate the writing movements. Specifically, three rules apply here:
   (a) Progress from large-scale to small-scale movements (scribbling and drawing exercises from large to small).
   (b) Progress from scribbling and drawing to tracing letters, such as retracing own writing.
   (c) Progress from numbers and single letters to short words (such as an, am, and). Once this is fluent, swift and automated, proceed to write texts.

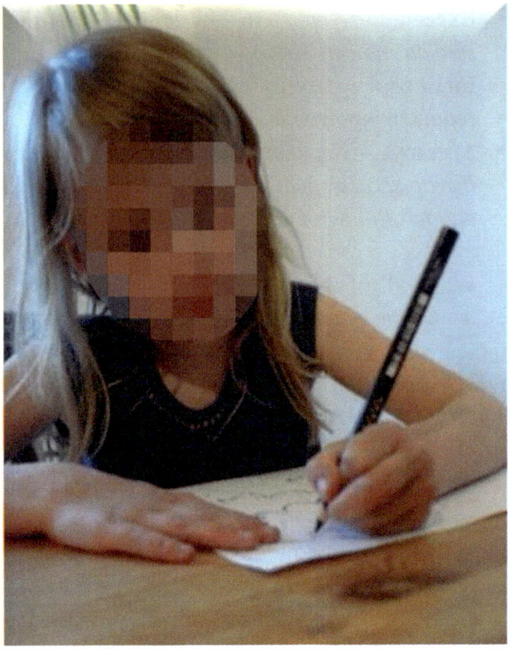

Fig. 11.9 A left-handed child during a tracing exercise

In clinical practice, a bottom-up approach might include the following fine motor exercises to support the reversion for children and adults. These activities are mostly bimanual and aim to strengthen both hands but also allow and encourage the left hand to lead:

- Drums—learn and practise different rhythms
- Finger dexterity courses—practise different movement patterns
- Marble games—in-hand manipulation with holding function of the ulnar side of the hand (i.e. ring and little fingers)
- Painting—finger paints, pavement drawings, paint brushes, coloured pencils, alternatives to pencils and pens used for writing
- Table games—Mikado, tearing and scrunching paper, stacking games
- Cutting with scissors—different shapes ranging from easy to challenging tasks
- Bead threading—making chains with large to tiny beads
- Handicrafts and craft activities—carpentry, ceramics, weaving, soapstone carving
- Finger hockey—playing on a table according to hockey rules, involving midline crossing
- Ball games—training eye-hand coordination and timing (table tennis, badminton)
- Relaxation exercises—targeting especially hands, arms, shoulders, back
- Massage—shaking, deep pressure, vibration, tapping.

However, these bottom up activities do not necessarily automatically lead to learning to write as an activity, so they should be followed up with some pencil-and-paper exercises. In addition, there are some specific ideas on supporting handedness reversion in the classroom. These measures are particularly important for the time taken to revert handedness, ranging between 2 and 8 months. It is important to involve the teachers in addition to the child and his parents/caregivers.

- *Designing the child's workspace* in the classroom. For example, left handers sit to the left of their neighbour; the light should come in from the right side.
- *Allow greater line spacing* when writing. This could be designated in the child's exercise books.
- *Offer partial dictations* (e.g. words instead of sentences) or oral exams. Allow more time for performance assessments.
- *Allow the child to write on a PC* or use a laptop at home and possibly at school.
- *Allow the child to complete texts at home.*
- *Let the child use a non-smudge rollerball* instead of a fountain pen, as this is easier and the writing looks neater.
- *Offer various assistive pencil grips* to ensure good ergonomic position and movement of fingers.
- *Provide left-handed equipment individually*, e.g. left-handed ruler, fountain pen or pencil sharpener. Take time to choose suitable pens.

To retrain writing letters, a *First Grade writing curriculum* can be used, since these are carefully graded in terms of how letters are formed, the order in which they are learnt and the complexity of writing (see Steinkopf 2014; Neumann 2014).

In addition, it can be helpful to do or learn *new activities* with left hand, particularly if they have not been performed and automated with the non-dominant hand. For example, learning a new instrument, working with a novel tool or doing a new sport can help revert to the left hand since no energy is required to "undo" the already automated movement sequences of the non-dominant hand (Sattler 1999).

The therapist should always work closely with the child, encouraging her/him to continuously *reflect on what feels good and what does not "fit"*. In this way, the individual handedness degree is taken into account and is free to unfold. It often seems to assist the reversion process if other activities are also performed with the left hand. The child should be the one to decide which activities these should be. We should refrain from generalising that "real" left handers should do everything with the left hand, since this is not the case in the typical population, especially not amongst left handers. Instead, the multitude of individual influences on hand formation are responsible for normal variability of hand use. This should be communicated to all who work with the child.

Finally, there are some **general tips and a summary of reversion training**:

- The child should be reverted *slowly and carefully*, preferably under the supervision of an experienced therapist or handedness expert. The reversion time frame could extend between 2 and 12 months, which must be communicated to the child, parents and teachers.
- It is important to inform the child and family members about *possible physiological and somatic side effects* such as nausea, dizziness or headaches. These symptoms are usually temporary (Kraus 2009; Sattler 2000; Willikonsky 2016). However, if these are severe and persistent, these physiological effects could indicate that the neurophysiological adaptation is difficult and may result in (more) switching repercussions. In this case, reversion should be discontinued.
- There is evidence that the *hands learn from each other* (e.g. "interlimb-transfer of learning;" (Sainburg 2002; Stöckel and Weigelt 2012). Some children seem to benefit when doing pre-writing exercises such as scribbling and drawing small circles with both hands in a mirror fashion. These exercises should not include writing letters or words, since these require parallel and opposite movement patterns.
- *Bimanual asymmetric activities* reinforce the role of the dominant hand (Kourtis et al. 2014) and should therefore be practised regularly. Asymmetric activities with role-differentiated actions include cutting with scissors, sewing, embroidering, gluing or hammering.
- *Coaching and communicating* with the child, parents and teachers remain an important part of the reversion training. Expectations that the reversion will solve all other school and home problems should be discouraged.
- *Negative sentences should be avoided* such as "do it faster" or "write more beautifully", as these negatively influence the child's motivation and attitude.

11.7.2 Refraining from Reversion Training

If several of the prerequisites for reversion training are not met, this option should be ruled out. In this case, intervention would focus on continuing to write with the non-dominant hand and on coping strategies for a converted left hander in a right-biassed world (see Sect. 4.5). As already mentioned, not all converted left handers exhibit problems. Low-degree left handers, and presumably those with good motor skills and other resources, appear to adapt to writing with the non-dominant hand more easily and compensate for any challenges or problems more effectively (see also Marcori et al. 2019; Meng 2007; Kraus and Nagele-Hiedl 2019). These converted handers appear to cope well in their everyday life and do not report that they experience problems. Therefore, the effort involved in handedness reversion may not pose a relevant option for them. In fact, they may not even realise that their handedness has been converted.

Other converted handers are more strongly lateralised and possibly lack effective **neurophysiological adaptability**. They may not have good motor skills or have motor planning problems, they may be "over-automated" on the non-dominant hand, or they have situational challenges that do not favour reversion. Consequently, these individuals remain converted left handers. Informing and coaching the child, parents and teachers is very important throughout the intervention. Here too, handedness conversion and possible switching repercussions need to be explained and clearly communicated, and the reasons for not reverting should be made transparent. Just knowing that handedness has been switched can prevent children from blaming themselves for problems that may arise and thinking they are "stupid". Furthermore, there is evidence that reversions can still occur later, regardless of age, when there may be better prerequisites (see Randolph 2007; Kushner 2012; Neumann 2014; Sattler 2000, 2002; Kraus 2009). It is crucial that the child be included in all decision-making processes.

Interestingly, experience in occupational therapy practice indicates that many children between the ages of 5 and 7 years usually **refuse to revert** (Kraus 2009, 2018b; Sattler 2002). This may have to do with the fact that most of these children generally struggling with fine motor tasks because of motor problems and have managed to draw and write with the non-dominant hand only with great effort and difficulty. When they finally succeed in writing their name, they are not motivated at all to start learning to write with the other hand all over again. Without the child's motivation, an essential prerequisite, reversion training will most likely fail. Experience shows that it often takes a certain amount of "suffering" with writing and other school subjects before a child may be motivated to undergo reversion training, frequently this happens in third or fourth grade when switching repercussions usually also become more severe as school demands increase.

As discussed in Sect. 4.5.3, certain **bimanual activities** such as playing **music** and **sports** seem to lessen switching repercussions significantly. For example, we know from the literature that musicians' motor cortex, cerebellum and corpus callosum differ from those of non-musicians. In addition, music seems to alter brain structures (Gaser and Schlaug 2003; Schlaug 2001). Similarly, sports seems to have a modifying influence on the brain's physical cortical structures and cognitive functions (Draganski et al. 2004; Thomas et al. 2012). Therefore, it stands to reason that activities such as music and sports inherently involve intensive and excessive interhemispheric exchange, strengthening the corpus callosum. Such increased interhemispheric interaction and communication may also benefit converted left and right handers through repetitive bimanual and bilateral activities when playing a musical instrument, swimming, running or climbing by reducing or even preventing switching repercussions (Kraus 2009, 2018b; Sattler 1999; Willikonsky 2016).

Similarly, the principle of **crossing the body midline** with both hands should be incorporated into the intervention programme since this also seems to strengthen the corpus callosum (van Hof et al. 2002). This can be achieved playfully by, for example, juggling beanbags or balls, since this involves both bilateral contralateral reaching on both sides as well as bimanual dexterity and coordination (see also Saidmamatov et al. 2022; Jacobs et al. 2018).

Here too, it may also be helpful to perform activities other than writing with the left hand to stimulate the dominant contralateral motor cortex. Converted left handers in self-help groups report that their well-being and specific motor and cognitive skills improve substantially due to such activities performed with their left hand (Kraus and Nagele-Hiedl 2019). Again, however, these experiences are very individual. Together with the child, one should find out what feels "right" and good for each child.

Last but not least, the option of *writing on a laptop or computer keyboard* with both hands avoids writing with the non-dominant hand. However, this is school-, teacher-, system- and age-dependent and can only be achieved by providing information and working closely with parents and teachers.

Incidentally, if the topic of switched handedness is frequently discussed in front of the child, s/he may *consciously steer which hand is used in activities*. There have been documented cases where the child deliberately uses a specific hand or displays alternating hand use instead of spontaneously because of social reasons, such as attracting attention, being oppositional or trying to fit in and live up to perceived expectations. Therapists should be aware of this possibility and try to ensure that the child is not consciously focussing on her/his hand use when performing preference items.

11.8 Concluding Remarks

This chapter has shown how different approaches relate to different types of variable hand use presents. In particular, we have looked at both bottom-up and top-down intervention approaches used by occupational therapists working with mixed-handed children who are compromised in their everyday participation in children who are compromised in their everyday participation and that have been found to be effective. These approaches are based on many years of practice and expertise by therapists specialising in remediating manual motor skills and handedness. Such documented case studies form the basis of developing an evidence-based approach. However, further research is required to examine these strategies in the context of practice-based evidence in order to ensure that the intervention measures are effective and that results can be generalised. We will now look at some real cases in the following chapter. These cases have all been assessed using a complete Handedness Profile with the HP Tools for analysis, so conclusions are drawn concerning the handedness type and variation.

References

Ayres AJ (1972) Sensory integration and learning disorders. Western Psychological Services, Los Angeles
Beery KE, Buktenica NA (1982) Administration, scoring, and teaching manual for the Developmental Test of Visual-Motor Integration. Modern Curriculum Press
Baumgarten A, Strebel H (2016) Ergotherapie in der Pädiatrie: klientenzentriert-betätigungsorientiert-evidenzbasiert. Schulz-Kirchner Verlag GmbH
Draganski B, Gaser C, Busch V, Schuierer G, Bogdahn U, May A (2004) Neuroplasticity: changes in grey matter induced by training. Nature 427(6972):311–312. https://doi.org/10.1038/427311a
Gaser C, Schlaug G (2003) Brain structures differ between musicians and non-musicians. J Neurosci 23(27):9240–9245
Gillon E (2007) Person-centred counselling psychology: an introduction. Sage
Grabowska A, Gut M, Binder M, Forsberg L, Rymarczyk K, Urbanik A (2012) Switching handedness: fMRI study of hand motor control in right-handers, left-handers and converted left-handers. Acta Neurobiol Exp 72(4):439–451
Jacobs J, Greef J, Heyman R (2018) Interactive game for children with difficulty crossing the midline. In: 2018 IEEE 6th International Conference on Serious Games and Applications for Health (SeGAH). IEEE, pp 1–8
Kisch A, Pauli S (2012) Die Ravensburger Feinmotorikkiste:(FeinMoKi). Verlag Modernes Lernen
Klöppel S, Vongerichten A, van Eimeren T, Frackowiak RSJ, Siebner HR (2007) Can left-handedness be switched? Insights from an early switch of handwriting. J Neurosci 27(29):7847–7853. https://doi.org/10.1523/JNEUROSCI.1299-07.2007
Kourtis D, de Saedeleer L, Vingerhoets G (2014) Handedness consistency influences bimanual coordination: a behavioural and electrophysiological investigation. Neuropsychologia 58:81–87. https://doi.org/10.1016/j.neuropsychologia.2014.04.002
Kraus E (2003) The handedness profile. The development of a normative profile to determine the extent of handedness in children. Doctoral thesis. La Trobe University, Melbourne
Kraus E (2009) Händigkeit bei Kindern Teil 2: Therapieansätze—Rückschulung als letztes Mittel der Wahl. Ergopraxis 2(1):22–25. https://doi.org/10.1055/s-0030-1254443
Kraus E (2018a) Manual zum Händigkeitsprofil. Manual for assessment
Kraus E (2018b) Theoretische Grundlagen zum Grundkurs des Händigkeitsprofils. Assessment manual
Kraus E (Hg.) (2019) Zwischen Links-& Rechtshändigkeit. Theorie, Diagnostik & Therapie bei Kindern mit wechselndem Handgebrauch. Springer, Berlin
Kraus E, Nagele-Hiedl U (2019) Ideen zur Intervention bei händigkeitsauffälligen Kindern. In: Kraus E (Hg.) Zwischen Links-& Rechtshändigkeit. Springer, pp 193–212
Kraus E, Sichert-Grinstead U (2013) Treffpunkt. Feinmotorische Grundlagen für das Malen & Schreiben. 2nd edn. Schulz-Kirchner Verlag, Idstein
Kraus E, Romein E, Weise U (2015) PEAP Pädiatrisches Ergotherapeutisches Assessment & Prozessinstrument. Schulz-Kirchner Verlag GmbH
Kushner HI (2012) Retraining left-handers and the aetiology of stuttering: the rise and fall of an intriguing theory. Laterality 17(6):673–693

Law M, Baptiste S, Mills J (1995) Client-centred practice: what does it mean and does it make a difference?. Can J Occup Ther 62(5):250–257

Mandich AD, Polatajko HJ, Macnab JJ, Miller LT (2001) Treatment of children with developmental coordination disorder: what is the evidence? Phys Occup Ther Pediatr 20(2–3):51–68

Marcori AJ, Monteiro PHM, Okazaki VHA (2019) Changing handedness: what can we learn from preference shift studies? Neurosci Biobehav Rev 107:313–319

May-Benson TA, Koomar JA (2010) Systematic review of the research evidence examining the effectiveness of interventions using a sensory integrative approach for children. Am J Occup Ther 64(3):403–414

McDougal B (2022) The happy Handwriter. The right was the first time. Internet. https://thehappyhandwriter.co.za/, zuletzt aktualisiert am 2022

Meng L-F (2007) The rate of handedness conversion and related factors in left-handed children. Laterality 12(2):131–138. https://doi.org/10.1080/13576500601005727

Mortenson WB, Dyck I (2006) Power and client-centred practice: an insider exploration of occupational therapists' experiences. Can J Occup Ther 73(5):261–271

Neumann M (2014) Natürlich mit Links. Zurück zur Linkshändigkeit - befreiter leben mit der starken Hand. Ariston, Berlin

Noonan VK, Kopec JA, Noreau L, Singer J, Dvorak MF (2009) A review of participation instruments based on the International Classification of Functioning, Disability and Health. Disability and rehabilitation 31(23):1883–1901

Pellegrini AM, Andrade EC, Teixeira LA (2004) Attending to the non-preferred hand improves bimanual coordination in children. Hum Mov Sci 23(3–4):447–460

Randolph SM (2007) Hidden handedness. The emerging story of handedness reversals. Foundation for Handedness Research

Roman-Liu D, Mockałło Z (2020) Effectiveness of bimanual coordination tasks performance in improving coordination skills and cognitive functions in elderly. PLoS One 15(3):e0228599. https://doi.org/10.1371/journal.pone.0228599

Saidmamatov O, Rodrigues P, Vasconcelos O (2022) Motor skills training program reinforces crossing the body's midline in children with developmental coordination disorder. Symmetry 14(6):1259

Sainburg R (2002) Evidence for a dynamic-dominance hypothesis of handedness. Exp Brain Res 142(2):241–258. https://doi.org/10.1007/s00221-001-0913-8

Sattler JB (1999) Linkshänder & umgeschulte Linkshänder in der Ergotherapie. Praxis Ergother 12(2):98–110

Sattler JB (2000) Der umgeschulte Linkshänder oder Der Knoten im Gehirn [The switched left-hander or the knot in the brain]

Sattler JB (2002) Linkshändige & umgeschulte linkshändige Kinder sowie Kinder mit wechselndem Handgebrauch in der Ergotherapie. Ergother Rehabil 41:21–29

Schlaug G (2001) The brain of musicians: a model for functional and structural adaptation. Ann N Y Acad Sci 930(1):281–299

Schmid PF (2002): Presence: immediate co-experiencing and co-responding. Phenomenological, dialogical and ethical perspectives on contact and perception in person-centred therapy and beyond, pp 182–203

Schönthaler E (2020) Die Händigkeit des Kindes. In: Schönthaler E (Hg.) Grafomotorik & Händigkeit. Ergotherapie bei Kindern. 2. Auflage. Thieme, Stuttgart, pp 188–220

Shumway-Cook A, Woollacott MH (2017) Motor control. Translating research into clinical practice. 5th edn. Wolters Kluwer, Philadelphia

Siebner HR, Limmer C, Peinemann A, Drzezga A, Bloem BR, Schwaiger M, Conrad B (2002) Long-term consequences of switching handedness: a positron emission tomography study on handwriting in "converted" left-handers. J Neurosci 22(7):2816–2825

Steinkopf F (2014) Schritt für Schritt mit links ins Glück. Jder zweite Mensch ist Linkshänder - meistens weiß er es nur nicht. Left Handers World, Heide

Stöckel T, Weigelt M (2012) Brain lateralisation and motor learning: selective effects of dominant and non-dominant hand practice on the early acquisition of throwing skills. Laterality 17(1):18–37

Sumsion T (2000) A revised occupational therapy definition of client-centred practice. Br J Occup Ther 63(7):304–309

Thomas AG, Dennis A, Bandettini PA, Johansen-Berg H (2012) The effects of aerobic activity on brain structure. Front Psychol 3:86

van Hof P, van der Kamp J, Savelsbergh GJP (2002) The relation of unimanual and bimanual reaching to crossing the midline. Child Dev 73(5):1353–1362. https://doi.org/10.1111/1467-8624.00476

Weinstock-Zlotnick G, Hinojosa J (2004) Bottom-up or top-down evaluation: Is one better than the other?. Am J Occup Ther 58(5):594–599

Willikonsky P (2016) Rückschulung—Ab jetzt mit links. Ergopraxis 8(1):26–29

Case Studies Using the Handedness Profile

12

Contents

I am five years old... In my right hand, I hold a yellow pencil... I can barely hold the pencil because my right arm and hand are too weak to do the job. It feels like something is wrong with my hand. It feels like it is numb or half-asleep and I can't wake it up... I don't have the strength to hold the yellow pencil with a grip that is firm enough to write. I try to push the pencil onto the lined paper, but I cannot develop enough pressure to write properly... The pencil seems like a tree and I am some kind of a worm wiggling at the roots. I am blushing with embarrassment, feeling hot and ashamed inside. (Account of a converted left hander reflecting on his early writing experience. Randolph 2007: 18–19.)

12.1 Introduction

Children with atypical handedness like the switched hander in the above quote experience stress and hardship in everyday activities. Handedness exists within a unique cosmos of traits, abilities, experiences, circumstances and attitudes, so real handedness cases are much more complex than the prototypical handedness profiles in Chap. 10 can display. Different types and variations often co-exist; they are dynamic and may change. For example, a variable left hander could also be converted *and* have motor problems. The proposed Handedness Typology is very helpful in understanding the complex patterns of variable hand use, and they can suggest a particular profile type, but real handedness profiles are unique, as are the children themselves.

This chapter presents the handedness behaviour of four children tested with the Handedness Profile in occupational therapy practice. Three of the cases illustrate the three handedness types: Degree-based (D-based), Motor-based (M-based) and Environment-based (E-based). The fourth case is more complex and includes two co-existing handedness types. **Zelda**[1] is a variable

[1] The cases are real but the names have been changed.

E. Kraus, *Beyond Left and Right Handedness*, https://doi.org/10.1007/978-3-031-24389-9_12

left hander (D-Type Variation); **David** a pathological right hander (M-type Variation); and **Bernard** a converted left hander (E-Type Variation) with motor deficits. **Hugo** is a variable left hander (D-type Variation) with more pronounced deficits on the left side, thus with elements of *pathological Right Handedness* (M-type Variation).

Each case starts with the reason for referral and a brief medical history, followed by the results of the different Handedness Profile (HP) subtests and the Category Profile. The cases are analysed using the HP Analysis Tools such as the Cluster Table with the HP Stairs. This tool helps to determine the largest clusters of applicable criteria that indicate particular handedness variations to be responsible for the variable hand use. The results are then interpreted and recommendations made. Except for the children's names, all information provided here is based on real cases.

12.2 Zelda: Variable Left Hander without Motor Deficiencies

♦**Handedness Code**[2] **VL.E0.M0/M00**[3]

12.2.1 Background Information

Zelda is 9 years old. According to her mother, she "swapps hands constantly depending on the situation". This unusual behaviour led to the referral to occupational therapy. However, apart from the tendency to reverse letters and a slight weakness in spelling, there are no indicators for atypical development or problems at participation level. Zelda's grades at school are good. She also has excellent fine and gross motor skills—she draws and paints a lot and performs very well at sports.

Zelda is the second of five children. The mother reports that pregnancy and birth were unremarkable. At 4 months, Zelda developed febrile convulsions and was hospitalised for 2 days without further complications. Zelda has an older 11-year-old brother, a 7-year-old sister and two younger brothers (5 and 2 years old). The older brother and sister are right handed, the 5-year-old brother seems more left handed and the youngest is still alternating hand use. Zelda's parents are both right handed, but some left handers are on the paternal side. Zelda's mother reports a decisive openness to *Left Handedness* in the family since the parents try to keep the environment neutral so that Zelda can experiment which hand to use for different activities.

Zelda presents as a friendly, cheerful child prepared to play along with the assessment "games" of the Handedness Profile (designed mainly for 4- to 7-year-olds), even though she is older. It is observed that she generally shows good motor skills with both hands.

12.2.2 Results of Handedness Profile

Functional Hand Preference Test (FHPT)

In the untrained FHPT, Zelda uses her left hand for half of the items and her right hand for the other half of unimanual activities. Six items are performed with the left hand, the others with the right. For 67% of items, she also shows ♦**internal consistency** (i.e. she always chooses the same hand for four performances).

The right hand performs only 8% more items than the left hand for the unimanual trained items. The bimanual untrained items are performed 36% more with the right hand. Interestingly, Zelda consistently executes four of the six items with her right hand and the other two only with her left, resulting in 100% internal consistency for the untrained bimanual items. Bimanual trained items were performed 28% more with the right hand, and only half of these showed internal consistency (Fig. 12.1).

[2] Handedness Codes of the Handedness Typology are used for quick reference of archived cases and for research purposes. They help identify at one glance the interplay between degree of handedness, environmental influences and motor abilities corresponding to the handedness types (see Sects. 10.2.1–10.2.11). The most prominent handedness type is coded first, followed by the second most prominent and the least prominent is placed last (see Sect. 8.7.2 for detail).

[3] Zelda's code summarises that it in the first instance, there is *Variable Left Handedness* (VL), with no deliberate rightward bias from the environment (E0), and average to above average motor abilities (M0/M00).

Ability (Untrained Proficiency): Hammering and Tapping

The Ability test shows that Zelda's untrained proficiency is 2% better when hammering with the right, whilst tapping is 2% better with the left hand. There is no difference between the hands when these two tasks are averaged for the Ability score. Since Zelda is older than 6 years, the available normative data is not applicable. However, her movement quality is good; she can perform the tasks quickly and efficiently, indicating that she has no motor deficits. The optical results of the Hammering and Tapping strikes are similar between the hands (Fig. 12.2).

Skill (Trained Proficiency): Tracing and Dotting

Zelda shows very good Skill with both hands during the tracing and dotting tasks. When comparing the two bear tracings, it is apparent that Zelda's performance is better on the left even though the right hand performs very well (Fig. 12.3). Zelda starts tracing with her left hand and achieves 10% better results compared to the right hand.

Zelda also starts dotting with her left hand and is faster and more accurate with this hand, outperforming the right hand by 18%. Overall, her average Skill is 14% better with the left hand. Zelda unambiguously states that the left hand felt better than the right.

Crossing the Body Midline

The Midline Crossing Test, shows predominantly right-handed responses: Zelda crosses four out of ten possible reactions with her right hand and picks up 80% of the centre Lego pieces with her right hand. She tends to have more ipsilateral reactions (i.e. picking up Lego pieces on the left side with the left hand and on the right side with the right hand).

Bimanual Cooperation

In the simultaneous bimanual circle drawing, the quality of circles and movements are very similar

Untrained unimanual (untr-uni)					
	Right (R)	Left (L)	Consistency	1. Hand	Atypical swaps
a2 Shaking box	4	0	R	r	0
a3 Teddy bear and soccer	3	1		r	0
b2 Putting pegs in pegboa	0	4	L	l	0
c1 Spinning top	0	4	L	l	0
d1 Building tower	3	1		r	0
d2 Rolling dice	2	2		l	0
Bonuspoints (R/L)	0,5	0,5			
Total (R/L)	12,5	12,5			
Use-Percentage	50	50			
IHD untr-uni (LQ)	0				

Trained unimanual (tr-uni)					
	Right (R)	Left (L)	Consistency	1. Hand	Atypical swaps
f1 Using toothbrush	3	1		l	0
f2 Eating with spoon	4	0	R	r	0
f5 Cutting with knife	2	2		r	0
g1 Writing in the air	0	4	L	l	0
h1 Drawing on paper	0	4	L	l	0
l1 Throwing ball	4	0	R	r	0
Bonuspoints (R/L)	0,5	0,5			
Total (R/L)	13,5	11,5			
Use-Percentage	54	46			
IHD tr-uni (LQ)	8				

Untrained bimanual (untr-bim)					
	Right (R)	Left (L)	Consistency	1. Hand	Atypical swaps
a1 Opening box	4	0	R	r	0
d3 Handbroom and dustpa	0	4	L	l	0
e1 Dealing cards	4	0	R	r	0
f3 Opening Tube	4	0	R	r	0
h2 Taking off stickers	0	4	L	l	0
k1 Tightening bolt and nut	4	0	R	r	0
Bonuspoints (R/L)	1	0			
Total (R/L)	17	8			
Use-Percentage	68	32			
IHD un-bi (LQ)	36				

Trained bimanual (tr-bim)					
	Right (R)	Left (L)	Consistency	1. Hand	Atypical swaps
b1 Sewing with lace	2	2		l	0
f4 Knife and fork	2	2		r	0
h3 Cutting with scissors	4	0	R	r	0
i1 Striking a match	3	1		r	0
j1 Putting key in lock	0	4	L	l	0
k2 Opening with screwdrive	4	0	R	r	0
Bonuspoints (R/L)	1	0			
Total (R/L)	16	9			
Use-Percentage	64	36			
IHD tr-bim (LQ)	28				

	Untrained	Trained	Uni- Bim
Unimanual	0	8	4
Bimanual	36	28	32
IHD (LQ)	18	18	
FHPT Total (LQ)	18		

Internal Consistency	
Right	38
Left	29
Total consistency	67
Number of atypical swaps	0

Fig. 12.1 Zelda's FHPT Test Results

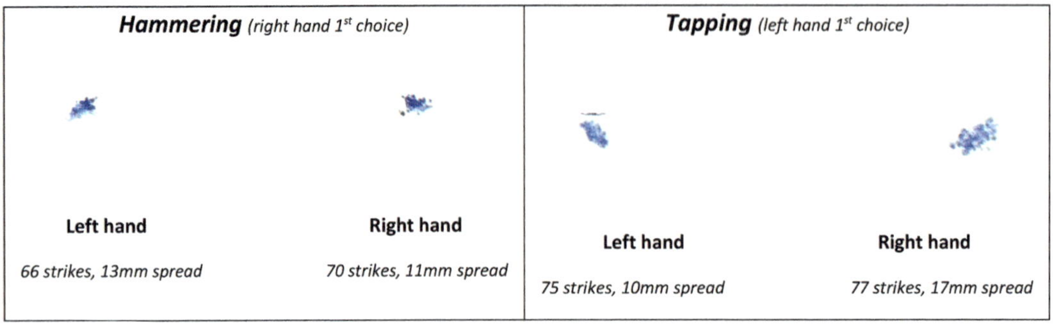

Fig. 12.2 Zelda's Ability Test: Hammering and Tapping results with the left and right hand

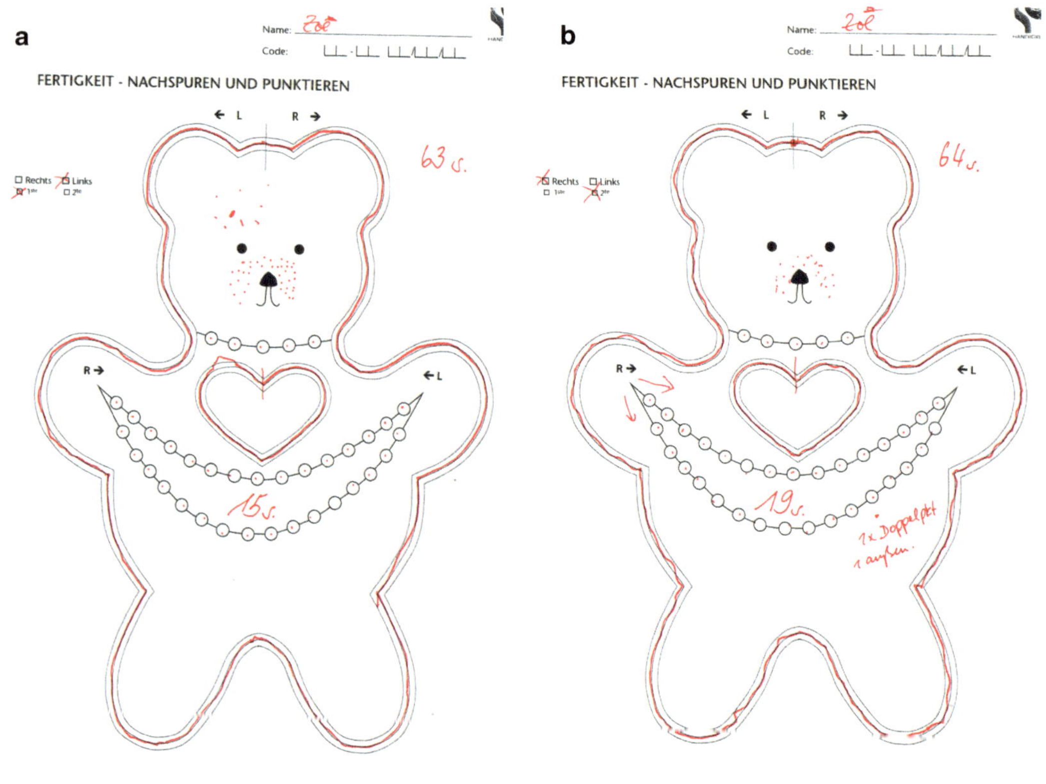

Fig. 12.3 Zelda's Skill Test: Tracing and Dotting Test results with left and right hands

and high on both sides, with the left hand leading marginally (Fig. 12.4).

Category Profile

The differences between the hands (also referred to as inter-hand differences or IHD) in the five subtests are summarised in the Category Profile based on laterality quotients of the subtests (Fig. 12.5).

Although Zelda always writes and draws with her left hand, her average preference values in the FHPT are slightly higher on the right. Also, in the Midline Crossing Test, a hand preference test, she used her right hand more often than the left. The Ability Test (Hammering and Tapping) shows no differences between the hands, whereas the Skill Test (tracing and dotting) displays a left-hand superiority. In the Bimanual Cooperation

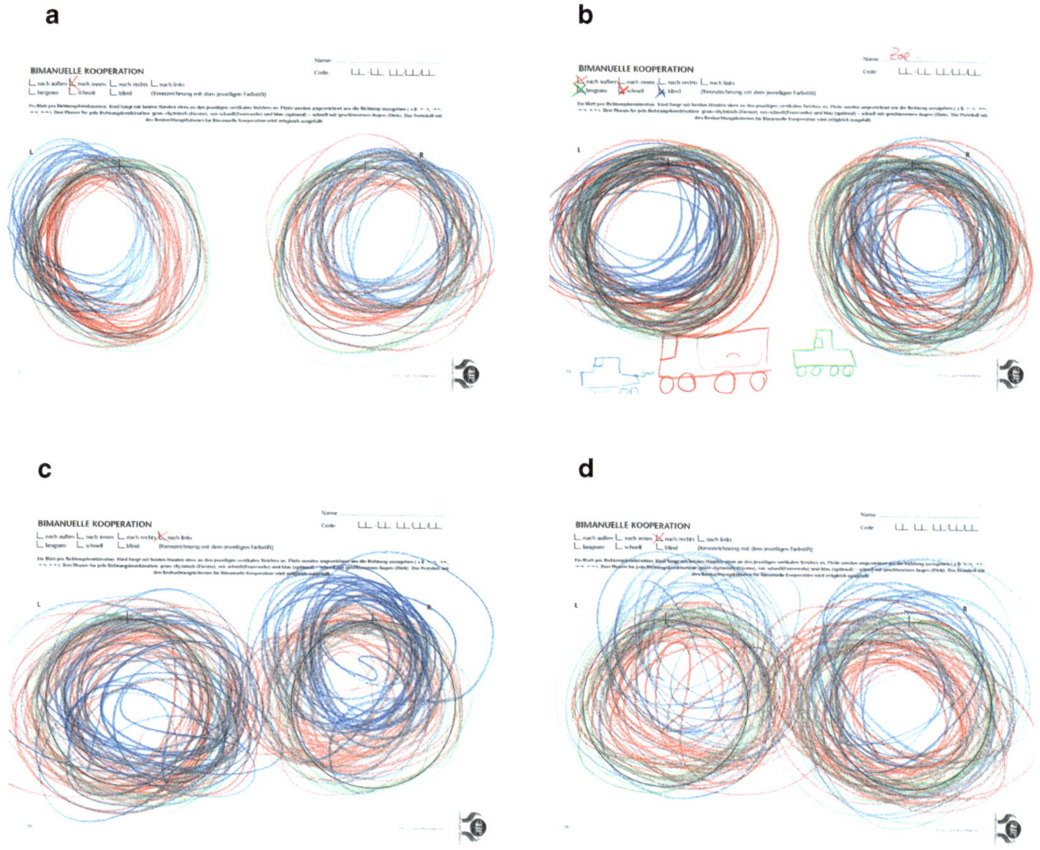

Fig. 12.4 Zelda's Simultaneous Bimanual Circle Drawings

Level of Proficiency				CATEGORY PROFILE	Degree of Handedness in 8 Categories												
Proficiency Categories			Proficiency values of L & R hands		Inter-Hand Difference (IHD) *(Laterality Quotient)*				large IHD			small IHD					large IHD
below average	borderline	average	*Percentage values*	Handedness dimensions	PARTIAL Laterality Quotients *(Inter-Hand Differences)*		TOTAL Laterality Quotients *(Inter-Hand Differences)*		L+ 75th-100th Percentile	L 25th-74th Percentile	L- 10th-15th Percentile	VL 1st-9th Percentile	No difference	VR 1st-9th Percentile	R- 10th-15th Percentile	R 25th-74th Percentile	R+ 75-100 Percentile
1	2	3	Category Values						1	2	3	4	4,5	5	6	7	8
		X	Internal consistency Total 67	***Preference:*** untrained FHP	Unimanual 0	Bimanual 36	Untrained 18	Total -21									
			Right 38 Left 29	***Preference:*** trained FHP	Unimanual 8	Bimanual 28	Trained 18										
		R L	Right 71 Left 71	***Motor Ability***	Hammering 2	Tapping -2	Total 0										
		R L	Right 66 Left 80	***Motor Skill***	Tracing -10	Dotting -18	Total -14										
	X		Contralat. Reaction 20	***Crossing the Midline***	Right 40 / Centre 80	Left 0	Total 40										
		X	Movement Quality 3	***Bimanual Cooperation***	Mirror -11	Parallel 7	Total -2										

Fig. 12.5 Zelda's Category Profile. **Degree of handedness** (columns on the right): Zelda's overall degree of preference and proficiency averages at 4.42 (5 + 5 + 4.5 + 2 + 6 + 4 = 26.5:6 = 4.42), i.e. almost in the "no difference" category. **Proficiency** (columns on the left): although performance is in the average range, it is not applicable since Zelda is too old for the normative data based on 6-year-old typically developed children. However, her motor skills appear good and at least age-appropriate at face value. Overall, her profile supports the D-based handedness type with the Variation *Variable Left Handedness* (VLH). *FHP* functional hand preference

Test, the left hand is slightly better. In all the motor tests, Zelda performs very well on both sides.

12.2.3 Interpretation and Summary

The ♦**Cluster Table** and the ♦**HP Stairs** (see Chap. 9) summarise quantitative and qualitative information from subtests (i.e. laterality quotients), questionnaires and checklists. They take into account relevant aspects of the complex individual background information, indicating possible causal factors for variable hand use. In Zelda's case, the largest (I) cluster aggregates around the D-based Variation *Variable Left Handedness* (65%) without motor deficiency. With 61%, the second-largest cluster (II) is the Variation *Ambidexterity*, with criteria for both hands performing equally well, including writing. However, this does not apply to Zelda, since she only writes with her left hand, so this variation can be excluded from the analysis (indicated by the bracket (II)). The third-largest cluster (III) with 26% on the variation *Left Handedness*, followed by (IV) *Variable Right Handedness* (21%). There will inevitably be an overlap between *Variable Left Handedness* and *Left Handedness*, explaining the third-largest cluster. *Variable Right Handedness* is arguably the variation that contains an unbeknown number of converted variable left handers that have adapted without significant problems. Some of the criteria of *Variable Left Handedness* would apply here too. However, Zelda is not a converted hander, so this cluster can also be excluded from analysis (IV). The other clusters are too small in comparison and can be neglected. Zelda's HP Stairs are shown in Fig. 12.6.

Overall, Zelda shows the profile of a *Variable Left Hander* with small inter-hand differences. Her motor skills and abilities are generally good and may even be above average, explaining the high cluster for *Ambidexterity*. The cluster under the Variation *Left Handedness* supports the direction of *Variable Left Handedness*. It is not surprising that *Variable Right Handedness* also emerges with a larger cluster since Zelda's shows a slightly higher *preference* for her right than her left hand. However, her proficiency is considerably better on the left, despite the very good performance of her non-dominant right hand.

12.2.4 Recommendations

Zelda continues to write with her left hand. There is no clear preference in some of her everyday actions since she equally uses her left or right hand. However, for several specific and more

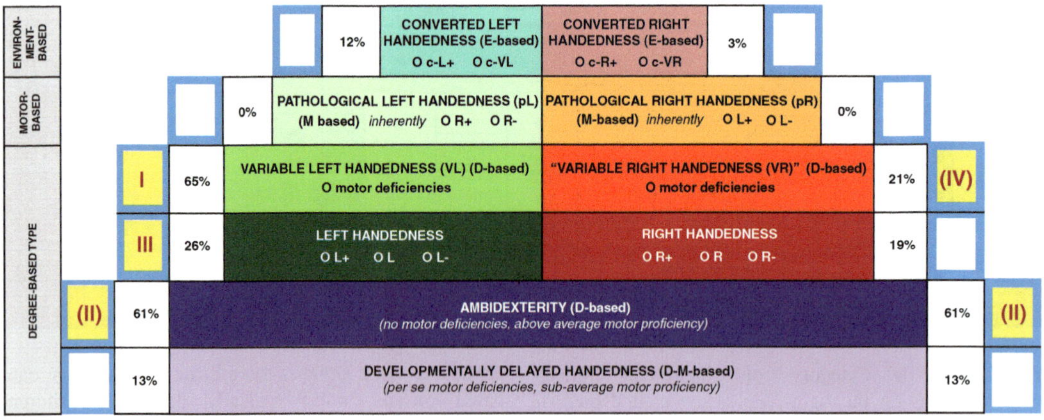

Fig. 12.6 Zelda's HP Stairs. Zelda's largest cluster is found in the D-based Variation *Variable Left Handedness*, followed by the variations *Ambidextrous Handedness* and *Left Handedness*. However, since she only writes with her left hand, Ambidexterity can be excluded from the analysis

demanding activities, she always uses her right hand (e.g. throwing a ball) or the left (e.g. writing).

Zelda copes very well with her variable hand use in her everyday life, showing high efficiency in her performance and no functional limitation or restriction in her participation. Thus, there is no need to make any changes or for intervention.

12.3 David: Pathological Right Hander

Handedness Code: M11(l).R.E1[4]

12.3.1 Background Information

David is in his first year of school and has fine motor skills and visual perception difficulties. He has been attending a particular occupational therapy practice for only 4 weeks. His mother is concerned because she suspects that David has been switched from left to right. His parents separated recently, and there is little contact with his father. A few months ago, David was tested at another occupational therapy practice, where the results showed a clear *Right Handedness*. However, the mother believes that David influenced the results by deliberately using his right hand. She reports that he often uses his left hand when he plays alone and then changes to the right when he feels being observed. She thus changed occupational therapy practice to obtain a second opinion and further clarification of David's handedness.

According to David's mother, there were no difficulties during the pregnancy. A caesarian delivered him at 38 weeks due to some problems of the uterus at the end of pregnancy. His Apgar scores were normal. David has exhibited fine motor problems since early childhood. His mother reports that Davide showed early left handed use, and she believes that his father caused him to switch handedness since he was not in favour of David being left handed. According to her, David changes hands during activities such as building and playing with cars, but he now consistently uses his right hand when drawing and writing.

During the assessment, David is friendly, if somewhat cautious initially, but he soon becomes more open and can be easily motivated. He seems frequently distracted by movement and sound but is willing to engage in the games of the FHPT. Towards the end of the test, his concentration wanes.

12.3.2 Results of Handedness Profile

Functional Hand Preference Test (FHPT)

The FHPT shows that David performs all *trained* activities exclusively with his right hand and thus achieves a very high internal consistency (overall with 96%). He also performs the unimanual untrained items exclusively with his right hand. David uses his left hand only in two bimanual items: He consistently opens the tube and removes the stickers with his left hand. Overall, he achieved an FHPT laterality quotient of 82% (see Fig. 12.7).

Ability (Untrained Proficiency): Hammering and Tapping

David hammers more accurately and quickly with his right hand, performing 24% better on the right than the left. Similarly, the right hand performs significantly better and more accurately in the tapping task. In 15 s, David manages 50 strikes with his right hand and only 37 with his left. Accordingly, the tapping laterality quotient is 20% better on the right. On average, his right score is superior to the left, with 22% better in the untrained proficiency Ability Test based on an average of the Hammering and Tapping tasks (see Fig. 12.8).

Skill (Trained Proficiency): Tracing and Dotting

David shows better right hand performance when tracing in the trained proficiency tasks. Although

[4] David's code summarises that major motor problems (M11) that have resulted in his an inherent *Left Handedness* (l), to be formed into a moderate *Right Handedness* (R), with the environment also having some influence (E1).

Untrained unimanual (untr-uni)					
	Right (R)	Left (L)	Consis-tency	1. Hand	Atypical swaps
a2 Shaking box	4	0	R	r	0
a3 Teddy bear and soccer	4	0	R	r	0
b2 Putting pegs in pegboa	3	1		r	2
c1 Spinning top	4	0	R	r	0
d1 Building tower	4	0	R	r	0
d2 Rolling dice	4	0	R	r	4
Bonuspoints (R/L)	1	0			
Total (R/L)	24	1			
Use-Percentage	96	4			
IHD untr-uni (LQ)	92				

Trained unimanual (tr-uni)					
	Right (R)	Left (L)	Consis-tency	1. Hand	Atypical swaps
f1 Using toothbrush	4	0	R	r	0
f2 Eating with spoon	4	0	R	r	0
f5 Cutting with knife	4	0	R	r	0
g1 Writing in the air	4	0	R	r	0
h1 Drawing on paper	4	0	R	r	0
l1 Throwing ball	4	0	R	r	0
Bonuspoints (R/L)	1	0			
Total (R/L)	25	0			
Use-Percentage	100	0			
IHD tr-uni (LQ)	100				

Untrained bimanual (untr-bim)					
	Right (R)	Left (L)	Consis-tency	1. Hand	Atypical swaps
a1 Opening box	4	0	R	r	0
d3 Handbroom and dustpa	4	0	R	r	0
e1 Dealing cards	4	0	R	r	0
f3 Opening Tube	0	4	L	l	0
h2 Taking off stickers	0	4	L	l	1
k1 Tightening bolt and nut	4	0	R	r	0
Bonuspoints (R/L)	1	0			
Total (R/L)	17	8			
Use-Percentage	68	32			
IHD un-bi (LQ)	36				

Trained bimanual (tr-bim)					
	Right (R)	Left (L)	Consis-tency	1. Hand	Atypical swaps
b1 Sewing with lace	4	0	R	r	0
f4 Knife and fork	4	0	R	r	0
h3 Cutting with scissors	4	0	R	r	1
i1 Striking a match	4	0	R	r	0
j1 Putting key in lock	4	0	R	r	0
k2 Opening with screwdrive	4	0	R	r	0
Bonuspoints (R/L)	1	0			
Total (R/L)	25	0			
Use-Percentage	100	0			
IHD tr-bim (LQ)	100				

	Untrained	Trained	Uni- Bim
Unimanual	92	100	95
Bimanual	36	100	68
IHD (LQ)	64	100	
FHPT Total (LQ)	82		

Internal Consistency	
Right	88
Left	8
Total consistency	96
Number of atypical swaps	8

Fig. 12.7 David's Results of the FHPT

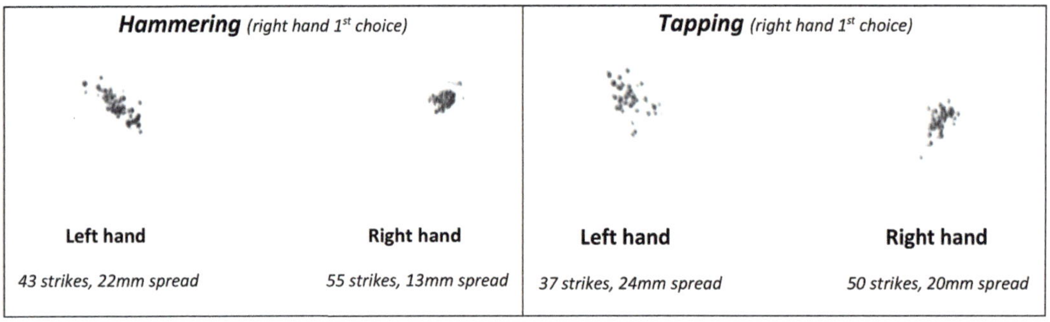

Fig. 12.8 David's Ability Test—Hammering and Tapping with the left and right hands

he needs the same amount of time for the left and right hands (31 s), his right hand is more accurate when staying on the centre line, resulting in an 11% superior performance compared to the left. The right hand also produces dots markedly faster (21 s) than the left hand (35 s). David places all dots into the circles with his right hand with good quality; the left hand seems to find this task difficult. The difference between the hands is stark: 32% better on the right. Overall, the Skill quotient for Tracing and Dotting is 22% better on the right (see Fig. 12.9).

Crossing the Body Midline

In the Midline Crossing Test (MCT), David shows a left handed phase but overall his right hand more often than the left two contralateral responses, six centre responses and four left ipsilateral responses. The right hand also crosses the midline more than the left (six times). Added together, the hands show an 80% midline crossing percentage. The left contralateral responses are subtracted from the right to calculate inter-hand differences, resulting in a midline crossing *quotient* of 40% shows

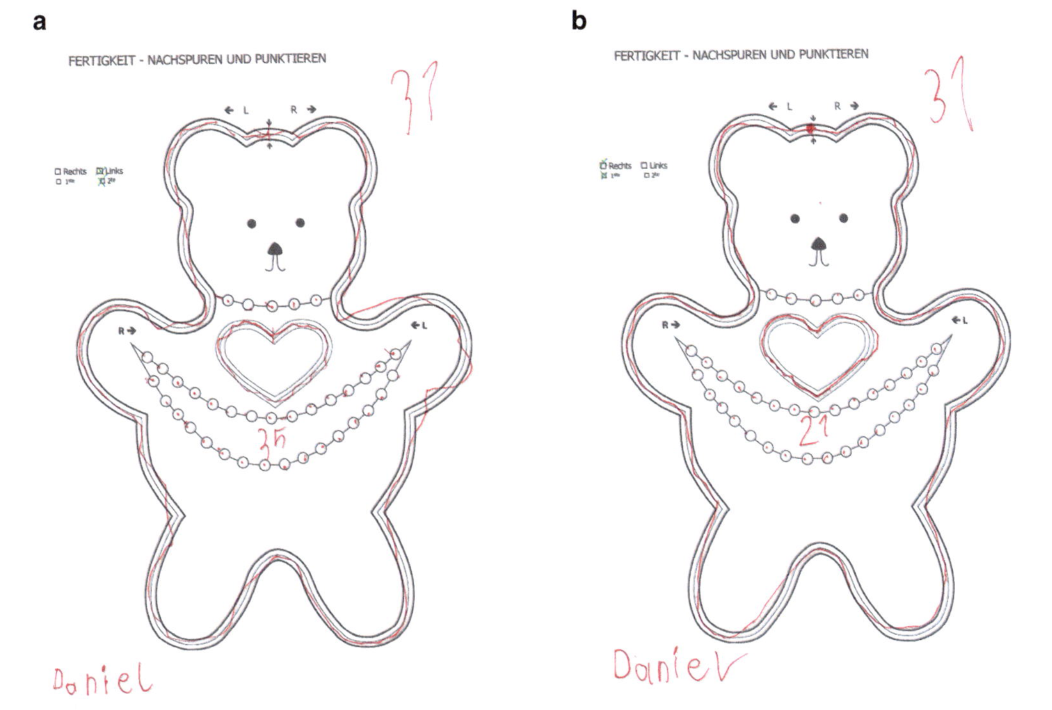

Fig. 12.9 David's Skill Test—Tracing and Dotting with the left and right hand

greater responses with the right hand. These results indicate that avoiding crossing the body midline is not responsible for his hand use variability.

Bimanual Circle Drawing

In the simultaneous bimanual circle drawing task, David could not maintain the direction with his left hand, even in slow and mirror-image movements. Accordingly, there is a very high difference between the hands: the right hand performs 71% better than the left. Furthermore, the quality of the circles is average to borderline on the right side, whilst it is below average on the left side (see Fig. 12.10).

Category Profile

The differences between the hands (inter-hand differences, IHD) in the five HP subtests are summarised in the Category Profile based on laterality quotients (see Fig. 12.11).

David shows a strong right-hand preference for untrained and, even more so, for trained items. He twice uses his left hand in bimanual untrained tasks and achieves an overall laterality quotient of 82% more right than left. In the untrained tasks, hammering and tapping his right hand performs in the average range and is much better than his left, which scores below average (below the tenth percentile). In trained proficiency, tracing and dotting (both of which show a high correlation with writing), the right hand also shows superior performance, with the left hand ranging below the 10th percentile.

David repeatedly crosses his body midline (an indication of neurological maturity)—but not consistently: he crosses over with both hands, more so with his right (60%) than with his left (20%). There seems to be a "left" phase during this test.

During the simultaneous bimanual circle drawing, David occasionally focuses on his left hand and then seemed to "forget" his right hand. His movement quality in the bimanual cooperation task is rated borderline, with a better performance clearly on the right.

David states in all motor tests that his right hand feels (a lot) "better" than the left.

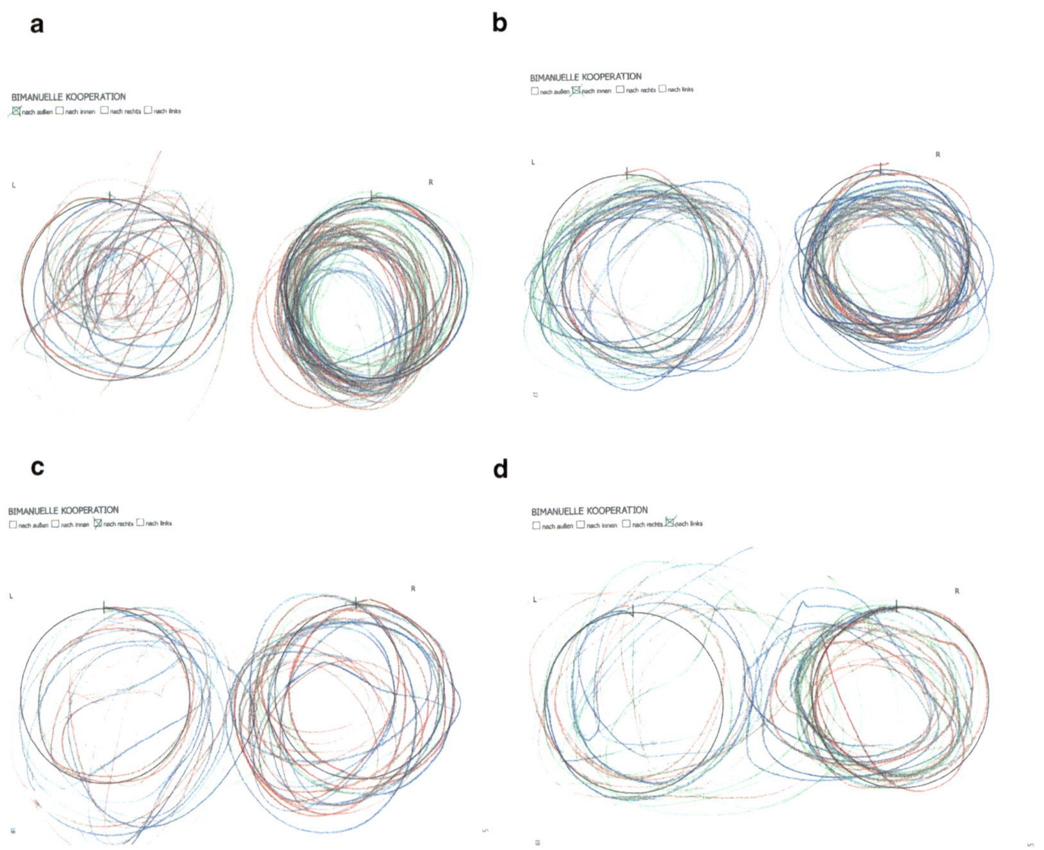

Fig. 12.10 David's Simultaneous Bimanual Circle Drawings

Level of Proficiency				CATEGORY PROFILE	Degree of Handedness in 8 Categories										
Proficiency Categories			Proficiency values of L & R hands		Inter-Hand Difference (IHD) *(Laterality Quotient)*		large IHD			small IHD					large IHD
below average	borderline	average	*Percentage values*	Handedness dimensions	PARTIAL Laterality Quotients *(Inter-Hand Differences)*	TOTAL Laterality Quotients *(Inter-Hand Differences)*	L+ 75th-100th Percentile	L 25th-74th Percentile	L- 10th-15th Percentile	VL 1st-9th Percentile	No difference	VR 1st-9th Percentile	R- 10th-15th Percentile	R 25th-74th Percentile	R+ 75th-100th Percentile
1	2	3	Category Values				1	?	3	4	4,5	5	6	7	8
		X	Internal consistency Total 96 Right 88 Left 8	***Preference:*** untrained FHP	Unimanual 92 / Bimanual 36	Untrained 64 / Total 82									
				Preference: trained FHP	Unimanual 100 / Bimanual 100	Trained 100									
L		R	Right 53 Left 31	***Motor Ability***	Hammering 24 / Tapping 20	Total 22									
L		R	Right 64 Left 42	***Motor Skill***	Tracing 11 / Dotting 32	Total 22									
		X	Contralat. Reaction 40	***Crossing the Midline***	Right 60 / Centre 60 / Left 20	Total 40									
	X		Movement Quality 2	***Bimanual Cooperation***	Mirror 72 / Parallel 69	Total 71									

Fig. 12.11 David's Category Profile. **Degree of handedness** (columns on the right): David's overall degree or extent of both preference and proficiency averages at 7.33 (7 + 8 + 8 + 8 + 6 + 7 = 42:6 = 7.33), i.e., is clearly on the right. **Proficiency** (columns on the left): this is in the average range for the right hand and the sub-average range for the left hand. Overall, his profile supports either a moderate to explicit right handedness, or the M-based handedness type with the Variation *pathological Right Handedness* (*p-RH*), with a left-sided motor weakness in particulart

12.3.3 Interpretation and Summary

As we can see from David's HP Stairs (Fig. 12.12), the largest cluster (I) aggregates around D-based variation *Right Handedness* with motor deficiencies (69%). Understandably, the third-largest cluster of *Variable Right Handedness* (54%) would share some of the same criteria as *Right Handedness* and thus supports the first cluster. This variation likely contains mild-degree converted left handers since right handers tend to have moderate to explicit degrees and form a more homogenous group. In David's case, however, the values for *Left Handedness* and *Variable Left Handedness* are so small that *Variable Right Handedness* as an explanation for alternating hand use does not seem convincing.

The second-largest cluster (II) indicates the M-based variation *pathological Right Handedness* (67%). This presumably means that a genetically predisposed left-handed person incurs some impairment to the contralateral dominant motor cortex resulting in motor deficiencies on the left. There should be evidence of pre-, peri- or postnatal stress for this variation. In addition, the Category Profile should show several large inter-hand differences, with sub-average motor performance, particularly on the left. Both criteria apply to David: He was delivered 2 weeks early by caesarean section due to premature labour and problems with the unterus. The difference between the hands is very large (R+) in hammering and tapping, and moderate in tracing and dotting. In addition, the observations of a left-handed phase during the Midline Crossing Test and also by his mother at home for undemanding tasks fit the variation of *pathological Right Handedness*. The left-handed phases also seem to be related to his occasional visual attention to the left side, which significantly worsened the motor performance of the right hand. The left hand deteriorated somewhat when he was focussing on the right. This indicates some deficiencies in bimanual cooperation.

The fourth-largest cluster (IV) of 31% aggregates around the E-based variation *converted Left Handedness*. The relatively high percentage is based on the mother's report that David's father converted his handedness in the early years when David used his left hand frequently at one year. After that, David started to prefer his right hand but repeatedly displayed left-handed phases. Since we know that handedness only becomes established after the age of 3, alternating left- and right-handed phases are to be expected within the first 2 years of life. Thus, early left-handed phases in the first year of life in isolation are not strong predictors of *Left Handedness*.

The D-based Variation *Developmentally Delayed Handedness* is the fifth-largest cluster

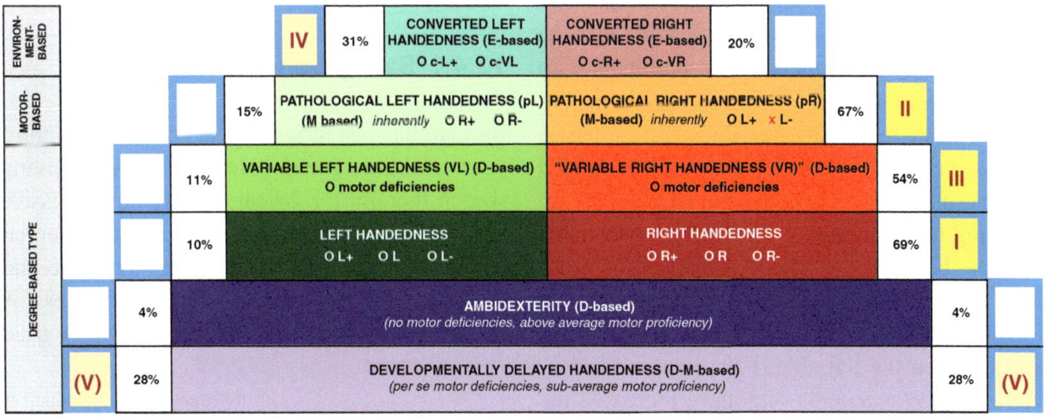

Fig. 12.12 David's HP Stairs. The largest cluster is seen in the Variation *Right Handedness*, followed by *pathological Right Handedness* and *Variable Right Handedness*. David's occasional use of his left hand during undemanding activities and his consistent use of the right hand for more complex and demanding tasks are typical for a pathological right hander with a left-sided weakness (Kraus and Nagele-Hiedl 2019)

(V) with 28%. This cluster is aggregated because of David's motor deficiencies, particularly on the left side. However, his hand use is unambiguously right, not comparable to children who have not established a preferred or more proficient hand due to developmental delay. For this reason, this cluster can be excluded from the analysis.

In David's case, a total of two main clusters emerge that would best explain his Handedness Profile. He shows a moderately pronounced *Right Handedness* with motor problems that primarily affect his bimanual coordination and his left hand's unimanual performance. Explicit *Right Handedness* with left-emphasised motor problems and large inter-hand differences verifies the second largest cluster of *pathological Right Handedness*. It would mean that David is originally a left-handed person whose motor areas of the right (dominant) brain hemisphere (dominant for him) were impaired possibly due to birth difficulties. As a result, the motor development on the right side developed better from the beginning. The observed left-handed phases could be due to an inherent *Left Handedness*, which is still occasionally revealed in motorically undemanding activities.

The third-largest cluster of *converted Left Handedness* may also have played a role, but this is unlikely to be the main cause of his alternating hand use. In conversation with the mother, it became clear that the separation from her husband was a great stress factor for her and that she feels rather overwhelmed by the problems with David's fine motor skills. She has read about converted handedness and possible consequences, she observes David's occasional left-handed actions, and she remembers his father insisting on using the right hand. So it is understandable that she believes that David's fine motor problems result from handedness conversion. Whilst this is plausible, it does not explain his inherent weakness on the left side. For this reason, *converted Left Handedness* may have increased the use of the right hand, but it is unlikely that it would be the main cause.

Concerns that David could have deliberately controlled his hand use during the test cannot be confirmed since he was very absorbed in the games, not realising that he was engaged in a handedness assessment.

12.3.4 Recommendations

Irrespective of whether we assign David's results to a right-handed person with some motor deficiencies or a pathological right hander, he should continue writing with his right hand. The left hand is significantly weaker, and David prefers to use the right unambiguously. Occupational therapy should primarily aim to improve writing skills with the right hand. Both David and his mother need to be informed about the results of his Handedness Profile.

Follow-Up

David continued writing with his right hand. The left-handed phases became rarer, even though therapy continued to focus on bimanual coordination and bimanual cooperation activities in addition to the handwriting programme.

12.4 Bernard: Converted Left Hander with Motor Deficiencies

Handedness Code: E1/E2.L-.M1[5]

12.4.1 Background Information

Bernard has just turned 5 years and is in his third year of kindergarten. He has been receiving speech therapy for 2 years due to an expressive speech disorder. The speech therapist observed Bernard frequently alternating his hand use and recommended clarification of his handedness. A decision is imminent on which hand will be used

[5] Bernard's code summarises that environmental influences (E1) led to a conversion of a mild left hander (L−) who has some motor problems (M1) and is currently reverting back to the dominant left hand (E2).

for drawing and writing once he starts the preparatory preschool programme.

Bernard's mother explains that he permanently v including drawing and cutting. According to her Bernard has become more unsure of his actions and no longer knows which hand he should use for certain activities. There are left handers on the maternal side. His two older siblings and his parents are right handed.

The mother reports that Bernard was born in the 40th week of pregnancy and delivered by caesarean section because the umbilical cord was wrapped around his neck. His weight and size were average. His birth cry was delayed, but the Apgar scores were normal. According to his mother, Bernard's general development was age-appropriate except for his speech. From age 3, he thus received speech therapy to address his expressive speech disorder, particularly to improve his vocabulary and reduce grammatical errors. She reports that Bernard can concentrate well and seems interested in his environment. He likes to imitate his older siblings and strives to be like them. His fine motor skills seem to have developed age-appropriately, and he can use both his left and right hand equally well. She believes that he does not experience difficulties in everyday activities and she thinks he is age-appropriately developed, except for his swapping-hands behaviour, which seems to affect spontaneous and trained activities. During drawing, he tends to work from right to left rather than from left to right (the direction of reading and writing). Whilst Bernard generally avoids drawing tasks, he frequently changes the pencil when he does draw, with an emerging preference for the right hand. He shows little initiative and imagination when drawing and doing crafts. His mother also notices that Bernard, unlike his siblings, always mounts his bike from the right side, and during a children's gymnastic course, he tends to perform the movement sequences and patterns the "other way round". Generally, she describes him as a child who strives to do everything correctly and who does not want to be different from other children.

The speech therapist reports that Bernard has recently developed better pencil grip and control on the right and seems to have consciously decided to use his right hand for drawing. However, she has observed that he tenses up during drawing and tends to swap hands, especially during other fine motor activities.

Bernard seems a little reserved at first but adapts well to the situation after a while. He generally avoids speaking, and his vocabulary, sentence structure and speech flow seem less age-appropriate. He only verbally expresses himself spontaneously when experiencing difficulties. Bernard is interested in activities with pen and paper and could write his name. Pencil grip and control have are not yet stable, fluent or automated.

12.4.2 Results of Handedness Profile

Functional Hand Preference Test (FHPT)

Bernard performs the trained unimanual activities (e.g. drawing, throwing, eating with a spoon) 16% more with his left hand. Also, the left hand is used more consistently within a specific activity. With trained bimanual tasks (e.g. using a fork and knife, cutting with scissors, lighting a match, opening a lock), he used the right hand 20% more than the left. Both hands are used equally for other activities, such as sewing with a shoelace. The untrained unimanual tasks (e.g. spinning tops, building a tower, throwing dice) are performed more with the left hand (28%), and in untrained bimanual tasks (e.g. opening the tube, dealing cards), he used the left hand predominantly (68%). Overall, Bernard uses his left hand 23% more than the right, particularly in untrained tasks (see Fig. 12.13).

Ability (Untrained Proficiency): Hammering and Tapping

Bernard's right hand manages 36 strikes in 15 s in the hammering task, being slightly faster than the left hand (33 strikes), but the left hand is more accurate with a 10 mm spread than 13 mm on the right. When tapping, the right hand is a little slower (35 strikes) than the left (38 strikes) but also more accurate (10 mm compared to 13 mm spread on the left). Notably, the right hand uses very little pressure, making the strikes hardly rec-

Untrained unimanual (untr-uni)					
	Right (R)	Left (L)	Consis-tency	1. Hand	Atypical swaps
a2 Shaking box	4	0	R	r	
a3 Teddy bear and soccer	0	4	L	l	
b2 Putting pegs in pegboa	0	4	L	l	
c1 Spinning top	2	2		r	
d1 Building tower	1	3		r	
d2 Rolling dice	1	3		r	
Bonuspoints (R/L)	1	0			
Total (R/L)	9	16			
Use-Percentage	36	64			
IHD untr-uni (LQ)	-28				

Trained unimanual (tr-uni)					
	Right (R)	Left (L)	Consis-tency	1. Hand	Atypical swaps
f1 Using toothbrush	0	4	L	l	
f2 Eating with spoon	0	4	L	l	
f5 Cutting with knife	0	4	L	l	
g1 Writing in the air	4	0	R	r	
h1 Drawing on paper	4	0	R	r	
i1 Throwing ball	2	2		r	
Bonuspoints (R/L)	0,5	0,5			
Total (R/L)	10,5	14,5			
Use-Percentage	42	58			
IHD tr-uni (LQ)	-16				

Untrained bimanual (untr-bim)					
	Right (R)	Left (L)	Consis-tency	1. Hand	Atypical swaps
a1 Opening box	0	4	L	l	
d3 Handbroom and dustpa	4	0	R	r	
e1 Dealing cards	0	4	L	l	
f3 Opening Tube	0	4	L	l	
h2 Taking off stickers	0	4	L	l	
k1 Tightening bolt and nut	0	4	L	l	
Bonuspoints (R/L)	0	1			
Total (R/L)	4	21			
Use-Percentage	16	84			
IHD un-bi (LQ)	-68				

Trained bimanual (tr-bim)					
	Right (R)	Left (L)	Consis-tency	1. Hand	Atypical swaps
b1 Sewing with lace	2	2		r	1
f4 Knife and fork	4	0	R	r	
h3 Cutting with scissors	2	2		l	
i1 Striking a match	2	2		r	
j1 Putting key in lock	2	2		r	
k2 Opening with screwdrive	2	2		r	
Bonuspoints (R/L)	1	0			
Total (R/L)	15	10			
Use-Percentage	60	40			
IHD tr-bim (LQ)	20				

	Untrained	Trained	Uni- Bim
Unimanual	-28	-16	-22
Bimanual	-68	20	-24
IHD (LQ)	-48	2	
FHPT Total (LQ)	-23		

Internal Consistency	
Right	21
Left	42
Total consistency	63
Number of atypical swaps	1

Fig. 12.13 Bernard's Results of the FHPT

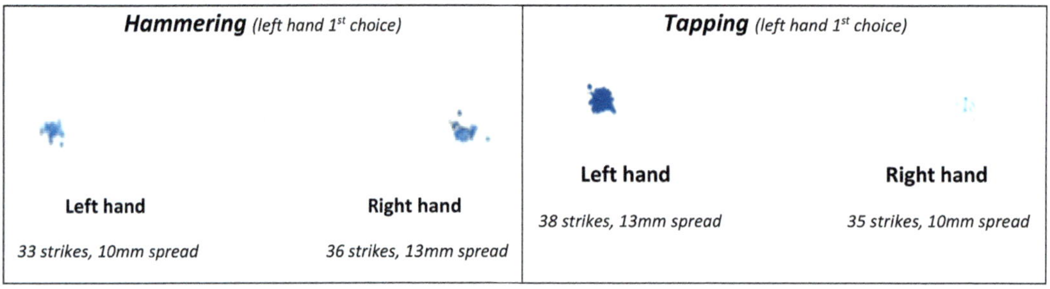

Fig. 12.14 Bernard's Ability test: Hammering and Tapping with the left and right hand

ognisable. On average, both hands perform similarly, but with a slight tendency (2%) to the left (Fig. 12.14).

Skill (Trained Proficiency): Tracing and Dotting

Bernard starts tracing with his right hand, taking 76 s to complete the task. His left hand performs the tracing task in only 49 s. Bernard is initially very motivated and tries very hard. However, the task seems particularly difficult for the right hand: he lifts the pen five times despite the explicit instructions not to do so, and he holds his breath during this concerted effort. Bernard seems much more relaxed with the left hand, and the movements are less laboured and more fluid. He lifts the pen only twice. There is no difference between the hands concerning his staying on the centre line. However, when dotting, the left hand is less accurate than the right, taking 44 s compared to the right hand with 29 seconds, and he shows clear signs of fatigue when dotting with the left hand (Fig. 12.15).

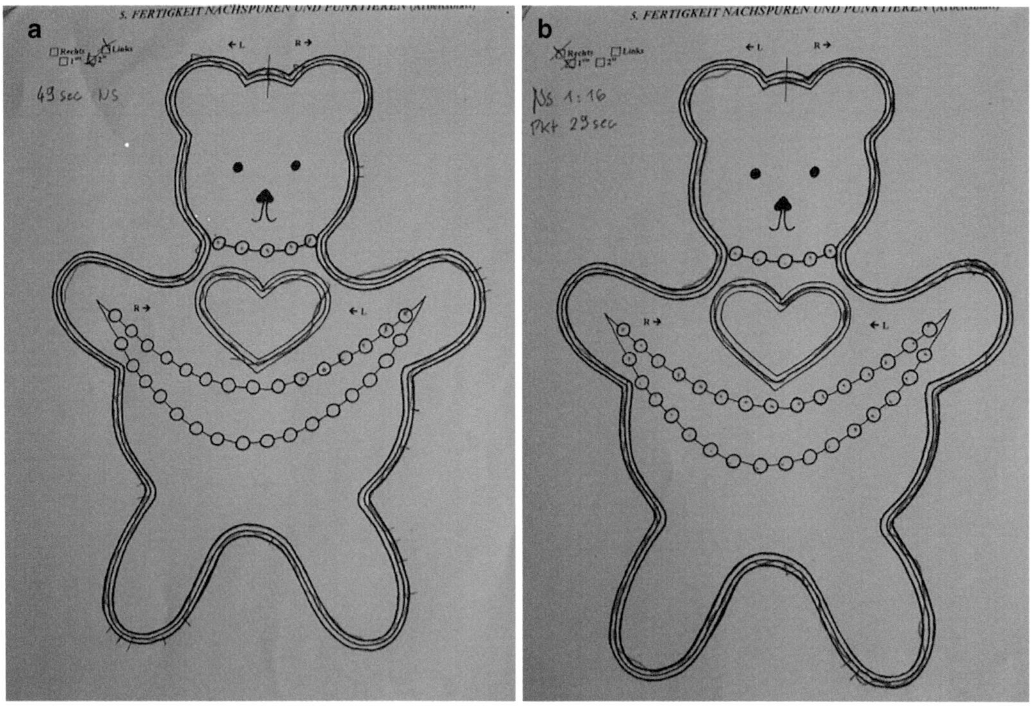

Fig. 12.15 Bernard's Skill Test: Tracing and Dotting with the left and right hand

Crossing the Body Midline

Bernard crosses the body midline 3 out of 20 times (twice with the left, once with the right), tending to avoid contralateral reaching. He picks up 9 out of 10 Lego pieces ipsilaterally (i.e. uses his right hand to pick up bricks on the right) and 8 of 10 Legos on the left side with his left hand. Bernard takes the Lego pieces in the middle exclusively with his right hand. Since he does not entirely avoid crossing over but reaches contralaterally with either hand, midline crossing avoidance is probably not the cause of his alternating hand use but rather a result.

Bimanual Circles

Bernard has great difficulty drawing the circles simultaneously with both hands and completes only a few cycles. Firm pressure can be seen on the right and the left depending on the direction, and the quality of circles is also better on the side with the firmer pressure. Bernard seems to visually fixate one hand, which then results in stronger pressure and better circles on that side. Overall, the left hand performed slightly better than the right. These discrepant results between the various movement directions indicate that the inter-hand difference may be caused by the direction of the circles rather than by an inherent weakness of one hand (Fig. 12.16).

Category Profile

Bernard shows a clear left-sided preference for the untrained items and a slight right-sided preference for the trained items. There are also differences between the trained and untrained motor tasks in the proficiency tests: the trained Skill (tracing and dotting) is better overall on the right, and the untrained ability (hammering and tapping) is slightly better on the left. The Midline Crossing Test and the Bimanual Circles, which are untrained, also show a slight left tendency (Fig. 12.17).

12.4.3 Summary and Interpretation

When looking at Bernard's HP Stairs (see Fig. 12.18), the value of the E-based Variation

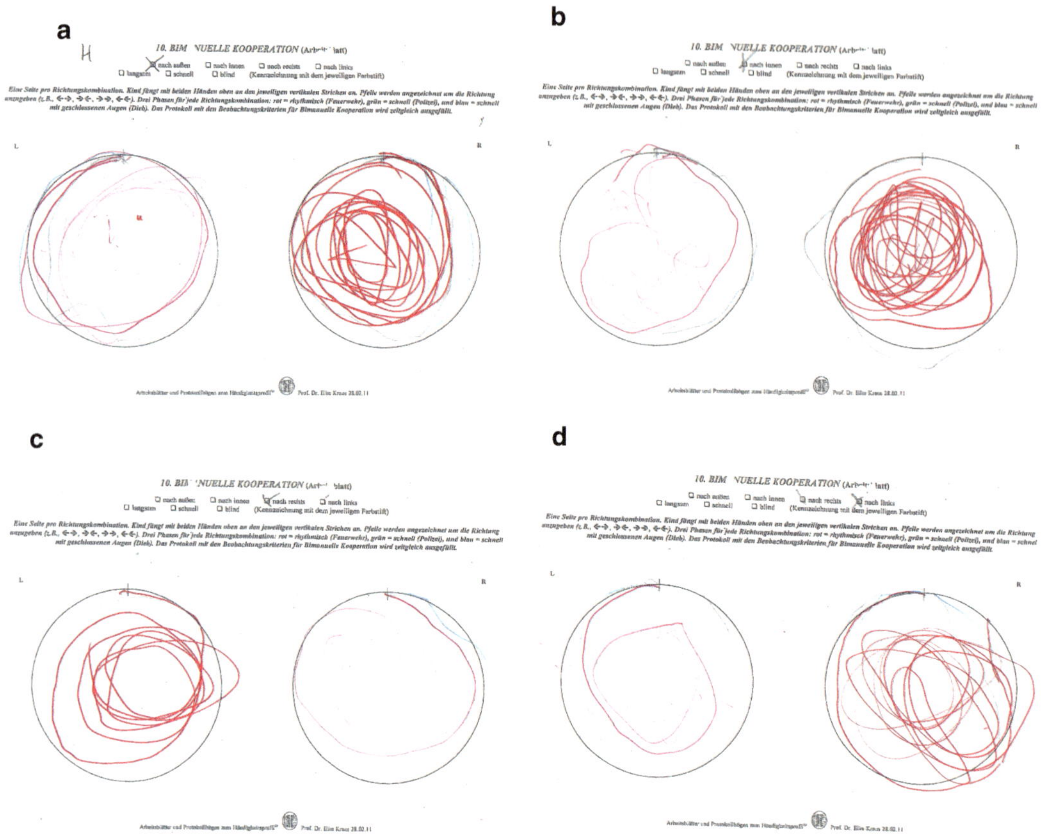

Fig. 12.16 Bernard's Simultaneous Bimanual Circle Drawings

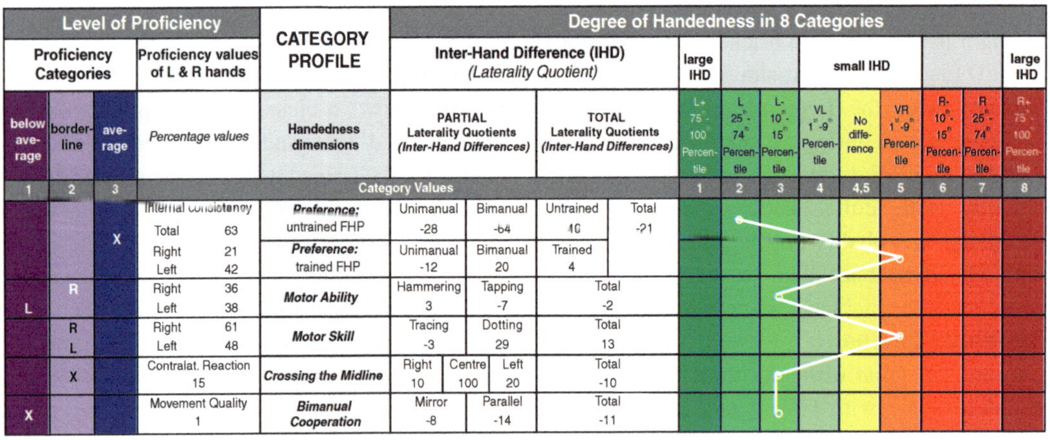

Fig. 12.17 Bernard's Category Profile. **Degree of handedness** (Columns on the right): Bernard's overall degree or extent of both preference and proficiency averages at 3.33 (2 + 5 + 3 + 6 + 3 + 3 = 22:6 = 3.33), i.e., clearly on the left. **Proficiency** (columns on the left): this is sub-average for both hands for Skill, and in ability, the left hand scores in the sub-average range. However, since Bernard is only 5 years, these sub-average results may relate to the normative data of six-year-olds. Overall, his profile supports the E-based and the M-based types with the variation *converted Left Handedness* (c-L) and a slight motor deficiency on both sides. *FHP* functional hand preference

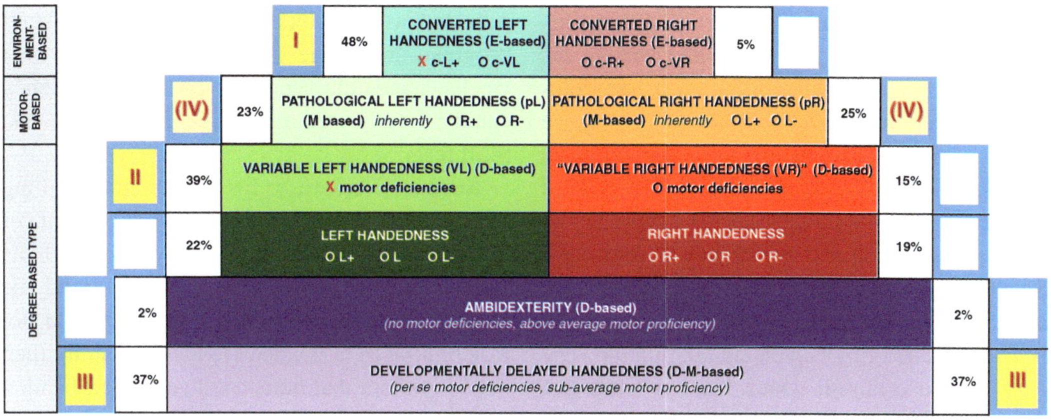

Fig. 12.18 Bernard's HP Stairs. Bernard's largest cluster is found in the E-based variation *converted Left Handedness*, followed by the D-based *Variable Left Handedness* with motor deficits and *Developmentally Delayed Handedness* (Kraus and Nagele-Hiedl 2019)

converted Left Handedness makes up the largest cluster (I) with 48%. Bernard has possibly started to copy other right handers around him since he wants to do things correctly and does not want to be different from other children (mother's report). The second- and third-largest clusters (II and III) are very close: D-based variations *Variable Left Handedness* (39%) and *Developmentally Delayed Handedness* (37%), typically involving motor deficits. Bernard shows mild but different motor deficiencies on either side, which apparently do not significantly affect his everyday activities. The E-based variation *converted Left Handedness* would indeed only make sense if there are higher values under *Left Handedness* or *Variable Left Handedness*—this is the case with Bernard. The fourth cluster (IV) indicates M-based *pathological Handedness*. However, since there is hardly any difference between left and right pathological handedness, this cluster does not make sense and can be disregarded as a causal explanation—the difficulties around birth reported by the mother are probably responsible for this enlarged cluster.

The combined results of the HP Stairs, incorporating background information, qualitative observation and the laterality quotients of the Category Profile, suggest that Bernard is a converted left hander with some sub-average fine motor skills. However, these may be due to his young age and lack of experience and fine motor activities and may be exacerbated by his increased use of his non-dominant hand for drawing. In addition, the slight deficiencies manifest differently on the two sides.

Possibly due to his recent increased use of the right hand, Bernard's performance is slightly better for drawing and writing. However, converted handedness may result in switching repercussions. In Bernard's case, two-handedness variations seem to contribute to his current ♦**Handedness Status**: he has *Variable Left Handedness* (D-Type) with some motor problems and is in the process of acquiring *converted Left Handedness* (E-Type) due to the right-handed environment since he presently draws and writes with his right hand. It is likely that his handedness degree is stronger than that of a variable left hander (e.g. a mild to moderate left hander), since he shows more left handed activitiy that would be typical for the variation VHL. His handedness conversion most probably contributes to a reduced asymmetry, and appears to be the main type responsible for his variable hand use.

12.4.4 Recommendations

Having classified Bernard as a *converted left hander* with slight motor deficiencies and a mild handedness degree, we need to establish if

Bernard could or should be reverted to using his dominant left hand for drawing and writing his name. It seems likely that the right-handed bias of the social and physical environments have contributed to Bernard using his right hand more frequently for these tasks. In addition, repeated practice (even if minimal) has probably led to greater automation and proficiency on the right. So when Bernard states that the right hand generally feels better when he draws, this could be because of emerging movement automation. The only way to establish which hand is better for drawing and writing would be to bring both hands to the same level of proficiency. If Bernard were to practise drawing exclusively with his left hand for a few weeks, automation on the left could probably be achieved at the same level as the right hand. The two sides would then be comparable, and a final decision for the writing hand can then be made. Since there are still almost 2 years before Bernard goes to school, there would be time for such an "experiment" (see Sect. 11.5.2).

The results of the Handedness Profile should be discussed with Bernard in age-appropriate language, and his parents should also understand the results. As an inherent left hander, it would be most advantageous for him to write with his left hand to avoid possible switching repercussions. Even though Bernard is still young, he should be empowered to become the agent for his hands: only he knows which hand feels the best for which activity. Also, it would be important to counter any possible negative attitudes towards *Left Handedness* by referring to the many prominent and famous left handers.

If Bernard is motivated to use his left hand for drawing and writing his name and if his family is supportive, the therapist could embark on an experimental left-handed phase for drawing and writing for a limited time period (see, for example, "Leon-Left-Week" above). In addition, Bernard can decide which other activities the left hand wants to perform consistently (e.g. brushing teeth). If he learns new and unfamiliar tasks, he should first try them out with the left hand. The experience with the left-handed activities during this experimental phase should be reflected weekly together with the therapist. If progress or change takes place over the next weeks, handedness preference and proficiency can be re-assessed using the HP Ability and Skill tests.

Suppose Bernard or his family are unwilling to engage in such a left-handed experiment, or Bernard was to clearly insists on writing with his right hand. In these cases, this should be respected. However, such a decision would not make him a right hander. He and his family then need to accept that he is a converted left hander. In that case, Bernard would then be encouraged to write exclusively with his right hand, knowing that he can revert to the left hand at any time. It is important to stress that he should not swap hands for writing and drawing since this would impede his ability to improve his writing skills. Furthermore, it may also interfere with hemispheric lateralisation and specialisation processes, which, in turn, may exacerbate problems and switching repercussions.

Follow-Up

Bernard was indeed motivated to try the left-handed experimental weeks. An individualised programme was implemented to increase the strength in his fingers particuarly on the left in order to develop a more consistent pressure when drawing. Through repeated practice, drawing and writing became more efficient and fluid on the left. Bernard started school with left-handed writing and managed this without great difficulties, even though his fine motor abilities remained below average.

12.5 Hugo: Variable Left Hander with an Affected Left Side and Subsequent Handedness Reshaping

Handedness Code: VL.M1(l).E0[6]

[6]Hugo's Handedness Code summarises that in the first instance he is a variable left hander (VL) with some motor problems (M1) particularly affecting his dominant left side (l), and a neutral environment (E0).

12.5.1 Background Information

Hugo is 5 years old. His parents report that he had refused to engage in drawing and other fine motor activities in kindergarten until a few months ago. He tends to use his left hand on the left side and his right hand on the right, and he alternates his hand use constantly. At another occupational therapy practice, his handedness had been assessed with another test, the HPT, 6 months previously, where results were inconclusive. However, the therapist who administered the test suspected that Hugo deliberately used either hand, as if deliberately showing that he is "ambidextrous". Hand preference of the HPT showed no clear difference between the hands, and also in the proficiency tasks, both hands performed below average. Current occupational therapy focuses on improving fine motor activities on both sides and he has the opportunity to freely experiment with his left and right hand without a bias towards a particular side. Recently, the right hand has improved considerably while the left-hand performance remained the same. Hugo has increasingly started drawing and writing with his right hand for a few months. As he is starting school this year, a final clarification of his writing hand is necessary.

Hugo's parents reported no difficulties during pregnancy, but he was 9 days overdue, and labour was induced. Hugo's father is an explicit left hander, and Hugo's paternal grandmother is a converted left hander. His parents ensured an open and neutral environment at home in order for him to develop his handedness "freely". Hugo is reported to have swapped hands for almost all activities since he was very young. He now cuts consistently with his left hand with scissors and always throws a ball with his right hand. Hugo himself remarks that his right hand is "more flexible" and that his left hand often "gets tired". Recently, Hugo has been using his right hand more during everyday tasks at home, and he presently almost always writes his name with his right hand.

Hugo presents as a self-confident, open and interested child with excellent verbal skills during the assessment. He spontaneously holds out his left hand when greeting with a handshake and seems to compensate for any weaknesses or difficulties verbally by excessive talking, explaining and asking questions. He proudly remarked when we met the first time "Did you know? I am ambidextrous!"

12.5.2 Results of Handedness Profile

Functional Hand Preference Test (FHPT)

Hugo's hand preference shows a significant difference between trained and untrained items. The untrained items are performed 40% more frequently with the right hand. Conversely, the trained items are performed 42% more left handed, particularly bimanual activities where he uses his left hand 84% more than the right. In unimanual untrained items, there is no difference between the hands. The internal consistency is fairly high overall (67%), and he is particularly consistent with the trained items. When all FHPT items are calculated together, the average laterality quotient is 1% more left. This means that across the 24 items, he performs about half with each hand, but within the trained items in particular, he consistently uses one hand (Fig. 12.19).

Ability (Untrained Proficiency: Hammering and Tapping)

In the Ability test, Hugo starts to hammer with his left hand but hammers slightly slower and less accurate than the right, resulting in a hammering quotient of 7% better on the right. When tapping, Hugo starts with the right hand but taps faster and more accurately with the left, achieving a laterality quotient of 6% better on the left. When hammering and tapping are averaged, Hugo's Ability quotient is 1% better on the right (Fig. 12.20).

Skill (Trained Proficiency): Tracing and Dotting

In the tracing task, Hugo beings the task with his right hand. However, whilst the right hand is notably more accurate than the left, it also takes twice as long. This brings down the score, so the difference is reduced to 4% better on the

Untrained unimanual (untr-uni)	Right (R)	Left (L)	Consistency	1. Hand	Atypical swaps
a2 Shaking box	4	0	R	r	
a3 Teddy bear and soccer	2	2		r	
b2 Putting pegs in pegboard	2	2		l	
c1 Spinning top	4	0	R	r	
d1 Building tower	3	1		r	
d2 Rolling dice	2	2		l	2
Bonuspoints (R/L)	1	0			
Total (R/L)	18	7			
Use-Percentage	72	28			
IHD untr-uni (LQ)	44				

Trained unimanual (tr-uni)	Right (R)	Left (L)	Consistency	1. Hand	Atypical swaps
f1 Using toothbrush	0	4	L	l	
f2 Eating with spoon	0	4	L	l	
f5 Cutting with knife	0	4	L	l	
g1 Writing in the air	4	0	R	r	
h1 Drawing on paper	4	0	R	r	
l1 Throwing ball	4	0	R	r	
Bonuspoints (R/L)	0.5	0.5			
Total (R/L)	12.5	12.5			
Use-Percentage	50	50			
IHD tr-uni (LQ)	0				

Untrained bimanual (untr-bim)	Right (R)	Left (L)	Consistency	1. Hand	Atypical swaps
a1 Opening box	4	0	R	r	
d3 Handbroom and dustpan	3	1		r	
e1 Dealing cards	4	0	R	r	
f3 Opening Tube	1	3		l	
h2 Taking off stickers	0	4	L	l	
k1 Tightening bolt and nut	4	0	R	r	
Bonuspoints (R/L)	1	0			
Total (R/L)	17	8			
Use-Percentage	68	32			
IHD un-bi (LQ)	36				

Trained bimanual (tr-bim)	Right (R)	Left (L)	Consistency	1. Hand	Atypical swaps
b1 Sewing with lace	0	4	L	l	#REF!
f4 Knife and fork	0	4	L	l	#REF!
h3 Cutting with scissors	0	4	L	l	1
i1 Striking a match	1	3		l	#REF!
j1 Putting key in lock	0	4	L	l	#REF!
k2 Opening with screwdriver	1	3		r	#REF!
Bonuspoints (R/L)	0	1			
Total (R/L)	2	23			
Use-Percentage	8	92			
IHD tr-bim (LQ)	-84				

	Untrained	Trained	Uni- Bim
Unimanual	44	0	22
Bimanual	36	-84	-24
IHD (LQ)	40	-42	
FHPT Total LQ	-1		

Internal Consistency	
Right	33
Left	33
Total consistency	67
Number of atypical swaps	2

Fig. 12.19 Hugo's Results of the FHPT

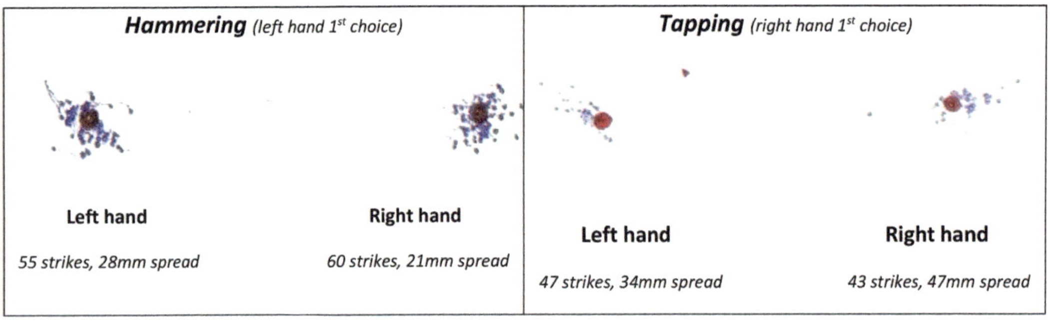

Fig. 12.20 Hugo's Ability Test: Hammering and Tapping with the left and right hands

right. Similarly, in the dotting task, the right hand shows fewer errors than the left, but both hands perform at similar speeds. Overall, the right hand performs 5% better than the left (Fig. 12.21).

Crossing over the Body Midline

The Midline Crossing Test, shows an overall left-handed tendency. Hugo crosses five times with the left and twice with the right. This result does not indicate avoidance of midline crossing. He picks up all but one of the Lego pieces in the centre with his left hand. If all the contralateral reactions were to be added, he would have crossed over 70% of the times. However, since the laterality quotient calculates the *difference* between the hands (R − L)/(R + L), the midline crossing quotient is 30% more left.

Bimanual Cooperation

Hugo shows mixed performance during the simultaneous bimanual circle drawing. The right hand mostly maintains direction in the fast movement variants and draws rounder circles. The pressure is the same on both sides and offers no distinguishing feature. During the slow bimanual movements, the hands lead alternatingly: sometimes it is the left, sometimes the right. The qual-

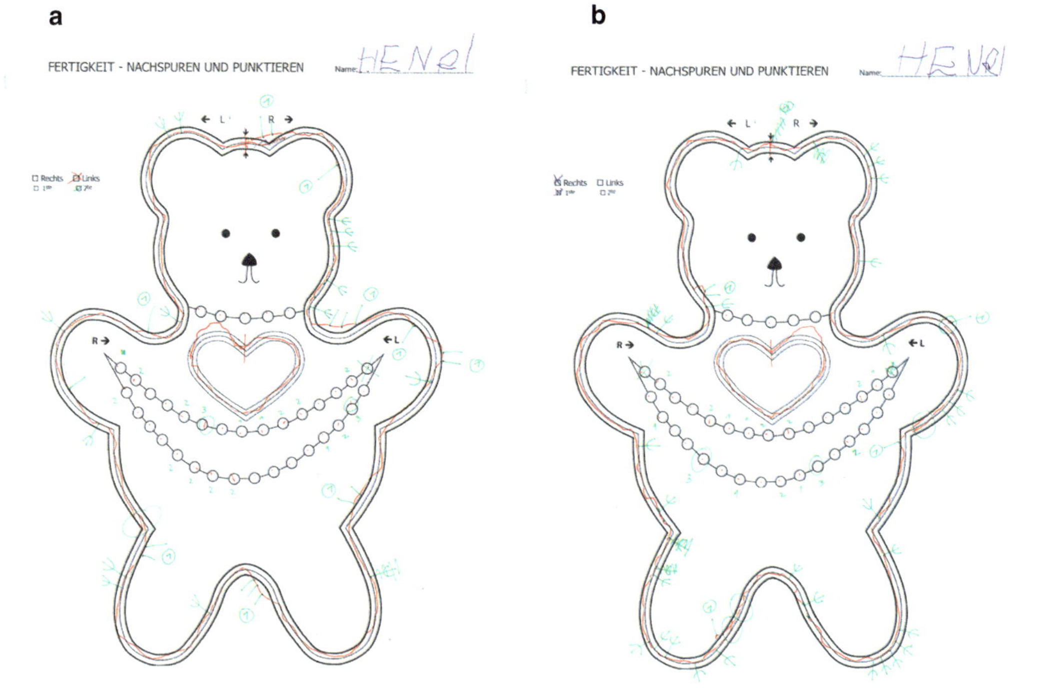

Fig. 12.21 Hugo's Skill Test: Tracing and Dotting with the left and right hands

ity of the circles is rated to be borderline on the right and sub-average on the left. Overall, the right hand performs 15% better than the left (Fig. 12.22).

Category Profile

The laterality quotients of all tests are summarised in the Category Profile and the suggests that his proficiency is better on the right, but his preference is more left (Fig. 12.23). The preference items show slightly more left-handed values, and the untrained ones show slight right-handed values—a typical characteristic of *Variable Left Handedness* (see Sect. 10.2.3). Hugo used his left hand predominantly in the Midline Crossing test. The proficiency tests show slightly better right-handed scores.

12.5.3 Interpretation and Summary

The clusters of Hugo's HP Stairs are relatively close together. The largest cluster, at 50%, aggregates under the variation *Developmentally Delayed Handedness*, followed by the variation of *Variable Left Handedness* at 45%, and in third place the Variation *pathological Right Handedness* with 35%. Together these variations suggest that Hugo is left handed with a very mild degree and shows motor deficiencies, particularly on the left side, causing him to increasingly use his right hand for motorically demanding tasks (Fig. 12.24).

For Hugo, the results relate quite clearly to the determining factors of handedness:

- *Genetic predisposition to hand preference:* It can be assumed that Hugo has the genetic predisposition of *Variable Left Handedness*, as his profile is typical of this variation. He performs untrained activities more with the right and trained activities more with the left hand. This pattern is not seen in *Variable Right Handedness*.
- *Pathological factors*: Hugo's mild motor deficiency is likely to have led to his avoidance of fine motor activities and subsequently to the referral to occupational therapy. Motor

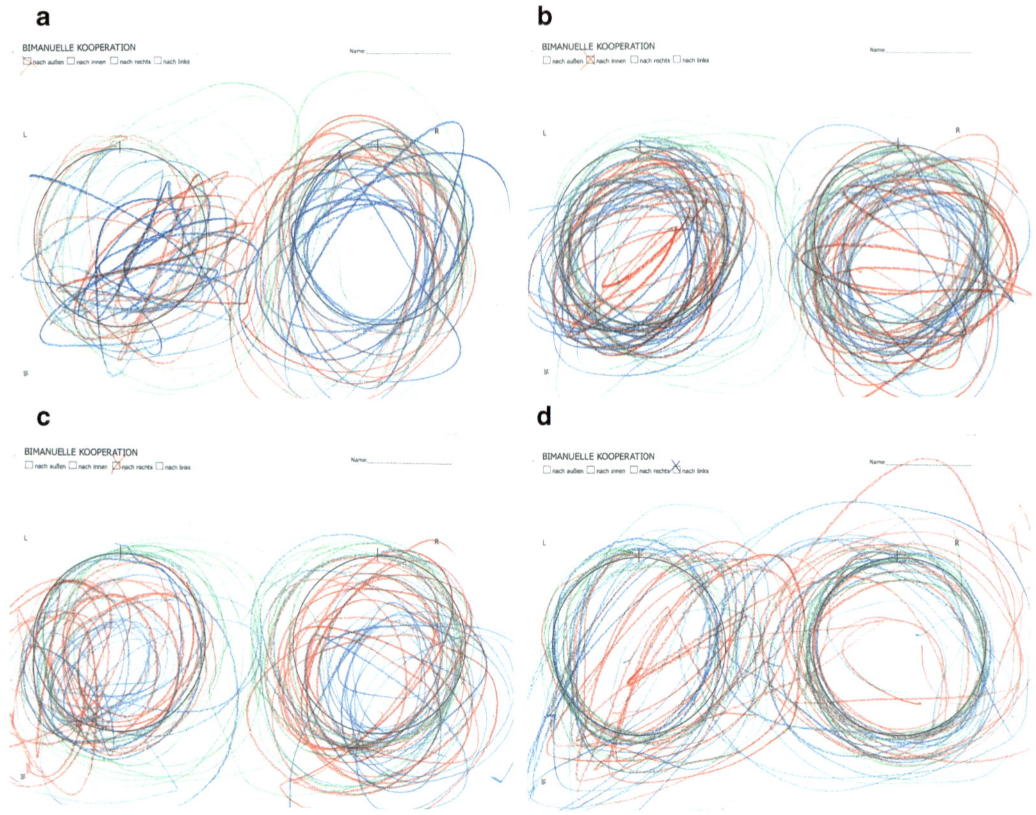

Fig. 12.22 Hugo's Simultaneous Bimanual Circle Drawings

Level of Proficiency				CATEGORY PROFILE	Degree of Handedness in 8 Categories										
Proficiency Categories			Proficiency values of L & R hands		Inter-Hand Difference (IHD) *(Laterality Quotient)*		large IHD			small IHD					large IHD
below average	borderline	average	*Percentage values*	Handedness dimensions	PARTIAL Laterality Quotients *(Inter-Hand Differences)*	TOTAL Laterality Quotients *(Inter-Hand Differences)*	L+ 75th-100th Percentile	L 25th-74th Percentile	L- 10th-15th Percentile	VL 1st-9th Percentile	No difference	VR 1st-9th Percentile	R- 10th-15th Percentile	R 25th-74th Percentile	R+ 75th-100th Percentile
1	2	3	Category Values				1	2	3	4	4,5	5	6	7	8
		x	Internal consistency Total 63 Right 33 Left 29	***Preference:*** untrained FHP	Unimanual [illegible]; Bimanual 36	Untrained 44; Total 3									
				Preference: trained FHP	Unimanual 0; Bimanual -76	Trained -38									
R		L	Right 41 Left 41	***Motor Ability***	Hammering 7; Tapping -6	Total 1									
	R	L	Right 57 Left 52	***Motor Skill***	Tracing 4; Dotting 6	Total 5									
	X		Contralat. Reaction 35	***Crossing the Midline***	Right 20; Centre -90; Left 50	Total -30									
X			Movement Quality 1	***Bimanual Cooperation***	Mirror 11; Parallel 19	Total 15									

Fig. 12.23 Hugo's Category Profile. **Degree of handedness** (columns on the right): Hugo's overall degree or extent of preference and proficiency averages 4.33 (6 + 3 + 5 + 6 + 2 + 6 = 26:6 = 4.33), i.e. slightly more left. **Proficiency** (columns on the left): Hugo's motor performance is slightly better with the right hand but borderline, whilst the left hand is average for a non-dominant hand. Overall, his profile supports the D-based and the M-based handedness types of *Variable Left Handedness* (*VLH*) and a motor deficiency, particularly on the left dominant side, which is particularly evident when drawing and writing. *FHP* functional hand preference

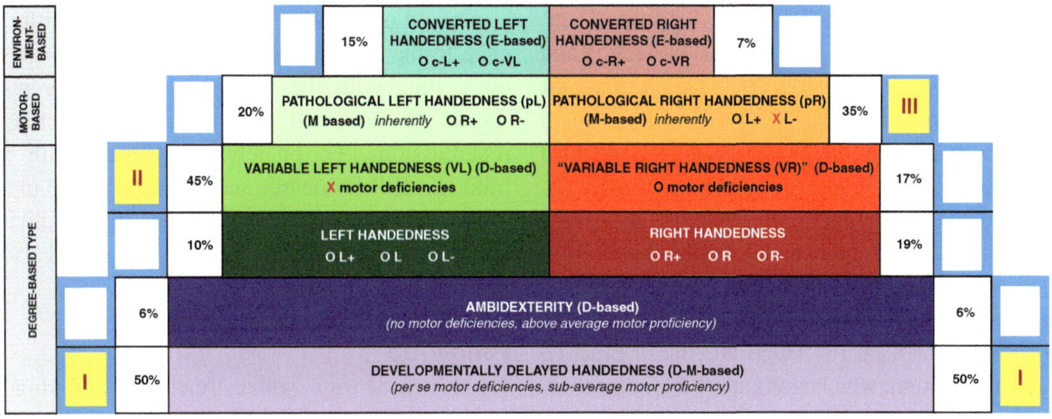

Fig. 12.24 Hugo's HP Stairs. Second to the largest cluster (*Developmentally Delayed Handedness*), *Variable Left Handedness* emerges, with *pathological Right Handedness* in third place

problems could be observed during testing. Although Hugo has already made significant progress in fine motor skills and can now hold the pencil with his fingertips, his pencil grip has not been automated and still changes often. In addition, a slight tremor is noted on both sides, but especially on the left. As a result, he compensates by performing the movements from his shoulder rather than his lower arm and hands so that there is little differentiated movement between the shoulder, elbow, wrist and fingers. It was also observed that he shows little strength and endurance and that he tires easily, particularly on the left side—something he also verbalises. The motor deficit may be attributed to the induced birth after being 9 days overdue. In any case, Hugo seems to have better fine motor skills and abilities on the right side, so his hand preference and his hand performance are not consistently on the same side.

- *Environmental influences on the development of handedness:* Apart from the general right-oriented environment we are all exposed to, it seems that Hugo has relatively optimal conditions at home to develop his handedness "freely". His strongly left-handed father and the openness for Hugo to experiment with the left and right hands have probably contributed to the high variability of his hand use. However, Hugo has had limited experience in drawing and writing since he has avoided fine motor activities until recently. Occupational therapy has made a difference in this respect over the last few months, and Hugo now seems to enjoy pencil work. In addition, the increased fine motor demands during activities have probably contributed to Hugo repeatedly trying out and choosing between his hands. As a result, he finds drawing and writing easier with his right hand. This is consistent with the observation that he begins a fine motor activity on the left (preference), then seems to tire and swap to the right.

Overall, the Handedness Profile suggests that Hugo's hand preference is that of *Variable Left Handedness*. However, because of sensory-motor deficits on his left side, it appears that his hand proficiency is developing better on the right side, and he shows a clear preference for using his right hand for drawing and writing. We refer to this as ♦**reshaping of handedness** rather than handedness conversion since, in his case, switching to the right due to socio-cultural influences can be ruled out (see environmental factors above). In this case, the decisive factor here seems to be Hugo's own motivation. Even though his preference is variable and he tends to perform untrained activities with the right and trained activities with the left, he twice wanted to change from the left to the right during the Skills tests, despite knowing that he should use his left hand.

In conclusion, it seems likely that several reasons are responsible for Hugo's variable hand use. (1) It is typical for persons with *Variable Left Handedness* to use the non-dominant right hand equally or more often than the left dominant hand for many everyday tasks (2) There is a discrepancy between his hand preference and hand proficiency, which, together with his predominantly left sensory-motor deficit, frequently leads to fatigue of the left hand. This causes him to then use his right hand (3) Hugo still lacks practice and automation, which also causes a kind of trial-and-error swapping. His preference for the right hand when writing becomes increasingly evident with more practice of fine motor activities within a relatively neutral environment.

12.5.4 Recommendations

As Hugo is about to start school, it is necessary to determine the writing hand as soon as possible. Given the above analysis and interpretation, it seems feasible that Hugo should write and draw consistently with the right hand, and his handwriting skills should be promoted on this side, particularly since he seems adamant about writing with this hand.

However, the sensory-motor deficits on the dominant left side are still relatively small compared to the right side. This is not a case of patholgocial *Handedness*, where there are large inter-hand differences. Early on, malalignment and asymmetry due to birth difficulties may be responsible for the observed left- and right-sided deficits. For this reason, it is advisable for Hugo to be assessed by an osteopath. Osteopathy has shown positive results in infants and children, restoring symmetry in osteopathic malalignments or blockage cases. Also, there is evidence that sensory-motor deficiencies may also be related (Fryman et al. 1992; Philippi et al. 2006; Rutte and Patijn 2015). Occupational therapists have repeatedly reported a change in handedness direction after osteopathic treatment. Should osteopathic treatment "free up" blockages, particularly on the left side, Hugo could commence left-handed writing as a variable left hander.

Should osteopathic treatment make no difference to the handedness status, and Hugo insists on writing with the right, he and his parents should be informed about possible switching repercussions. Fortunately, individuals with a mild-handedness degree seem to be affected to a lesser extent by such repercussions than explicit and moderate handers. Hopefully, this would also be the case with Hugo.[7]

Follow-Up

There was no osteopathic treatment, and Hugo continued to write with his right hand. He was discharged from occupational therapy after his fine motor and writing skills had improved. Even though his handwriting is not very neat and tends to be laborious, he seemed to be coping well overall and performing age-appropriately in his second year of school.

12.6 Concluding Remarks

This chapter looked at four real handedness cases as they presented in clinical occupational therapy practice, using the Handedness Profile and Handedness Typology. We could see the effect when motor deficiencies are superimposed on one or both sides, together with the varying degree of handedness *and* the effect of the right-biassed environment. Such combinations increase the complexity of a handedness status. By measuring different dimensions of handedness in a systematic and standardised way, we could unpack the complexity and comprehensively analyse patterns of mixed handedness. From a practice-based perspective, instruments such as the Handedness Profile and the Handedness Typology help us understand the likely causes for a child's variable hand use and pave the way for targeted and informed intervention with mixed-handed children.

[7] Hugo had more time before going to school, treatment could have been invested to improve and prepare the left hand sufficiently for writing. But in this case it is important to be pragmatic and ensure that Hugo can enter school writing with the better hand that he seems to prefer.

In the final reflection, I consider the implications of the assessment and typology on practice and research.

References

Fryman VM, Carney RE, Springall P (1992) Effect of osteopathic medical management on neurologic development in children. J Osteopath Med 92(6):729

Kraus E, Nagele-Hiedl U (2019) Fallbeispiele aus der Praxis. In: Kraus E (Hg.) Zwischen Links-& Rechtshändigkeit. Springer

Philippi H, Faldum A, Schleupen A, Pabst B, Jung T, Bergmann H et al (2006) Infantile postural asymmetry and osteopathic treatment: a randomized therapeutic trial. Dev Med Child Neurol 48(1):5–9

Randolph SM (2007) Hidden handedness. The emerging story of handedness reversals. Foundation for Handedness Research

Rutte S, Patijn J (2015) Biomechanics and laterality in musculoskeletal medicine: an additional approach? In: Oxford textbook of musculoskeletal medicine, p 111

Synopsis of Part III

Once again I resort to a visual summary of the chapters in Part III, which brings together the theory and research of the first two parts and culminates in clinical practice. Chapter 11 presents guidelines for intervention for children with atypical handedness. The guidelines are determined by the type and variation of handedness using the multidimensional Handedness Profile, Tools for Analysis and the Handedness Typology. Chapter 12 presents four cases across the three Types (D-based, E-based and M-based), displaying examples of the assessment results and interpretation and making recommendations for clinical practice. This application of the Handedness Profile and the Handedness Typology would not have been possible if these had not been based on research findings and developed as described in the previous chapters (Fig. 1).

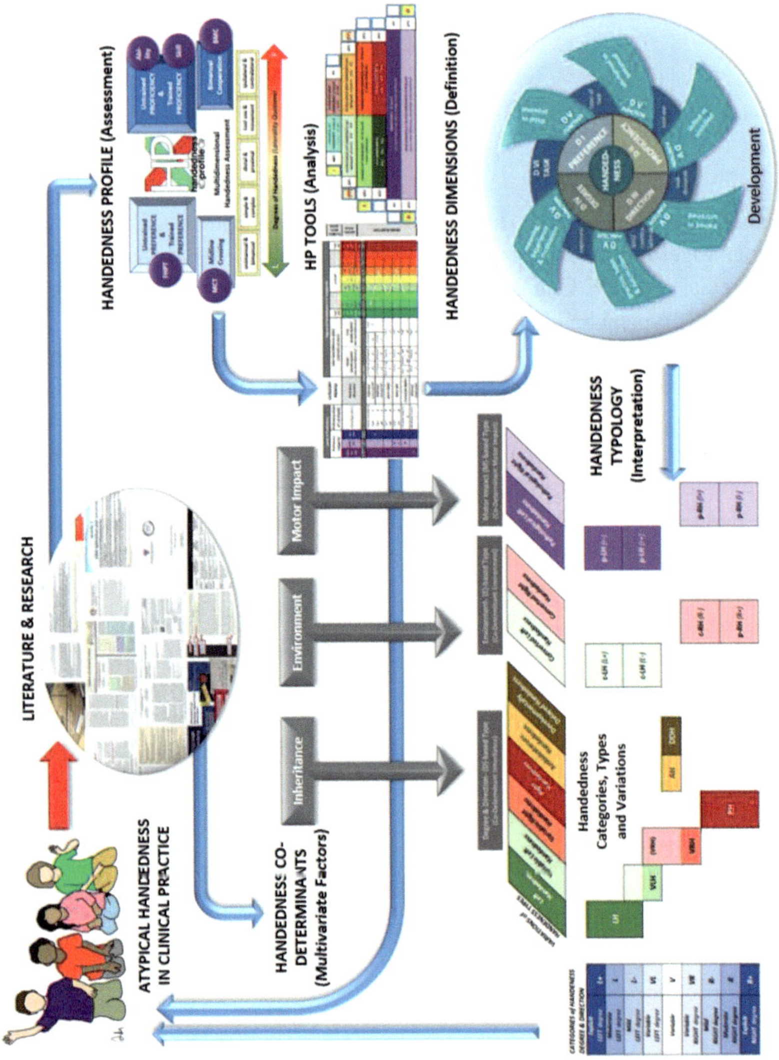

Fig. 1 Synopsis for Part III

Reflections: Implications for Practice, Theory and Research

Handedness research in the twentieth century produced not only promising pathways of understanding but also a number of dead ends. The heavy dependence on incidence rate studies produced extended controversies and rampant inconsistencies in the attempts to connect left handedness to both pathological and non-pathological traits.... A post on a Facebook page...asked the question 'What if left handed people are actually normal?' The answer to that question is that they actually are normal. (Porac 2016: 201)

Having worked for 30 years in the field of handedness as an occupational therapist, researcher and academic, I look back on this exhilarating journey so far. It has taught me an immense amount about handedness and related fields, specifically, the importance of a clear need for a comprehensive and systematic evaluation of handedness in practice, research and theory. In these reflections, I return to my original point of departure and research question: when is variable hand use normal in developing children, and when is it problematic? This is important knowledge for occupational therapists and other practitioners working with the so-called mixed-handed children. In many ways, I can answer this question today. I have developed instruments, tools and systems to assess, analyse and interpret handedness, based on the findings and recommendations from the literature. These have enabled me to capture variable handedness in a differentiated way that is indeed useful and practicable for clinical practice. So on the one hand, there is a sense of closure. However, whilst some questions have been resolved, many more have emerged. I indeed suspect that this extraordinary journey may well continue.

Feeding on the multifaceted knowledge and insights explored in this book, similar questions can be posed from a wider practice-based perspective reaching beyond *left* and *Right Handedness* of individuals. In particular, when is a particular handedness status typical or atypical across the life span and across conditions, particularly in the light of different handedness degrees and cascade of developmental processes? Or put differently: when is variable hand use normal and efficient, and when is it indicative of problems or associated with disorders on a continuum ranging from a typical human trait to a feature related to a medical condition? We assume that every person has a genetically based predisposition to be a left- or right-handed person with a certain degree of handedness (i.e. hand dominance). This is initially established in the first 6 years of life (handedness development). Beyond this, multiple factors continue to influence the *degree* of handedness spanning the entire life span (this process is referred to as handedness formation). Together, these processes are part of the normal hand formation that continues across the life span and is typical for all humans. However, certain circumstances, predispositions, interventions or medical conditions can also significantly influence and change the direction of handedness. The non-dominant hand is used for complex tasks that require practice and training to become proficient. Indeed, genetic predisposition, environmental factors and possible pathological impacts are considered to be the three major handedness co-determinants in the process of handedness formation.

E. Kraus, *Beyond Left and Right Handedness*, https://doi.org/10.1007/978-3-031-24389-9

Against this background, we could conceptualise main factors on a continuum with seven posts: *inheritance, environment, child development, infantile cortical insult, infantile subcortical insult, adult cortical damage* and *clinical conditions* (see Fig. A.1). Whilst the first two factors can be considered typical or normal since they apply to all people, child development and cortical infantile insult may be medically diagnosed if they are severe enough. If the impact of an early brain injury in infants and children is relatively mild, developmental delay may or may not be diagnosed, again depending on the severity. Pathological handedness in its mild form is also not part of medical diagnoses but when there is severe asymmetrical hemispheric damage, hemiplegic cerebral palsy is ascertained. When the affected hemiplegic side is the inherently dominant one, atypical handedness will also be a feature of this disorder since there is a change in handedness direction and degree. Finally, subcortical trauma might make it impossible or very difficult to use the dominant hand, such as fractures, burns or amputation of the dominant arm. Similarly, on a cortical level, traumatic brain injury or stroke can cause hemiplegia in adulthood and prevent the efficient use of the dominant hand. In these cases, too, a forced direction in handedness will result and affect the individual. The impact of these changes has not received much research attention.

These proposed groups, *typical ("normal")*, *possible medical diagnosis* (depending on the severity) and *medical diagnosis* are contrived. In real life, it is likely that these factors would overlap or co-exist, not only concerning the degree of handedness and the right-biassed environment but also the disorders (e.g. developmental and pathological conditions). Whilst such overlaps and concurrences add to the high complexity of the handedness status, differentiating between them may help us to contextualise mixed handedness. When grouping handedness according to the typical-atypical continuums, it becomes apparent that specific research is required to better understand handedness also in relation to medical conditions and disorders.

Let us now return to the individual handedness status of children to reflect implications for practice in the paediatric context. We can conclude from this book that the more comprehensive and accurate diagnostic measures and

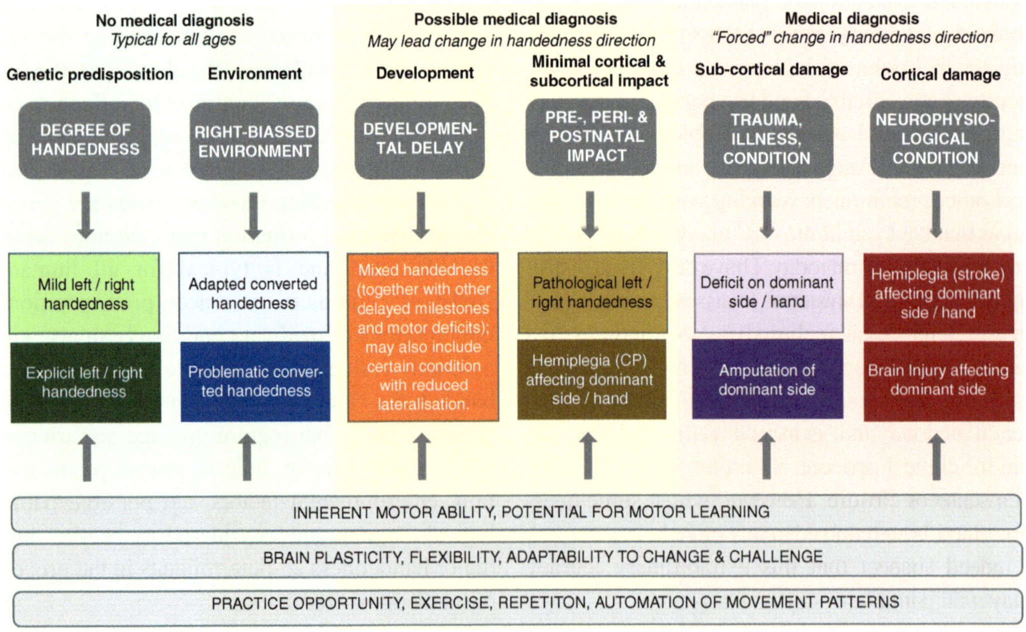

Fig. A.1 Continuum of typical to atypical Handedness Formation with and without medical diagnosis

assessments we use, the more specific and relevant the subsequent focus in therapy and intervention. Valid and reliable assessments are essential to evidence-based practice since they show if, and to what extent, the intervention has been effective. With handedness assessments, we need multidimensional and multivariate measures based on quantitative and qualitative data. The latter remains somewhat subjective data is often based on rating scales. Prospectively, digitised measures could measure qualitative aspects of motor performance far more accurately and reliably, such as pressure, steadiness and fluency. Thus, there is a great potential in digitising handedness assessment measures, particularly since normative data for both children and adults could provide more information on handedness categories, types and variations. In addition, normative data can create a differentiated benchmarking with precise and detailed data of inter-hand differences in motor proficiency. Such data might also generate new insights and expand our understanding of handedness as a phenomenon.

As we have seen throughout this book, current research and literature reveal many new and exciting aspects of handedness, such as gaining more profound insight into inter-hemispheric brain activity through MRI studies, understanding the polygenetic and environmental determinants of handedness and how these influence its development in a dynamic and cascade-like manner. However, these findings are often not directly relevant to clinical practice. The practice-based approach to researching handedness prompted me initially to develop comprehensive instruments for practitioners to assess and understand mixed handedness in children. Now the practice-orientated perspective raises further relevant questions with a clear need for research to help reach beyond and expand the current research landscape of handedness. In particular, using the Handedness Profile and its tools as well as the proposed Handedness Typology would establish a good basis for praxis-based handedness research. Here are some very specific research questions, with some ideas on the rationale and methodology.

1. **What is the normal distribution of Handedness Profiles in typically developed adults and children? What are the differences across various handedness degrees and categories, age groups and gender?**

   Rationale: The Handedness Profile is used as a normative benchmark for assessing various handedness dimensions across all age groups. Ideally, the Handedness Profile should first be fully digitised as piloted in the manDAAD study (Kraus and Hufnagl 2020; Kraus and Schübl 2020).

   Methodology: Normative studies across all age groups are conducted based on all subtests of the Handedness Profile to measure various handedness dimensions. Normative data is generated using means and standard deviations based on laterality quotients and analysed according to degrees (categories), age and gender. Relevant background information should be included.

2. **What is the relationship between motor proficiency and hand preference in typically developed adults and children of different age groups?**

   Rationale: The relationship between preference and proficiency as handedness dimensions remains unclear. This is investigated using the detailed data of the multidimensional Handedness Profile.

   Methodology: Normative data from preference and proficiency subtests of the Handedness Profile are analysed according to degrees (categories), gender and age.

3. **Can normative handedness profiles of typically developed populations be analysed according to the proposed Handedness Types and variations? Do individuals with a particular handedness variation indeed present with the proposed criteria of the Handedness Typology?**

   Rationale: The proposed handedness types and variations are based on literature and clinical practice. This needs to be verified and validated.

   Methodology: Handedness profiles and background information of subjects with *Converted Handedness*, *Pathological*

Handedness and *Variable Handedness* are generated. These empirical profiles are compared to the criteria of the Cluster Table defining the current handedness types.

4. **How do degrees of handedness based on the Handedness Profile relate to different conditions characterised by reduced lateralisation (e.g. Autism, Schizophrenia)? Do individuals with these conditions display specific handedness profiles? How do these profiles compare to the proposed Handedness Typology?**

   Rationale: The Handedness Profile generates detailed standardised data across various handedness dimensions that can be compared to groups of individuals with reduced lateralisation.

   Methodology: Handedness profiles of subjects with conditions characterised by reduced lateralisation are tested with the Handedness Profile and possibly other measures to establish possible associations between variables.

5. **What is the relationship between degrees and dimensions of handedness and degrees and dimensions of laterality in typically developed adults?**

   Rationale: Many of the typically used laterality measures do not correlate highly with handedness in terms of *direction.* It has not finally been established to what extent the *degree* of handedness correlates with laterality or whether the different aspects or dimensions of handedness and laterality are associated.

   Methodology: The Handedness Profile and the Laterality Profile are conducted with typically developed adults, and data is analysed for possible correlations.

6. **How does the performance of the Functional Hand Preference Test (FHPT) of the Handedness Profile compare to a self-evaluation (or third-party evaluation) questionnaire version with the same items? How do the 10-item EHI compare to the 24-item FHPT?**

   Rationale: If it is confirmed that there is a high correlation between the two types of performance, the questionnaire version could be used for adults in research and practice, thereby saving time and potentially accessing more subjects. Since the EHI is the most frequently used and best-validated preference test for handedness, a comparison can be made between the EHI and the FHPT items since the EHI items are part of the FHPT.

   Methodology: Adult subjects complete the FHPT questionnaire as well as the FHPT performance test. Possible correlations are examined. The laterality quotients of the 10 EHI items are compared to those of the 24 FHPT items.

7. **Which treatment or intervention approaches are effective for children with a specific handedness type or variation? Are there general interventions that facilitate lateralisation in children with atypical handedness?**

   Rationale: There is a lack of research on evidence-based practice in treating children with mixed handedness.

   Methodology: The Handedness Profile and the HP-Axes are used for children's atypical handedness before and after intervention to assess changes in hand preference and hand proficiency.

Defining and categorising degrees of *Left* and *right handedness* consistently across various dimensions allows us to create profiles that can be interpreted and compared in *clinical practice*. Similarly, a differentiated, systematic and standardised procedure can help divide handedness into clear categories, which enables us to use them as controlling variables, such as investigating relationships between handedness and specific traits or disorders in *research*. Finally, both practice and research are needed to further develop postulates on handedness in our quest to better understand handedness in *theory*.

I indeed hope that the Handedness Profile, its tools of analysis and the Handedness Typology may contribute to a practice-based perspective in future handedness research. Furthermore, I also hope that these instruments will assist more practitioners to assess handedness in a systematic and comprehensive manner to understand

and differentiate atypical variable hand use successfully. This will prevent switched handedness and allow specifically tailored handedness intervention, which in turn will help improve and optimise the participation of these children in everyday life.

References

Kraus E, Hufnagl P (2020) manDAAD—Manuelle Fertigkeiten: Digitalisiertes Assessment, Analyse & Dokumentation. Abschlussbericht (Final Report). Unter Mitarbeit von Alice Salomon University of Applied Sciences & Hochschule für Technik & Wirtschaft Berlin. Hg. v. IFAF. Institut für Angewandte Forschung. Berlin, 2

Kraus E, Schübl C (2020) Digitalisierung in den Gesundheitsberufen: Therapeutische Diagnostik durch den Einsatz digitaler Technologien. Alice SoSe 2020:98–99

Porac C (2016) Laterality. Exploring the enigma of left-handedness. Elsevier Science, Amsterdam. http://www.sciencedirect.com/science/book/9780128012390

Glossary[1]

ABILITY *(SUBTEST of the HANDEDNESS PROFILE)* The inherent disposition to motor proficiency in the context of inherited and/or acquired sensory-motor capacity. In the context of the Handedness Profile, Ability is assigned to the untrained motor proficiency tasks as seen during the tasks of ♦**Hammering** and ♦**Tapping**.

Ability Quotient The laterality quotient represents the difference between the right and left hand (R-L) as an inter-hand difference (IHD) concerning motor ability (based on the average of Tapping and Hammering).

AMBIDEXTERITY **(A)** *(VARIATION of the D-BASED HANDEDNESS TYPE)* Both hands perform equally well, and the motor skills are average or above average on both sides. It is a rare phenomenon that affects individuals with excellent motor skills who have learnt to write with both hands and do complex activities equally well on both sides. Arguably, the vast majority of individuals of this Variation are mild or variable left handers.

Atypical handedness It is used as a term used synonymously with other terms describing handedness as being "variable", "alternating", "inconsistent", "unclear", "uncertain", "unsure" and "ambiguous". It is used similarly to ♦mixed handedness, a fabricated category for undefined handedness, as a collective term, but in addition to mixed handedness it also encompasses defined handedness such as ♦***Variable Left Handedness*** or ♦**Ambidexterity**, which is identifiable but atypical.

Ambilaterality Both *sides* (excluding handedness) are equally good—footedness, eyedness and earedness are equally good on both sides, and therefore, there is no clear side preference.

Asymmetry See **functional asymmetry**.

Automation This is achieved with practice and repetition when motor sequences and patterns are learnt and automated so that they are eventually carried out "automatically", as can be seen by activities such as running, writing and cycling.

Bimanual It refers to movement patterns, tasks or activities involving both hands simultaneously. This could involve different patterns: simultaneous or sequential, symmetrical or

---

[1]This glossary defines and standardises key terms within the context of this book. These terms relate to the conceptual handedness framework, the Handedness Profile and its tools and the Handedness Typology. It is based on a combination of definitions (references for the definition by researchers and authors are found in the subsequent chapters.) from experts in the field, some of which were adapted, others were newly developed. Therefore, the purpose of these definitions is to establish a uniform, consistent and comprehensive use of the terms used in this book to improve readability and reduce ambiguity. In the chapters, the terms cited in the glossary are written in bold and marked with the symbol ♦.

Terminology used in the HANDEDNESS PROFILE and HP TOOLS are underlined with a single line, and the terminology of the HANDEDNESS TYPOLOGY are *UNDERLINED WITH A DOUBLE LINE* for easier reference. The other terms describe handedness relating to its causes, definition, processes of change, state or outcome and categories are used consistently. For a better overview, the taxonomy in the introduction summarises some of the main terminologies (Fig. 1).

Fig. 1 Taxonomy of Handedness Terminology

E. Kraus, *Beyond Left and Right Handedness*, https://doi.org/10.1007/978-3-031-24389-9

parallel (opposite) movements, or asymmetric division of roles between the hands (see also ♦**Role Differentiated Bimanual Movement/ Manipulation RDBM**). The latter involves an active, leading hand and a holding, stabilising hand, so each hand has a role (movement pattern) that is very different from the role of the other hand.

Bimanual coordination It refers to the way both hands work together in a coordinated, cooperative and complementary manner. Good bimanual coordination is evident when the movement execution in both hands is smooth, efficient, effective and speedy, without delay, excessive movements or pressure.

Bimanual cooperation It is considered to be an aspect of bimanual coordination and specifically refers to the interaction of both hands in movement patterns where the movement of one hand relates to that of the other hand. These patterns could mirror each other, perform opposite or parallel patterns or they could be role differentiated (see also ♦**Role Differentiated Bimanual Movement/ Manipulation RDBM**). The emphasis is not on smooth coordination between the hands (see ♦**bimanual coordination**) but on comparing the performing hands, such as: which hand leads, is faster or performs better?

BIMANUAL COOPERATION TEST (BCT) (SUBTEST of the HANDEDNESS PROFILE) It assesses the principle of bimanual cooperation by drawing circles simultaneously in four different directions: outward, inward, to the right and the left. The demands of the bimanual circle drawing tasks are accentuated by increasing the speed and eliminating visual feedback.

Bottom-up approach It assumes that basic bodily functions such as muscle strength or concentration need to be improved before higher and more complex functions, activities or occupations such hand handwriting can be performed. Consequently, a bottom-up therapy approach incorporates training and practising of such basic bodily functions. It contrasts the ♦**top-down approach**.

CAT-PROFILE See ♦**CATEGORY PROFILE**

Categorisation of handedness It is based on the grade 8 categories of the Handedness Profiles (see ♦**CATEGORY PROFILE** Together with a further category, variable (V), this categorisation is also used in the ♦**HANDEDNESS CODE.**

***CATEGORY PROFILE (HP TOOL)* (abbreviated to Cat-Profile)** It refers to the graph depicting the inter-hand differences through laterality quotients of all the various subtests of the Handedness Profile as a summary. It profiles the degree of handedness of each subtest in eight handedness categories: explicit *Left Handedness* (L+), moderate *Left Handedness* (L), mild *Left Handedness* (L−), *Variable Left Handedness (VLH)*, *Variable Right Handedness (VRH)*, mild *Right Handedness* (R−), moderate *Right Handedness* (R), and explicit *Right Handedness* (R+). In addition, the level of proficiency is broadly established for each of the subtests to complement the eight categories, grouping them into average/typical, borderline and sub-average/atypical. The ♦**proficiency level** is based on normative data for 6-year-olds and provides a rough estimate for older age groups.

***Category Profile Score** (HP TOOL)* Also called the Profile Score. It refers to the average of all laterality quotients calculated across the seven subtests of the Handedness Profile and categorised according to eight categories on an assigned ordinal scale: explicit *Left Handedness* (L+ = 1), moderate *Left Handedness* (L = 2), mild *Left Handedness* (L− = 3), *Variable Left Handedness* (VL = 4), *Variable Right Handedness* (VR = 5), mild *Right Handedness* (R− = 6), moderate *Right Handedness* (R = 7) and explicit *Right Handedness* (R+ = 8). The average of all eight categories comprises the overall Category Profile Score.

***Checklist** (HANDEDNESS PROFILE)* All motor proficiency subtests of ♦**Handedness Profile** are supplemented with checklists (identical for both sides) in order to systematically compare the movement quality of the hands in a more standardised manner. They include the ♦**Tracing** and ♦**Dotting** tasks (♦**Skill** subtest), the ♦**Hammering** and ♦**Tapping** tasks (♦**Ability subtest**) and bimanual simultaneous circle drawing (♦**Bimanual Cooperation Test**).

Classification of handedness See ♦**categorisation of handedness**.

Client-centred approach The person or child (client) and her/his needs and aspirations are placed at the centre of the approach. S/he is enabled and supported to engage and participate in everyday life, with the focus on what the individual can and wants to do, her/his perspective, needs and goals are central, informed by the unique circumstances and context.

Clinical conditions They relate to those conditions that present with a reduced laterality and lesser degree of handedness. They include: Schizophrenia, mental disability, Autism, Down's Syndrome and development delay.

CLUSTER TABLE *(HP TOOL)* It is a tool for analysis where the qualitative and the quantitative data of the Handedness Profile are combined and formulated into criteria, which relate to a particular ♦**handedness variation**. The qualitative data is derived from the parent questionnaire, observation protocol and checklists of the different subtests. There are 25 criteria for each handedness variation which can be graded on a 5-pt scale, representing typical aspects thereof. Those variations with the highest percentage of applicable criteria (i.e. clusters) are assumed to also indicate the greatest probability that this Variation is responsible for the observed variable hand use. The Cluster Table is summarised graphically by means of the ♦**HP Stairs** and helps to structure the diverse multivariate information for clinical reasoning and decision-making.

Co-determinants of handedness They refer to the three origin factors that "cause" and form handedness. These include *Inheritance* and Genetics related to the direction and degree of handedness, *Environmental influences* and *Motor-pathology* Factors. The three ♦**Handedness types** were derived from these co-determinants.

♦**Compound handedness dimensions** They consist of ♦**Function Dimension** and ♦**Task Dimension.** In addition, there are two ♦**defining handedness dimensions**, ♦**Hand Preference**, ♦**Hand Proficiency**, ♦**Handedness Direction** ***and*** ♦**Handedness Degree**.

Consistency See external and internal consistency.

Contralateral hand use/reaching/response It is synonymous with crossing the midline and is performed when one hand reaches across the body midline to pick up an item or perform a task on the opposite visual side. It is the opposite of ♦**ipsilateral hand use**, where a hand is used on the same side of the body and the body midline is not crossed.

CONVERTED LEFT HANDEDNESS c-LH *(VARIATION of the ENVIRONMENT-BASED HANDEDNESS TYPE)* It refers to switching and training the non-dominant right hand for handwriting in particular, often due to direct and indirect socio-cultural influences, as well as the right-biassed physical environment. Consequently, the right hand becomes automated for writing and other skills.

CONVERTED RIGHT HANDEDNESS c-RH *(VARIATION of the ENVIRONMENT-BASED HANDEDNESS TYPE)* It refers to the training of the non-dominant left hand for handwriting in particular. There are three typical reasons for switched *Right Handedness* (which is rare compared to ♦*converted Left Handedness*): imitation of a left-handed "hero" or idol; pressure from left-handed family members; or incorrect assessment of handedness. Consequently, the left hand is automated for writing and other skills.

Crossing the body midline See ♦**midline crossing**

D-CC hypothesis It relates the ♦**handedness degrees** (D) as a behavioural measure of the extent of hemispheric specialisation to the efficiency of the ♦**Corpus Callosum (CC)** and interhemispheric communication, using ♦**bimanual cooperation** as a behavioural measure. It is proposed that different combinations of the various degrees of handedness (D) and different levels of bimanual cooperation (CC) could explain why the mixed handed group is so heterogenous and the contradictory research results.

♦**Defining handedness dimensions** They consist of ♦**Hand Preference**, ♦**Hand Proficiency**, ♦**Handedness Direction** ***and*** ♦**Handedness Degree**. In addition, there are two ♦**compound handedness dimensions**, ♦**Function Dimension** and ♦**Task Dimension**.

DEGREE-BASED HANDEDNESS TYPE (D-BASED TYPE) *(HANDEDNESS TYPOLOGY)* It relates to the inheritance and the genetic aspects relating to the direction and the degree of handedness. For example, variable hand use may exist because of an inherited mild ♦**Handedness Degree** or strength of hand preference and performance. This means that the non-dominant hand is used more often in persons with a lesser degree or mild extent of handedness, compared to those with an explicit or strong degree or extent of handedness. There are six Variations of the D-based Type: (1) ♦***Left Handedness*** (***LH***), (2) ♦***Right Handedness*** (***RH***), (3) ♦***Variable Left Handedness*** (***VLH***), (4) ♦***Variable Right Handedness***, (5) ♦***Ambidexterity*** (***A***) and (6) ♦***Developmentally Delayed Handedness*** (***DDH***). The ♦**Laterality Quotient** is used to measure the degree of handedness.

Degree of handedness See **Handedness Degree.**

Deliberate hand use It refers to individuals who do not engage in preference activities spontaneously and unintentionally, but instead deliberately control which hand they use to pick up or use items.

Developmental delay It may affect various developmental aspects and milestones, as the child is not performing age-appropriately in those areas, including coordination of fine and gross motor movement, visual-spatial perception, ♦**handedness development**, etc. Often these delays are apparent from early on as the child does not achieve the appropriate developmental milestones. However, in contrast to ♦**developmental disorders**, developmental delay is defined as being less severe and not affecting all areas of development.

Developmental disorders They severely affect numerous developmental milestones and the child performs clearly below his/her age. Development disorders usually affect more than one of these areas: *physical* (e.g. substantial fine and gross motor incoordination), *cognitive* (including language, memory, processing speed, etc.) and *socio-emotional* (including communication, interaction, etc.). It is often used as an umbrella term and may include medical conditions such as Autism and Down's Syndrome. In contrast to ♦**developmental delay**, developmental disorders are defined as being more severe and affecting all or most areas of development.

DEVELOPMENTALLY DELAYED HANDEDNESS (DDH) *(VARIATION of the D-BASED HANDEDNESS TYPE)* It belongs to the ♦**D-based Type**, but it also overlaps with the ♦**M-based handedness type**, since it is by default associated with motor abnormalities and problems. There should be evidence of ♦**developmental delay** in the early history (♦**Parent Questionnaire**) and usually some other delayed developmental milestones that could explain the variable hand use. Typical criteria of this variation are the avoidance of crossing the body midline and internal inconsistency (i.e. changing hands within the same activity).

Differential Check (Diff-Check) *(HP TOOL)* A brief version of most of the variations of the ♦**Cluster Table** based on the three most important criteria. In addition, it features additional criteria for other reasons that reduce lateralisation, such as certain medical conditions.

Digital Scoring Template *(HANDEDNESS PROFILE)* Digital format of the ♦**Handedness Profile (HP)** which digitally calculates the ♦**Laterality Quotients** measuring the ♦**Inter-hand Differences (IHD)** for the different subtests of the Handedness Profile. It also automates the construction of the ♦**Category Profile**, which visually summarises the dimensions of handedness across the subtests, based on the quantitative data of the HP.

Direction of handedness See ♦**Handedness Direction.**

Distal It refers to parts of the body and movements that are further away from the body centre (e.g. hand and fingers). Distal musculature and movements are more strongly lateralised than ♦**proximal** body parts and movements, which have a closer proximity to the body centre (e.g. neck and shoulder).

Dominance It refers to the inherited, polygenetic disposition of manual (handedness) and hemispheric specialisation (see also ♦**hand dominance**). Although the term has been considered to be outdated in the literature because it insinuates that one side is dominant over the other, this is not the implication of the term dominance in this book. Rather, it refers to the *inherited* tendency to be left or right handed.

Dominance Index (DI) The DI expresses the ratio of the right-hand performance concerning the overall motor performance. A DI of 100 stands for a very strong degree of *Right Handedness*, a DI of 0 for a very strong degree of *Left Handedness*, and a DI of 50 means that both hands achieved the same test results. The DI is thus not used in the ♦**Handedness Profile**. Instead, the ♦**Laterality Quotient** for ♦**Handedness Degrees** and ♦**Proficiency Level**.

Dotting *(Task of the SKILL SUBTEST of the HANDEDNESS PROFILE)* It is a task in proficiency subtest ♦**SKILL** in the ♦**Handedness Profile** assessing *trained* motor performance together with the Tracing task. The average between the two tasks makes up the Skill score, whereby the ♦**Inter-hand Differences (IHD)** are measured with the ♦**Laterality Quotient**. This subtest requires a quick stop-start and accurately targeted movement. It correlates highly with writing.

Enablement It is used in the context of therapists empowering or enabling the child/client/person to set goals or solve problems themselves and act effectively.

ENVIRONMENT-BASED HANDEDNESS TYPE (E-BASED TYPE) *(HANDEDNESS TYPOLOGY)* It refers to the type of handedness formation based on the physical and (mostly right-biassed) socio-cultural environmental influences. In particular, if the ♦**handedness direction** is changed as a result of the environment and no longer coincides with the innate dominant hand, one of two variations manifest: either ♦*converted Left Handedness* (*c-LH*) (most common), **or** ♦*converted Right Handedness* (*c-RH*) (much rarer).

Established handedness See ♦**handedness establishment**.

Experimentation phase If the handedness assessment does not yield clear results and there is the possibility of switched handedness, the less automated (possibly the inherently dominant) hand is consistently and repeatedly used for drawing and writing for a specified time (e.g. Leon-Leftie Week). This can provide valuable information needed for the decision for the writing hand and requires close supervision.

Explicit left (L+)/right (R+) handed Category These are the categories based on the top 25% (75th–100th percentile) in the ♦**Category Profile,** consisting of individuals with a very strongly lateralised hand use.

External consistency/inconsistency It refers to the consistency *across* a variety of different activities or actions. High external consistency would be noted if the individual always uses the same hand for different activities, and the overall ♦**Laterality Quotient** would be high, showing large ♦**Inter-hand Differences**. External inconsistency (i.e. low consistency) would mean that some activities would be performed with the one hand and other activities with the other hand. However, external consistency does not provide information on how consistent a hand is used within an activity (♦**internal consistency**) since this requires several trials of the same activity.

Family ***Left Handedness*** See Family Sinistrality.

Family sinistrality (FS) The occurrence of *Left Handedness* in close family members (parents, siblings, children) is referred to as FS+; the occurrence of *Left Handedness* in the wider family circle of relatives (grandparents, grandchildren, uncles, aunts, cousins) is referred to as FS−.

Functional asymmetry It indicates that each hemisphere adopts different and independent functions, such as controlling aspects of a task whereby the certain aerials of the one hemisphere are activated. In contrast, other aerials in the other hemisphere are inhibited. This process is reflected in the role division of the hands during bimanual activities.

Function dimension One of the two proposed *compound dimensions* of handedness as defined for the ♦**Handedness Typology**. This dimension refers to the individual performing manual actions. It differentiates the tasks according to several dual characteristics that differ in their extent of lateralisation (the first always being more lateralised and the second less): distal and proximal; unimanual and bimanual; skilled and unskilled, as well as trained and untrained. In addition, repeated execution through practice forms automated movements, habits and routines within the context of meaningfulness and experiences and are subject to motivational factors. This dimension is unique to every person. The other proposed compound dimension is the Task Dimension. The compound dimensions complement the four proposed *defining dimensions* of ♦**Hand Preference,** ♦**Hand Proficiency,** ♦**Handedness Direction** and ♦**Handedness Degree**.

FUNCTIONAL HAND PREFERENCE TEST (FHPT) *(SUBTEST of the HANDEDNESS PROFILE)* It consists of 24 items (12 unimanual, 12 bimanual) that are further divided into 6 ♦**trained** and 6 ♦**untrained** items. Each item is performed at least four times to obtain an indication of the ♦**internal consistency** to observe to what extent the same hand is used consistently within the same activity. 10 of the 24 items are derived from the Edinburgh Handedness Inventory (EHI).

Hammering *(Task of the ABILITY SUBTEST of the HANDEDNESS PROFILE)* One of the two tasks in the ♦Ability subtest of the ♦**Handedness Profile** to assess untrained motor proficiency, the other task being ♦**Tapping**. The motor control for Hammering is located ♦**proximally** since it generated from the shoulder and elbow when the child hammers as fast as possible into a target dot.

Hand dominance It refers to the inherited, polygenetic disposition of manual specialisation of being left or right handed (see also ♦**dominance**). This differentiation allows the possibility of an individual having a certain hand dominance, but his/her ♦**Handedness Formation** or ♦**Handedness Status** might be different.

Hand preference It refers to one of the four defining dimensions of handedness, where one hand is preferred over the one (i.e. how *often* is the hand used in tasks of varying difficulty). In the ♦**Handedness Profile (HP),** preference is differentiated into trained and untrained tasks, whereby training incorporates practice with a specific hand (usually the right hand because of the right-biassed environment). The other three defining dimensions are ♦**Hand Proficiency,** ♦**Handedness Direction** and ♦**Handedness Degree**.

Hand proficiency It refers to one of the four defining dimensions of handedness, pertaining the level of motor performance (i.e. how *good* is the hand). In the ♦**Handedness Profile (HP)**, Proficiency is differentiated into *trained proficiency* that has been practised with a specific hand (Skill subtest consisting of Tracing and Dotting tasks) and *untrained proficiency* (Ability subtest consisting of Hammering and Tapping tasks). In the HP, Proficiency always combines speed and accuracy in its measurement, and it is expressed in a percentage of the maximum performance possible. The other three defining dimensions are ♦**Hand Preference,** ♦**Handedness Direction** and ♦**Handedness Degree**.

Hand use It refers to the frequency of an action, a task or activity performed by one hand or both hands.

Hand use percentage It is used in the calculations in the ♦**Functional Hand Preference Test (FHPT)** to denote the percentages of the left and right hands separately. The ♦**Laterality Quotient** is used to calculate the difference between the two Hand Use Percentages, using the formula R − L/R + L. This records how much more one hand is used, or how much better it is compared to the other hand.

Handedness The clearest and strongest form of human laterality. It is a polygenetic and multidimensional phenomenon, subjected to multivariate influences, and can be broadly divided into preference and performance whereby the contralateral motor cortex controls the movements of the arms and legs. It is also revealed in both its direction (*Left* or *Right Handedness*) and its degree, strength or extent. See also ♦**defining handedness dimensions** and ♦**compound handedness dimensions.**

Handedness categories It is the classification of the degree of handedness according to eight categories. See ♦**categories** and ♦**Category Profile (Cat-Profile).**

Handedness criteria It refers to the specific criteria or characteristics of the various handedness types. In the ♦**Cluster Table,** the criteria differentiate the handedness types from one another. Each criterion can be rated on a scale of 0–4 to see which handedness type obtains the highest aggregation or cluster, which systematically supports the clinical decision-making of the therapist.

Handedness degree It proposed to be one of the four *defining dimensions* of handedness and refers to the extent, "strength", "consistency" or "stability" of handedness—the more one hand is used and the better it performs in relation to the other hand, the greater its degree of handedness. The other three defining dimensions are ♦**Handedness Direction,** ♦**Hand Preference** and ♦**Hand Proficiency**. In addition, there are two proposed compound dimensions, ♦**Function Dimension** and ♦**Task Dimension**.

Handedness determinants See ♦**co-determinants of handedness**

Handedness development It refers to the first 6 years of life when handedness develops as one of many developmental milestones. It is part of the process of handedness establishment formation, which traverses the entire life span.

Handedness dimensions The two main dimensions are preference and performance. Each can be accentuated, resulting in further dimensions: *crossing the body midline* is a more challenging form of hand preference since it involves the contralateral visual hemispace; and *bimanual cooperation* is a more challenging form of motor performance since it involves the simultaneous collaborative action of both hands together.

Handedness direction It proposed to be one of the four *defining dimensions* of handedness and refers to being either left or right handed. The other three defining dimensions are ♦**Handedness Degree,** ♦**Hand Preference** and ♦**Hand Proficiency**. In addition, there are two proposed *compound dimensions*, ♦**Function Dimension** and ♦**Task Dimension**.

Handedness establishment It refers to the process of how handedness is developed and established, encompassing the entire life span, including ♦**handedness development** as well as ♦**handedness formation**, but also other reciprocal and influencing factors. Handedness establishment differs from ♦**handedness status** (the state or outcome of handedness status at a particular point in time) since it refers to the dynamics, change and process of handedness development.

Handedness formation It refers to the process of how handedness continues to be established and changes in degree, after the phase of ♦**handedness development**, which ends at the age of 6 years. This may include the non-dominant hand being used for proficient and highly skilled tasks, including handwriting, mostly because of motor deficiencies on the dominant side (see ♦**pathological handedness**).

<u>HANDEDNESS PROFILE</u> A standardised, validated and partially normed assessment to determine the direction and the degree (extent) of handedness in individuals with swapping hand use. It takes into account the handedness dimensions ♦**Hand Preference** and ♦**Hand Proficiency**, and it differentiates between trained, untrained, unimanual and bimanual activities or actions. It also offers a range of interpretation tools that can help to determine the ♦**handedness type**, which could explain the varying hand use.

Handedness reversion It refers to the "unswitching" or reverting to the original dominant hand in individuals with switched handedness. They practice writing with their dominant hand during reversion training, thereby undoing their switched handedness.

HANDEDNESS CODE *(HP Tool)* It is a code comprised of three sets of numbers and letters that describe handedness in terms of its degree, motor abilities and environmental influences. The set of numbers and letters with the primary influence makes up the beginning of the code. The ***degree of handedness*** is depicted by one of nine categories (**L+, L, L−, VL, V, VR, R−, R** and **R+).** The **E*nvironment (E)*** is coded as **E0** = no environmental influence to change handedness; environment consolidates dominant hand), **E1** = environmental influence converts or switches dominant hand (for writing) to non-dominant hand, or **E2** = converted hander reverts back to dominant hand (for writing). ***Motor abilities*** are coded as **M0** = no motor problems, average to good motor abilities, **M00** = excellent, above-average motor abilities, extensive practice, very good bimanual coordination/cooperation and motor planning skills, **M1** = motor problems, borderline to sub-average motor abilities and **M11** = severe motor problems, including significant motor planning problems and bimanual incoordination/in cooperation. Examples of handedness codes are cited with each handedness type variation in the glossary.

Hemispheric asymmetry See hemispheric lateralisation.

Hemispheric lateralisation It is the process resulting in ♦**hemispheric asymmetry**, enabling the hemispheres to work independently of, and complementary to, each other. These lateralisation processes are a prerequisite for ♦**hemispheric specialisation** of each hemisphere to take place, whereby specific functions, processes and abilities are specialised in one of the hemispheres in the context of development, interaction with the environment, practice and repetition.

HP AXES *(HP TOOL)* It serves as a visual summary tool to depict the three broad determinants of handedness: degree or extent of handedness (inheritance), the performance of motor abilities (motor skills) and effect of exercise (environment). As part of the Handedness Profile, the HP Axes serve to concisely document a ♦**Handedness Status,** and it can quickly and clearly portray changes in any of these three areas.

HP STAIRS *(HP TOOL)* A visualisation tool that summarises the aggregations of the Cluster Table, depicting the largest clusters and the probability that the handedness types with the largest clusters are responsible for the swopping hand use.

Handedness status It refers to the presentation, state or constellation of handedness at a particular time, with all its presenting dimensions and aspects. In contrast to the processes of ♦**handedness development** and ♦**handedness formation**, of handedness constellation is static, like a condition or a state.

HANDEDNESS TYPE *(HANDEDNESS TYPOLOGY)* A form of handedness composition based on several sources: the ♦**Category Profile** depicting the inter-hand differences (laterality quotients), parent questionnaire or case history and the Cluster Table. There are three main types of handedness corresponding to the three broad constellations of influences on handedness: ♦**Degree-based handedness type** based on the genetically determined degree of handedness; ♦**Motor-based handedness type** where pathological influences affect the inherently dominant hand and ♦**Environment-based handedness type** where the physical and social contexts influence the handedness formation. Each handedness type has two or more ♦**handedness variations**.

HANDEDNESS TYPOLOGY It is a system or structure to differentiate systematically between different profiles compositions and thus types of handedness, based on the cluster of applicable criteria referring to the *Categorisation Profile*, background information and structured observations during the assessment. The Handedness Typology offers probable explanations as to why an individual has varying (inconsistent, mixed, swopping) hand use and facilitates the analysis and interpretation of the *Handedness Profile*.

HANDEDNESS VARIATION *(HANDEDNESS TYPOLOGY)* Each ♦**handedness type** has two or more variations. For more information, see ♦**Degree-based handedness type** (D-based variations); ♦**Motor-based handedness type** (M-based Variations) and ♦**Environment-based handedness type** (E-based variations).

Hemispheric specialisation It refers to the specialisation of the hemispheres where certain functions are lateralised and then specialised. It is a defining characteristic of how the human brain is organised. The higher the task demand, the greater the need for hemispheric specialisation interhemispheric communication.

Incongruence It refers to a discrepancy the ♦Handedness Direction between the subtests of the ♦**Handedness Profile**, so that some subtests feature left-handed values and others right-handed values (e.g. preference and performance are not on the same side).

Inter-hand difference (IHD) It is the disparity between the hands, both in terms of preference and performance. The laterality quotient measures the IHD by using the formula R − L/R + L × 100.

Internal consistency/inconsistency It refers to the consistency or constancy *within* an activity when it is performed several times. A high internal consistency would be noted if the individual *always* uses the same hand for that activity. This might not be reflected in the overall laterality quotient, which is usually based on a variety of different tasks. For example, an individual may use the left hand for half the tasks, and the right hand for the other half, so the difference between the hands would be 0 (see ♦**external consistency**). However, if the left and right hands are always used for the specific tasks, the internal consistency could still be very high.

Internal constancy/inconstancy See **internal consistency/inconsistency.**

Ipsilateral hand use It is performed when one hand is used on the same side of their body and the body midline is not crossed. It is the opposite of ♦**contralateral hand use/reaching/response**, where one hand reaches across the body midline to pick up an item or perform a task on the opposite visual side.

Lateralisation See ♦**hemispheric lateralisation** and ♦**manual lateralisation.**

Laterality It is synonymous with "sidedness", including the preference of the foot (footedness), eye (eyedness), ear (earedness) and other lateralised behaviour, such as crossing arms and turn around the body axis. Handedness is considered to be a highly specialised and complex form of laterality, and these terms are not used synonymously.

Laterality Quotient (LQ) It measures the inter-hand difference (IHD) in *preference* items to portray as a percentage how much more frequently one hand is used compared to the other: LQ = (R − L)/(R + L) × 100. In the Handedness Profile, the LQ is also used to measure IHDs in ♦**proficiency** by calculating R−L about the perfect performance.

LEFT HANDEDNESS (LH) (VARIATION of the D-BASED HANDEDNESS TYPE) It is part of the ♦**Degree-based handedness type** in the ♦**Handedness Profile**. It includes explicit, moderate and mild degrees of *Left Handedness*, where the average ♦**Laterality Quotient** for preference and performance remains on the left.

Manual asymmetry See manual lateralisation.

Manual lateralisation It is the process resulting in ♦**manual asymmetry**, enabling the hands to work independently of, and complementary to, each other. ♦Manual specialisation takes place once the hands are lateralised can work independently from one another. Specialisation requires opportunity and practice for one of the hands to become consistently better at a certain task. These lateralisation processes are a prerequisite for the development of ♦**Role Differentiated Bimanual Movement (RDBM),** whereby each hand performs specific leading or assistive actions in the context of development, active interaction with the environment, practice and repetition.

Midline crossing It refers to one hand reaching spontaneously across the midline of the upper body, for example, to pick up an item on the opposite visual and physical space of the body (see also ♦**contralateral hand use**). Midline crossing is thought to be more demanding than ♦**ipsilateral** reaching and it is usually preferred with the ♦**dominant hand**. The stronger the ♦**Handedness** Degree, the more frequent the midline crossing and the further the distance in the crossing.

Midline Crossing Quotient It refers to the laterality quotient based on the difference between the hands in crossing the body midline (♦**contralateral response**). Children with developmental delay and other conditions typically avoid spontaneous midline crossing. It is thought to indicate neuro-physiological immaturity.

Mild left (L−)/right (R−) handed category These are the categories based on the 10th–25th percentile of ♦**Handedness Degrees** in the ♦**Category Profile,** consisting of individuals with a mildly lateralised hand use. It is likely that there are "successfully" converted mild and variable left handers in the mild and *Variable Right Handedness* categories.

Mixed handedness It is used as a fabricated category and comprises an umbrella term to incorporate all terms used to describe an undefined ♦**Handedness Status**, including ♦**inconsistent**, ♦**ambiguous**, "♦**unestablished** and ♦**variable** handedness. It is used synonymously with ♦**variable hand use**, which refers to the alternating hand use between the left and right hands in everyday activities. It also incorporates other terms such as "non-right", "non-left", "confused", "uncertain" and "less lateralised". Once a particular ♦handedness variation has been assigned to the Handedness Status, the term "mixed handedness" is no longer used.

Modalities It refers to the lateralised body parts, such as like feet, eyes and ears.

Moderate left (L)/right (R)-handed category These are the categories based on the middle 50% (25th–75th percentile) of ♦**Handedness Degrees** in the ♦**Category Profile,** consisting of individuals with a moderately lateralised hand use.

MOTOR-BASED HANDEDNESS TYPE (M-BASED TYPE) *(HANDEDNESS TYPOLOGY)* It refers to the motor aspects that interfere with the development and establishment of handedness. Typically, suppose there is evidence of early damage to the hemisphere with the dominant motor cortex. In that case, the non-dominant side is used for proficiency tasks and becomes more skilled than the dominant hand. This type has two variations: ♦***pathological Left Handedness*** and ♦***pathological Right Handedness.***

Motor disability/disorder It refers to the standard term to mean severe motor problems to the extent that they disable function and below-average or atypical motor performance. Disability and disorder are the strongest levels of motor problems implicating a medical diagnosis/condition (e.g. cerebral palsy).

Motor dysfunction It refers to the standard term to mean motor problems and below-average conspicuous or atypical motor performance. Dysfunction is a milder version of ♦**motor disorder**, which implicates a disability or medical diagnosis/condition, but it is more potent than ♦**motor deficiency**.

Motor deficiency It is used as the standard term to mean mild motor problems (i.e. less severe than ♦**motor dysfunction**) with borderline or atypical motor performance that might also be below average in some aspects. Deficiency is a much milder version of ♦**motor disorder**, which implicates a disability or medical diagnosis/condition.

Observation protocol *(HANDEDNESS PROFILE)* It is used to systematically document qualitative influencing factors that could skew or unduly influence the outcome of the assessment, such as a lack of concentration or insufficient language ability. Whilst these factors may determine the outcome of the assessment, they are independent of, or have nothing to do with handedness.

Parent questionnaire *(HANDEDNESS PROFILE)* It is used to collect qualitative information on possible determinants for handedness construction/development and influencing factors. It includes, for example, the incidence of left-handed family members, an early history of possible pre-, peri- and postnatal impact factors around birth. These factors might be responsible for causing minimal brain damage and developmental delay, of social influences that might have resulted in switched handedness (e.g. training a left hander to write with the right hand).

PATHOLOGICAL LEFT HANDEDNESS (p-LH) *(VARIATION of the MOTOR-BASED HANDEDNESS TYPE)* It refers to innately right-handed individuals with early damage (pre-, peri- or postnatal) to the left (dominant) hemisphere and motor cortex. Typically, such insults occur early, before or whilst handedness is being developed, based on a form of motor pathology on the ♦**dominant hand**. Consequently, the non-dominant left side (hand) is used for proficiency tasks and becomes more skilled than the inherently dominant right hand. The damage could be cortical (at brain level affecting the dominant motor cortex) or subcortical (injury to the dominant upper limb). The other variation of this handedness type is ♦***pathological Right Handedness,*** which is much rarer.

PATHOLOGICAL RIGHT HANDEDNESS (p-RH) *(VARIATION of the MOTOR-BASED HANDEDNESS TYPE)* It refers to innately left-handed individuals with early damage (pre-, peri- or postnatal) to the right (dominant) hemisphere and motor cortex. Typically, such insults occur early, before or whilst handedness is being developed, based on a form of motor pathology on the ♦**dominant hand**. Consequently, the non-dominant right side (hand) is used for proficiency tasks and becomes more skilled than the inherently dominant left hand. The damage could be cortical (at brain level affecting the dominant motor cortex) or subcortical (injury to the dominant upper limb). The other variation of this handedness type is ♦***pathological Left Handedness***, which is much rarer.

Performance This term is used synonymously in the literature with ♦**Hand Proficiency**. In this book, the term "performance" is used in a general way to indicate that tasks are performed particularly refers to performing ♦**Hand Preference** tasks, rather than just rating it in a questionnaire or ♦**third-party handedness assessment,** ♦**performance assessment** or ♦**self-assessment**.

Performance assessment of handedness It is based on the ratings of the observation of a test administrator when the child/individual performs preference or proficiency tasks.

Practice-based approach to handedness It refers to handedness as a phenomenon, its assessment and interpretation within everyday life as well as the clinical, therapeutic or educational setting. It informs subsequent research in a pragmatic and outcome-orientated way.

Practice effect (extent) It refers to the extent to which one hand has been exercised, trained and thereby automated for certain activities through repetition.

Preference See ♦**Hand Preference**.

Preference score It refers to the score of the laterality quotient portraying the inter-hand difference. The difference in hand use is based on the number of actions with each hand, calculated by the *Laterality Quotient* (LQ = R − L/R + L × 100). In the Handedness Profile, LQs are generated for trained and untrained items as well as unimanual and bimanual items.

Proficiency See ♦**Hand Proficiency**.

Proficiency level It is part of the ♦**Category Profile** and supplements the eight ♦**Handedness Degrees** by broadly indicating the level of motor proficiency in each of the subtests. It is based on normative data for 6-year-olds. The average or by grouping them into *average/typical* (25th–100th percentile), *borderline* (10th–24th percentile) and *sub-average/atypical* (1–9th percentile). For older age groups, the movement quality is estimated according to typical/efficient/smooth movement patterns and scored as *typical*, *borderline* and *atypical*.

Proficiency score It refers to the score of the ♦**Laterality Quotient** R − L/100%, portraying the ♦**Inter-hand Difference** based on the maximum (ideal or perfect 100%) performance.

Profile score See ♦**Category Profile Score**

Prototypical profile This is an exemplary ♦**Category Profile** to illustrate a specific handedness variation. It can serve as a reference or anchor example of what handedness profiles in this variation tend to look like. An individual Handedness Profile will be unique and differ somewhat from the prototypical profile, but the similarity should be clear.

Proximal It refers to parts of the body and movements that are a closer proximity to the body centre (e.g. neck and shoulder). Proximal musculature and movements are less strongly lateralised than ♦**distal** body parts and movements, which are further away from the body centre (e.g. hand and fingers).

Re-education of handedness See ♦**Handedness Reversion**.

Reverting handedness See ♦**Handedness Reversion**.

RIGHT HANDEDNESS (RH) (VARIATION of the D-BASED HANDEDNESS TYPE) It is part of the ♦**Degree-based handedness type** in the ♦**Handedness Profile**. It includes explicit, moderate and mild degrees of *Right Handedness*, where the average ♦**Laterality Quotient** for preference and performance remains on the right.

Role differentiation It refers to task distribution between the hands during bimanual activities, where one hand assumes a leading, more active role (typically the dominant hand), and the other an assisting, stabilising role (typically the non-dominant hand).

It is a term describing ♦**Role differentiation in terms of a movement or manipulation patterns.**

Self-assessment of handedness It is based on the estimation of which hand is used in the preference tasks listed, as rated by the person him/herself.

SKILL *(SUBTEST of the HANDEDNESS PROFILE)* It refers to the level and development of motor proficiency through repeated practice and training. It is subject to practice and automation. In the context of the ♦**Handedness Profile**, Skill is considered a *trained* motor performance, based on the subtests ♦**Tracing** and ♦**Dotting**, which correlate highly with writing.

Skill quotient It is the laterality quotient representing the difference between the right and left hand (R – L) as the inter-hand difference (IHD) concerning motor skill (based on the subtests Tracing and Dotting).

Specialisation See ♦**hemispheric specialisation.**

Stamina test It is a stress test performed when there is no clear handedness yet , but the decision on the writing hand is imminent (e.g. the child at school entry). Each hand colours and writes for 10–15 min, and the results are then compared.

Switching repercussions It refers to typical consequences, side effects, or symptoms that can occur when handedness is switched or converted from the dominant to the non-dominant hand, in particular for writing. Switching repercussions include concentration problems, memory retention, language problems (e.g. stuttering), dyslexia, dyscalculia, fine and gross motor coordination problems, psychosomatic symptoms (stomach and headaches, bedwetting), socio-emotional problems (e.g. aggressive outbursts or low frustration tolerance).

Tapping *(Task of the ♦ABILITY SUBTEST of the HANDEDNESS PROFILE)* One of the two tasks in the ♦Ability subtest of the ♦**Handedness Profile** to assess untrained motor proficiency, the other task being ♦**Hammering**. The motor control for Tapping is located more distally and is generated from the wrist that rests on the table whilst the child taps as fast as possible into a target dot.

Task dimension One of the two proposed *compound dimensions* of handedness as defined for the ♦**Handedness Typology**. This dimension includes those aspects that influence hand use and hand function externally, including what type of task needs to be performed, what tools and other demands are required, the placement of an item (ipsilaterally or contralaterally), exposure to items and availability of tasks are available, and to what extent this is the case. This dimension is more related to environmental factors and represents the external demands for performance. The function and task dimensions are referred to as the compound dimensions since they consist of several subdimensions that form unique constellations in every individual. The other proposed compound dimension is the ♦**Function Dimension**. The compound dimensions complement the four *defining dimensions* of ♦**Hand Preference,** ♦**Hand Proficiency,** ♦**Handedness Direction** and ♦**Handedness Degree**.

Third-party handedness assessments They are based on the estimation of which hand is used in the preference tasks listed, as observed by a third party such as parents, teachers or relatives.

Top-down approach It focuses on an individual's daily life and what she/he does (occupations) in terms of participation—his/her functional status is considered only concerning the daily activities and occupations, and their multidimensional context. It is contrasted by the ♦**bottom-up approach**, the activity and skills of the client. This contrasts with the *Bottom-up approach.*

Tracing *(Task of the SKILL SUBTEST OF THE HANDEDNESS PROFILE)* It is a task in proficiency subtest ♦**SKILL** in the ♦**Handedness Profile** assessing *trained* motor performance together with the Dotting task. The average between the two tasks makes up the Skill score, whereby the ♦**Inter-hand Differences (IHD)** are measured with the ♦**Laterality Quotient**. This subtest requires continuous, evenly graded and smooth movement. It correlates highly with writing.

Trained tasks They refer to activities or movement sequences that have been subjected to a particular side-biassed influence or training and were thus practised with a specific hand (e.g. shake hands or write with the right hand). With repeated practice, movements are automated. Such trained activities have a high cultural value, and they do not necessarily demand a high level of skill.

Trunk rotation It refers to movements of the body core that involve the thoracic and lumbar vertebrae and surrounding muscles (e.g. the upper torso rotates to one side whilst the pelvis/hips remain stable).

Typology of handedness *(HANDEDNESS TYPOLOGY)* See ♦**Handedness Typology**.

Unestablished handedness It refers to the incomplete process of establishing handedness (which either be ♦**handedness development** or ♦**handedness formation**). It is used synonymously with ♦**mixed handedness** (umbrella term).

Unimanual It refers to activities that involve one hand and are thus usually less complex than bimanual activities. Unimanual actions are more easily learnt and automated through exercise and repetition.

Unpractised tasks They refer to new or unfamiliar activities that have not been carried out or practised and thus are not automated. Such unfamiliar activities can be complex or simple. With a few repetitions, individuals manage to learn new tasks fairly quickly unless there are problems with their motor planning ability.

Untrained tasks They refer to activities or movement sequences that have not been subjected to a particular side-biassed (right) influence or training. They may be spontaneous or automated, depending on the amount of repetition. Particularly left-handed individuals with a moderate to strong degree of handedness are likely to use their left hand for untrained tasks.

Variable left (VL)/right VR–) handed category *(HP TOOL)* These are the categories based on the bottom 10% (1st–9th) percentile of ♦**Handedness Degrees** in the ♦**Category Profile,** consisting of individuals with highly variable hand use. It is likely that there are "successfully" converted mild and variable left handers in the mild and variable right-handed categories. If there is no tendency of left or right, only "variable (V)" is used (i.e. there is no difference between the hands, or an ♦**Inter-hand Difference** of 0%).

Variable hand use It refers to changing hand use across and within activities, typical of individuals with a low degree of handedness with a clear and consistent writing hand and no functional limitations. If this is not the case, the term ♦**mixed handedness,** indicative of unclear or unestablished handedness, is used in which case alternating hand use limits the functionality of a person and delays the establishment of the dominant hand.

VARIABLE LEFT HANDEDNESS (VLH) *(VARIATION of the DEGREE-BASED HANDEDNESS TYPE)* It differs significantly from the other left ♦**handedness variations** since it shows an incongruent ♦**Category** Profile whereby some values of the subtests are on the left, and others on the right. Typically, variable left handers perform more proximal and spontaneous movements, actions or activities with their right hand (e.g. playing tennis), whilst more distal and complex actions (e.g. writing) are executed with their left hand, despite the socio-cultural influences of the right-biassed environment.

VARIABLE RIGHT HANDEDNESS (VRH) *(VARIATION of the DEGREE-BASED HANDEDNESS TYPE)* This variation is not the mirror image of ♦***Variable Left Handedness*** since all values of the ♦**Category Profile** are congruent and on the right side. It is likely that this variation contains an unknown number of switched variable left handers that may "successfully" write with their non-dominant right hand, who may or may not have ♦**switching repercussions.**

Variable hand use It refers to the alternating hand use between the left and right hands in everyday activities, with a ♦**Handedness Status** that has not yet been defined yet. Used synonymously with ♦**mixed handedness**, which is a fabricated category. Normal variability is unique to a person, depending on his/her culture, habits, experiences, practice effects, environment, occupation, etc. Variable hand use is especially seen in *bimanual activities,* which is more complex and requires a *division of roles* between the hands.

Writing and pre-writing skills Drawing and writing are specialised fine motor skills that are extensively practised and improved with exercise and become automated. They are usually performed with the preferred hand that is also more skilled.

Index

E. Kraus, *Beyond Left and Right Handedness*, https://doi.org/10.1007/978-3-031-24389-9